Infections of the Cornea and Conjunctiva

Sujata Das • Vishal Jhanji

Editors

Infections of the Cornea and Conjunctiva

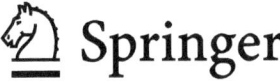 Springer

Editors
Sujata Das
Cornea and Anterior Segment Service
L V Prasad Eye Institute
Bhubaneswar, Odisha
India

Vishal Jhanji
Department of Ophthalmology
University of Pittsburgh School
of Medicine
Pittsburgh, PA
USA

ISBN 978-981-15-8810-5   ISBN 978-981-15-8811-2   (eBook)
https://doi.org/10.1007/978-981-15-8811-2

This Springer imprint is published by the registered company Springer Nature Singapore Pte Ltd.
The registered company address is: 152 Beach Road, #21-01/04 Gateway East, Singapore 189721, Singapore

Foreword 1

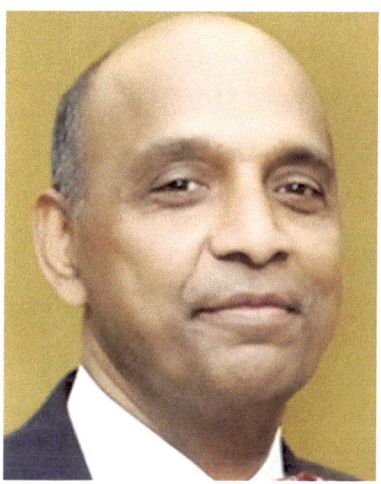

Infections of the ocular surface area constitute a common problem for ophthalmologists everywhere, particularly higher in the developing countries. The plethora of microbes that cause infections is ever increasing creating challenges for early diagnosis and treatment with drugs that are specifically effective against different organisms. An understanding of the causative organism and appropriate therapy is key to prevent worsening of the disease that can lead to corneal blindness.

The various sections in this book are authored by individuals with considerable experience and expertise in the respective areas and hence present the current knowledge related to the problem.

Both the groups of ophthalmologists, ones in practice and the ones in training, will find this book to be a valuable resource on the subject of corneal and conjunctival infections. The coverage is quite comprehensive and the presentation is very lucid.

Overall, the content, the galaxy of authors who have contributed various chapters and editors with vast expertise make this book a worthy addition to any library and an excellent reference for all ophthalmologists.

I compliment the editors for this valuable addition for the education of ophthalmologists.

Gullapalli N. Rao
L V Prasad Eye Institute
Hyderabad, Telangana, India

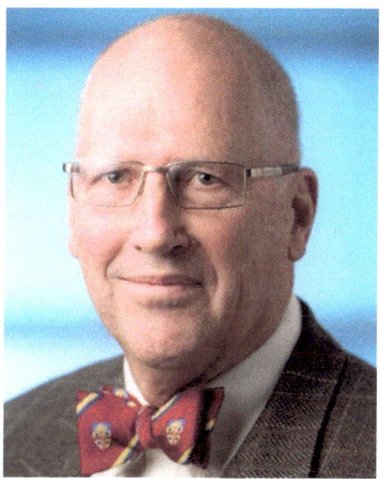

It is a distinct pleasure to write a foreword for this important and impressive book. Not only is it a very good, up to date and clear review of what is known and is the best practice for managing infections of the cornea and conjunctiva, but it is also written by two of my former fellows and this makes me feel very proud. They have brought together experts from around the world who have contributed their knowledge and understanding.

Infections of cornea continue to be the leading cause of visual impairment and blindness worldwide. The book includes chapters of each of the major causes of corneal infections including those due to bacteria, fungi, amoeba and parasites, and there are specific chapters on Herpes simplex and Herpes zoster keratitis. It also has chapters on conjunctivitis due to bacteria, virus and chlamydia, with a specific chapter on conjunctivitis of the newborn.

Proper diagnosis of the causative organism is critical, and although culture remains the prevailing diagnostic tool, newer techniques such as in vivo confocal microscopy are helpful for diagnosing fungal and acanthamoeba infections. Next-generation nucleic acid sequencing holds the potential to improve diagnosis both for common causes and for those that currently are more difficult to diagnose. Given the importance of an accurate diagnosis to help guide the correct management, the book includes chapters on the clinical assessment of corneal ulcers and the various diagnostic methods.

Although we can successfully manage many patients presenting with infectious keratitis and conjunctivitis, the outcomes as sometimes poor, with complications such as perforation or severe scarring. Adjuvant therapies aimed at improving clinical outcomes are discussed throughout this excellent book by experts from around the world who build on their extensive experience.

I recommend this book most highly and without reservation. It will be of immense help for comprehensive ophthalmologists when they are confronted by these often-challenging cases. It is also a superb and authoritative update for those who specialise in the management of these complex corneal infections.

Hugh R. Taylor
Harold Mitchell Chair of Indigenous Eye Health
Melbourne School of Population and Global Health
University of Melbourne
Carlton, VIC, Australia

Preface

Although the idea for this book has been brewing for a long time, the real work started about 2 years ago. The foremost need was to come up with topics for each chapter. Thankfully, it was not difficult. Having worked with cornea specialists around the globe, we knew what exactly bothers all of us when it comes to the management of our patients. We had a list of authors in our minds, stalwarts in the world of cornea and external eye diseases, colleagues who have inspired us since forever. These were expert clinicians and academicians who we started approaching in meetings, talking about the possibility of a book on infections of the ocular surface. Soon, the discussions started taking form. Fortunately, we were able to rope in authors from our wish list whom we wanted to be part of this task force.

Microbial keratitis is a leading cause of ocular morbidity in both the developed and developing world. This book is a compilation of real-world experience from busy clinics. Each chapter presents a step-by-step approach towards the management of patients with ocular surface infections. We hope that the readers will benefit from a wide variety of topics that have been covered in the chapters. This book is designed from a practitioner's viewpoint. Our inspiration for this work is our patients, colleagues and mentors. We realise that this book, like all the other books, will need updates from time to time, and trust us, will be on it. For now, we plan to live in the present and absorb what this book must provide.

Bhubaneswar, Odisha, India   Sujata Das
Pittsburgh, PA   Vishal Jhanji

Contents

About the Editors

Sujata Das is a faculty member at the L V Prasad Eye Institute (LVPEI), Bhubaneswar, India, and the Medical Director of Drushti Daan Eye Bank at Bhubaneswar. She received her basic medical degree and postgraduate training in Ophthalmology from Berhampur University, Odisha, India. She completed her subspecialty training in Cornea and Anterior Segment from LVPEI, Hyderabad, India. She also completed her ICO Fellowship in Cornea at the University of Erlangen-Nürnberg, Germany, and Clinical Fellowship in Cornea at the Royal Victorian Eye & Ear Hospital and CERA, Melbourne University, Australia. She has pursued an Advanced Management Program for Healthcare from the Indian School of Business, Hyderabad, India, and received a D.Sc. (honoris causa) from the Ravenshaw University, Odisha, India. She is a recipient of the Developing Country Eye Researcher Award from the ARVO Foundation, and an Achievement Award from the AAO. She is also the recipient of numerous awards from the All India Ophthalmological Society. She has served as a member of the ORBIS faculty for the evaluation of subspecialty education programme in Cornea. Dr. Das is presently involved in research encompassing corneal infections, eye banking and genetic analysis of Fuchs' Endothelial Corneal Dystrophy.

Vishal Jhanji is a Professor of ophthalmology at the University of Pittsburgh of Medicine, USA. He completed his ophthalmology training from the All India Institute of Medical Sciences, New Delhi, India. He was fellowship trained in cornea and refractive surgery in India and Melbourne, Australia. Dr. Jhanji is presently involved in research encompassing keratoconus, dry eyes, infectious keratitis and corneal imaging. He is an Honorary Professor at the Chinese University of Hong Kong and Visiting Professor at the Joint International Eye Center of Shantou University, China.

Contributors

Eduardo C. Alfonso, MD Bascom Palmer Eye Institute, Miller School of Medicine, University of Miami, Miami, FL, USA

Bhupesh Bagga, FRCS Cornea & Anterior Segment Service, L V Prasad Eye Institute, Hyderabad, Telangana, India

Maneesha M. Bellala, DNB Cornea & Anterior Segment Service, L V Prasad Eye Institute, Hyderabad, Telangana, India

Amar Bhat, MD The Eye & Ear Institute, University of Pittsburgh School of Medicine, Pittsburgh, PA, USA

Kara M. Cavuoto, MD Bascom Palmer Eye Institute, Miller School of Medicine, University of Miami, Miami, FL, USA

James Chodosh, MD, MPH Infectious Disease Institute and Department of Ophthalmology, Massachusetts Eye and Ear, Harvard Medical School, Boston, MA, USA

Sujata Das, MS, FRCS (Glasg.), AMPH, DSc Cornea and Anterior Segment Service, L V Prasad Eye Institute, Bhubaneswar, Odisha, India

Prashant Garg, MS Cornea & Anterior Segment Service, L V Prasad Eye Institute, Hyderabad, Telangana, India

Jamila G. Hiasat, MD, MRCSEd Division of Pediatric Ophthalmology, Strabismus, and Adult Motility, UPMC Children's Hospital of Pittsburgh, University of Pittsburgh School of Medicine, Pittsburgh, PA, USA

Bennie H. Jeng, MD Department of Ophthalmology and Visual Sciences, University of Maryland School of Medicine, Baltimore, MD, USA

Vishal Jhanji, MD, FRCS(Glasgow), FRCOphth The Eye & Ear Institute, University of Pittsburgh School of Medicine, Pittsburgh, PA, USA

Prafulla K. Maharana, MD Cornea, Cataract and Refractive Surgery Services, Dr. Rajendra Prasad Centre for Ophthalmic Sciences, All India Institute of Medical Sciences, New Delhi, India

Beeran B. Meghpara, MD Wills Eye Hospital, Thomas Jefferson University, Philadelphia, PA, USA

Darby D. Miller, MD, MPH Mayo Clinic, Jacksonville, FL, USA

Darlene Miller, DHSc, MPH, MA, CIC Bascom Palmer Eye Institute, Miller School of Medicine, University of Miami, Miami, FL, USA

Dilip K. Mishra, MD Ophthalmic Pathology Service, L V Prasad Eye Institute, Hyderabad, Telangana, India

Isa S. K. Mohammed, MD Department of Ophthalmology and Visual Sciences, University of Maryland School of Medicine, Baltimore, MD, USA

Somasheila I. Murthy, MS Cornea & Anterior Segment Service, The Cornea Institute, L V Prasad Eye Institute, Hyderabad, Telangana, India

Ken K. Nischal, MD, FAAP, FRCOphth Division of Pediatric Ophthalmology, Strabismus, and Adult Motility, UPMC Children's Hospital of Pittsburgh, University of Pittsburgh School of Medicine, Pittsburgh, PA, USA

Dipika V. Patel, BA, MA, BM.BCh, PhD, MRCOphth Department of Ophthalmology, Faculty of Medical and Health Sciences, University of Auckland, Auckland, New Zealand

Smruti Rekha Priyadarshini, MS Cornea and Anterior Segment Service, L V Prasad Eye Institute, Bhubaneswar, Odisha, India

Jaya Rajaiya, PhD Infectious Disease Institute and Department of Ophthalmology, Massachusetts Eye and Ear, Harvard Medical School, Boston, MA, USA

Christopher J. Rapuano, MD Wills Eye Hospital, Thomas Jefferson University, Philadelphia, PA, USA

Aravind Roy, MS Cornea & Anterior Segment Service, L V Prasad Eye Institute, Vijayawada, Andhra Pradesh, India

Pranita Sahay, MD, DNB Department of Ophthalmology, Lady Hardinge Medical College & Smt Sucheta Kriplani Hospital, New Delhi, India

Berthold Seitz, MD, ML, FEBO Department of Ophthalmology, Saarland University Medical Center, Homburg/Saar, Germany

Savitri Sharma, MD Jhaveri Microbiology Centre, L V Prasad Eye Institute, Hyderabad, Telangana, India

Namrata Sharma, MD, DNB Cornea, Cataract and Refractive Surgery Services, Dr. Rajendra Prasad Centre for Ophthalmic Sciences, All India Institute of Medical Sciences, New Delhi, India

M. Srinivasan, MS Cornea & Refractive Surgery Services, Aravind Eye Hospital, Madurai, Tamil Nadu, India

Zeba A. Syed, MD Wills Eye Hospital, Thomas Jefferson University, Philadelphia, PA, USA

Nóra Szentmáry, MD, PhD Dr. Rolf M. Schwiete Center for Limbal Stem Cell and Aniridia Research, Saarland University, Homburg/Saar, Germany

Department of Ophthalmology, Semmelweis University, Budapest, Hungary

Sonal S. Tuli, MD Department of Ophthalmology, University of Florida Health Eye Center, Gainesville, FL, USA

Lawson Ung, MD Infectious Disease Institute and Department of Ophthalmology, Massachusetts Eye and Ear, Harvard Medical School, Boston, MA, USA

Geeta K. Vemuganti, MD School of Medical Sciences, University of Hyderabad, Hyderabad, Telangana, India

Amar Bhat and Vishal Jhanji

1.1 Introduction

Bacterial conjunctivitis is a relatively common infection that affects the bulbar and palpebral conjunctiva. Most often, bacterial conjunctivitis is treated empirically by general practitioners rather than ophthalmologists. Presenting symptoms usually include redness and discharge, and the time course of the condition can vary from hyperacute to chronic. Treatment usually consists of topical antibiotic drops, which facilitate resolution and decrease morbidity; some atypical causes of bacterial conjunctivitis may require additional treatment.

1.2 Epidemiology

Patients with bacterial conjunctivitis most often present initially to their primary care provider (PCP) rather than an ophthalmologist. Ocular problems comprise 1–4% of consultations to PCPs, and bacterial conjunctivitis was the most common diagnosis that providers made [1–3]. It is difficult to know the true incidence of bacterial conjunctivitis as cultures are not routinely obtained before topical antibiotic therapy is instituted. It is likely that PCPs over-diagnose bacterial conjunctivitis, as topical antibiotics are prescribed in most cases of suspected acute infective conjunctivitis, of which only half may be bacterial [4]. Bacterial culture results from a tertiary care center demonstrated that the most common bacterial isolates in bacterial conjunctivitis were *Staphylococcus aureus*, coagulase-negative *Staphylococcus*,

A. Bhat
The Eye & Ear Institute, University of Pittsburgh School of Medicine, Pittsburgh, PA, USA

V. Jhanji (✉)
Department of Ophthalmology, University of Pittsburgh School of Medicine, Pittsburgh, PA, USA
e-mail: jhanjiv@upmc.edu

© Springer Nature Singapore Pte Ltd. 2021
S. Das, V. Jhanji (eds.), *Infections of the Cornea and Conjunctiva*,
https://doi.org/10.1007/978-981-15-8811-2_1

Streptococcus pneumoniae, and *Haemophilus*; other bacteria, including *Chlamydia*, made up a minority of the cases [5, 6].

1.3 Risk Factors

The ocular surface is generally resistant to infection due to a multitude of natural defense mechanisms. Utilization of the innate and adaptive immune system in combination with the anatomically protective ocular surface contributes to the natural resilience of the conjunctiva [7]. Tears not only flush the eye of pathogens, but they also contain other protective components such as immunoglobulins, lysozyme, and lactoferrin [8–9]. The normal flora of the conjunctiva includes *Staphylococcus epidermidis*, *Propionibacterium acnes*, *Streptococcus*, and *diphtheroids*, and these bacteria may serve a protective role by secreting antibiotic-like substances or acidic metabolic waste products [2, 10].

Interruptions of the normal ocular surface appear to be a risk factor for bacterial conjunctivitis. Ocular surface disease such as dry eye, deep fornix syndrome, ectropion and entropion, defective tear film, systemic immunosuppression, prior infections, ocular trauma, history of hospitalization, and cosmetic application practices (in females) have been associated with ocular bacterial infections [11–14].

1.4 Classification

Bacterial conjunctivitis should be classified by its time course (hyperacute, acute, or chronic), exudation (mucoid, mucopurulent, or purulent), and other remarkable features (membranes, pseudomembranes, granulomas). Classically, hyperacute purulent conjunctivitis would suggest *Neisseria gonorrhoeae* as the pathogen, while chronic conjunctivitis in a patient with deep fornices could suggest *Staphylococcus aureus* in many cases. Due to the variability of duration and symptoms with which patients may present, the gold standard of pathogen determination remains Gram stains and conjunctival cultures.

1.5 Symptoms

Patients with bacterial conjunctivitis frequently present with bilateral symptoms, though unilateral disease is not uncommon. Patients with unilateral risk factors may be more prone to developing unilateral disease. Symptoms of bacterial conjunctivitis commonly include redness, foreign body sensation, discharge, and itching. Eyelids feeling "stuck" together in the morning is another common symptom. If symptoms are initially unilateral, they may develop contralateral symptoms within a couple of days. Lid swelling, fullness, or erythema may also be present, especially in cases of blepharoconjunctivitis. It is difficult to discern between bacterial and viral conjunctivitis using symptomatology alone [15–16].

The duration of bacterial conjunctivitis in combination with clinical findings may point towards a specific causative organism. Hyperacute conjunctivitis typically presents with severe purulent discharge and has rapid onset and progression. Acute conjunctivitis is defined as an onset of less than 4 weeks, whereas chronic conjunctivitis is defined as longer than 4 weeks in duration.

1.6 Signs

Findings in bacterial conjunctivitis may include injection, tearing, discharge, papillae, follicles, membranes, granulomas, or cicatricial changes. Conjunctival injection, a nonspecific sign caused by dilation of the conjunctival blood vessels, is useful in monitoring the progression of disease or response to treatment (Fig. 1.1). Reflex tearing is common due to irritation of the ocular surface. In early stages of bacterial conjunctivitis, more serous discharge may be noted. Accumulation of dead tissue, degenerated white blood cells, and bacteria contribute to the purulence of the discharge (Fig. 1.2). As goblet cells begin secreting more mucus, discharge can become more

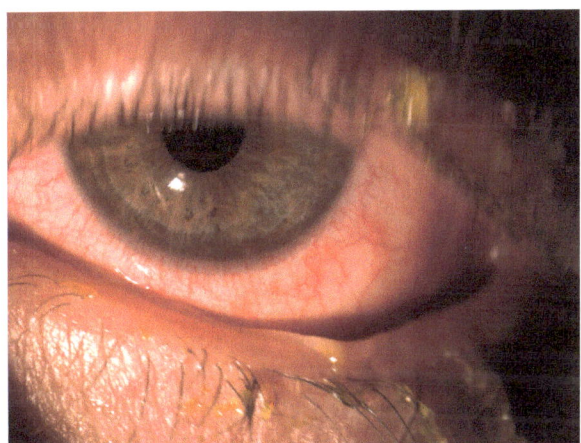

Fig. 1.1 Slit lamp photograph showing conjunctival congestion in a patient with bacterial conjunctivitis

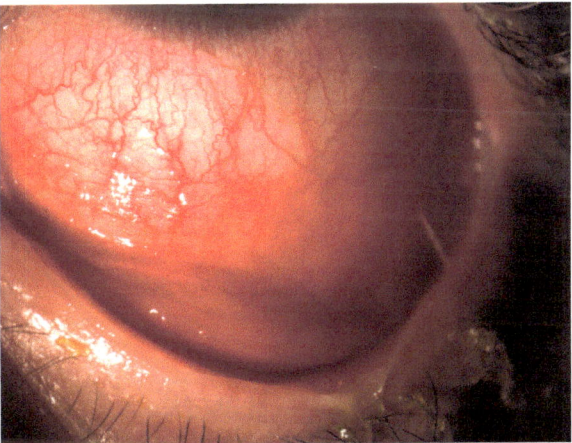

Fig. 1.2 Slit lamp photograph showing purulent ocular discharge in the lower fornix in a patient with bacterial conjunctivitis

Fig. 1.3 Slit lamp photograph showing copious conjunctival discharge in *Neisseria* conjunctivitis

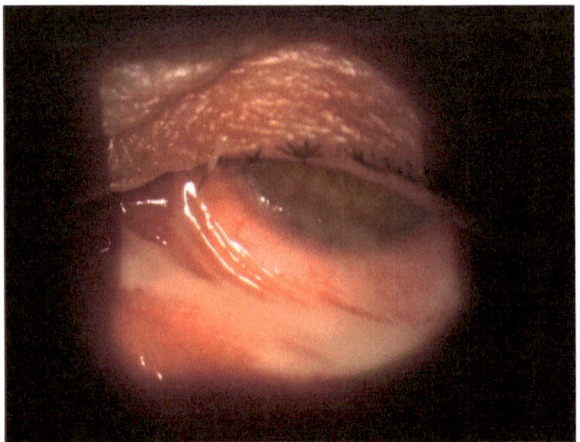

Fig. 1.4 Slit lamp photograph showing papillary response on everted upper lid in bacterial conjunctivitis

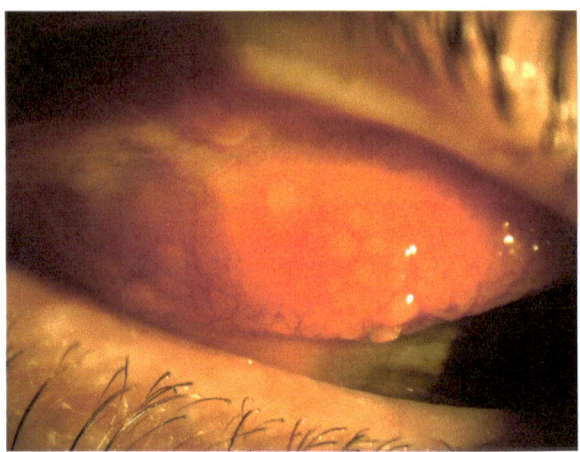

mucopurulent. Purulent (rather than mucopurulent) discharge is classically seen with *Neisseria* conjunctivitis, though other causes have been reported (Fig. 1.3) [17].

1.6.1 Papillae

Papillae are elevations in the conjunctiva with a central fibrovascular core. Papillae occur where the conjunctiva is anchored to underlying tissue by septae, which are fibrous connections of the conjunctival epithelium to the underlying substantia propria. The fibrous connections are the microscopic structural guides that allow the formation of individual papillae, usually less than 1 mm in diameter. With slit lamp examination, papillae are visible as small elevations, usually with a flat-top, with central pinpoint red dots which represent their central blood vessels (Fig. 1.4). Arborization of the blood vessels is also sometimes seen at the surface. The normal palpebral conjunctiva has blood vessels arranged in a radial pattern, extending from

Fig. 1.5 Follicular response in lower fornix in *Chlamydial* conjunctivitis

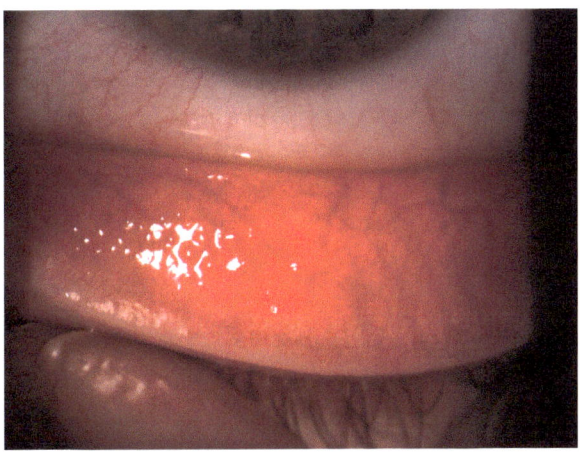

the fornix to the lid margin. Due to the hypertrophy of the superficial layers of the palpebral conjunctiva in papillary conjunctivitis, the normal underlying vasculature of the palpebral conjunctiva is often obscured. The presence of papillae is a nonspecific marker of conjunctival inflammation (acute or chronic) [17].

Giant papillae are formed when there is breakdown of intervening septae between papillae, allowing the smaller papillae to coalesce. Giant papillary conjunctivitis usually occurs as a result of chronic inflammation and is commonly seen in vernal keratoconjunctivitis, atopic keratoconjunctivitis, or secondary to chronic exposure to foreign bodies (contact lenses, loose sutures, prostheses). Bacterial conjunctivitis does not classically cause giant papillae.

1.6.2 Follicles

Follicles are dome-shaped elevations in the conjunctiva without a central blood vessel and are usually more whitish or translucent than papillae (Fig. 1.5). Follicles often have a surrounding, circumferential blood vessel in contrast to papillae. Similar to lymph node follicles, the histology of conjunctival follicles demonstrates aggregates of lymphocytes; germinal centers and a surrounding mantle zone can also be seen. Follicles can be seen normally in children without conjunctivitis or other pathologies. The presence of follicles is more specific than that of papillae, though bacteria are not a classic cause of acute follicular conjunctivitis. However, *Chlamydia*, *Moraxella*, and Lyme disease from *Borrelia burgdorferi* have all been reported to cause a chronic follicular conjunctivitis [13, 18–20].

1.6.3 Membranes and Pseudomembranes

Membranes and pseudomembranes are pale-colored sheets of fibrin and inflammatory debris that occur when discharge coagulates on the conjunctival surface. Histologically, a true membrane also incorporates the conjunctival epithelium with the growth of capillaries into the membrane; this results in bleeding when the membrane is peeled [21–22]. Although it is classically taught that pseudomembranes do not bleed when peeled, bleeding is still often observed with pseudomembrane peeling due to the severe inflammation and friability of the underlying conjunctiva. Bacterial causes of membranous and pseudomembranous conjunctivitis include beta-hemolytic streptococci, *Neisseria*, *Corynebacterium*, and *Chlamydia*. Noninfectious causes most commonly include chemical burns, Stevens-Johnson syndrome, and ocular cicatricial pemphigoid. Pseudomembranous conjunctivitis has also been reported in giant fornix syndrome [14].

1.6.4   Granulomas

Granulomas appear as nodular changes of the conjunctival stroma which can sometimes be confused with follicles. Granulomas can be necrotizing or non-necrotizing and be caused by infectious or noninfectious causes. Noninfectious causes of conjunctival granulomas include sarcoidosis and foreign bodies, whereas infectious causes can include syphilis, tuberculosis, *Bartonella henslae*, *Francisella tularensis*, and *Sporothrix shenckii* [23]. The diagnosis of Parinaud oculoglandular syndrome is made when there is a unilateral granulomatous and follicular conjunctivitis with a swollen preauricular lymph node. Clinical history is important to help determine the likely etiology if biopsy cannot be performed.

1.6.5   Cicatricial Changes

Cicratrization of the conjunctiva can occur in various conjunctival pathologies. Cicatricial changes can include formation of symblepharon or ankyloblepharon, cicatricial entropion, shortening of the fornices, and linear or stellate conjunctival scars [24]. Over time, loss of goblet cells contributes to keratinization of the conjunctiva and cornea. Classical causes of cicatricial conjunctivitis are noninfectious or autoimmune, though bacterial cicatricial conjunctivitis has been seen with *Chlamydia*, *Corynebacterium*, and *Streptococcus*.

1.7   Acute Bacterial Conjunctivitis

Bacterial conjunctivitis is most often seen in the acute setting, with an estimated annual incidence rate of 135 per 10,000 in the United States [25]. Most acute bacterial conjunctivitis is seen by providers who are not eye specialists, and topical antibiotics are frequently prescribed for treatment. Topical antibiotics have demonstrated to speed the resolution of symptoms and infection and were not shown to have any serious side effects [26].

Acute bacterial conjunctivitis in children is most commonly due to *Haemophilus influenzae*, although *Streptococcus* and *Staphylococcus* conjunctivitis is common as well [15]. *Moraxella* conjunctivitis has also been reported with a high incidence in some studies, and one study showed transmission among multiple students in a Navajo boarding school [13, 27]. Clinical history may provide important clues to the etiologic agent, though it is not nearly specific enough to replace conjunctival cultures. Children with concurrent otitis and conjunctivitis were more likely to have *Haemophilus* conjunctivitis, while concurrent pharyngitis and conjunctivitis may hint at an adenoviral conjunctivitis [28]. In newborns, chlamydial conjunctivitis is one of the most common causes of ophthalmia neonatorum and may develop in 30–50% of infants born to mothers with proven exposure to chlamydia [29].

In adult conjunctivitis, *Staphylococcus aureus*, coagulase-negative *Staphylococcus*, and *Streptococcus pneumoniae* are seen more frequently than *Haemophilus* [5, 6]. *Moraxella* conjunctivitis, although less common, may present with an acute or chronic conjunctivitis with or without follicles [6, 13]. The frequency and etiology of conjunctivitis may vary based on a number of factors, from climate to hygiene. Seasonal changes may contribute to the frequency of bacterial conjunctivitis, with two studies demonstrating that bacterial conjunctivitis was more common in winter [28, 30].

Spirochetes have been known to cause conjunctivitis as well. *Borrelia burgdorferi*, the spirochete that causes Lyme disease, may cause a follicular conjunctivitis in around 10% of patients with early Lyme disease [19–20]. Keratitis with nummular infiltrates and uveitis or neuro-ophthalmic manifestations will often occur months later in Lyme disease. *Treponema pallidum*, the spirochete responsible for syphilis, may rarely present as a papillary conjunctivitis [31].

Chlamydia trachomatis serotypes D-K are the cause of inclusion conjunctivitis in neonates and sexually active individuals. In sexually active individuals, the conjunctivitis often presents in a chronic setting, although sometimes it may be misdiagnosed if seen acutely. In neonates, ophthalmia neonatorum is the broad name for various conjunctivitis conditions that may occur within a few weeks after birth [29]. Mothers with chlamydial cervicitis who undergo vaginal delivery have a 50–75% chance of passing the *C. trachomatis* to their newborn. Incubation takes approximately 1 week, though onset of neonatal inclusion conjunctivitis may occur earlier if there was premature rupture of membranes. Typical onset for neonatal inclusion conjunctivitis is 5–14 days after birth. Symptoms may vary from mild (mild injection and watery discharge) to severe (eyelid edema, pseudomembrane formation, severe mucopurulent discharge). Newborns diagnosed with chlamydial conjunctivitis require 14 days of systemic erythromycin to prevent vision loss. Additionally, the mother of the baby and any sexual partners of the mother should be treated as well [29]. Trachoma and non-neonatal inclusion conjunctivitis will be discussed further in the Sect. 1.10.

The clinical course of conjunctivitis will vary depending on the virulence of the pathogen, though most cases of bacterial conjunctivitis are self-limited. In general, there will be a short incubation period followed by beginning of symptoms (redness, irritation, sticky eyelids in the morning). The conjunctivitis will worsen and often spread to the contralateral eye within the first week. The peak of the conjunctivitis is usually within 2–3 days of symptom onset. Without treatment, most bacterial conjunctivitis will resolve within 2 weeks, although topical antibiotics can speed up the resolution of the infection [26]. Exact treatment regimens vary, and success has been reported using a variety of different topical antibiotic drops and ointments. Ointments may blur vision, so use of ointments is often not preferred by patients. Many providers often begin treatment with broad-spectrum topical antibiotics and tailor treatment if the conjunctivitis is refractory. One point of concern is the potential for antibiotic resistance; topical surgical prophylaxis has possibly contributed to an increase in quinolone-resistant *Staphylococcus* from endophthalmitis samples [6]. Bacteria can develop resistance to second- and third-generation quinolones with a single mutation, and resistance to fourth-generation quinolones requires an additional mutation, so repeated or extended treatment with topical antibiotics should be avoided if possible.

1.7.1   Complications

Although the course of most acute bacterial conjunctivitis is self-limited, there is a theoretical risk in increasing the bacterial burden on the eye. Potential complications of bacterial conjunctivitis include preseptal cellulitis, corneal ulceration, corneal perforation, symblepharon formation, cicatricial entropion, and xerosis. Blood cultures should be considered in children with *Haemophilus* conjunctivitis due to the possibility of septicemia, especially if there are any other concurrent issues like otitis media.

1.8   Hyperacute Bacterial Conjunctivitis

Conjunctivitis that rapidly progresses with copious purulent discharge, conjunctival injection, chemosis, and lid swelling is known as hyperacute purulent conjunctivitis. The purulent discharge will rapidly reappear after saline lavage or debridement. Lid swelling may be so severe that it can mimic preseptal cellulitis and even orbital cellulitis if ocular motility appears limited. A preauricular lymph node may be palpable. The most common causes of hyperacute purulent conjunctivitis are the gram-negative diplococci *Neisseria gonorrhoeae* and *Neisseria meningitidis*. *N. gonorrhoeae* affect newborns and sexually active people, whereas *N. meningitidis* may occur in patients of any age exposed to meningococcus [32–33]. Less commonly, other pathogens that typically cause mucopurulent conjunctivitis may produce a hyperacute purulent conjunctivitis in the setting of immunosuppression.

  In neonates, gonococcal conjunctivitis most often presents 2–7 days after birth with copious purulent discharge. The incidence of gonococcal conjunctivitis is significantly lower than chlamydial conjunctivitis in the newborn, but 30–42% of infants born to mothers with *N. gonorrhoeae* may develop gonococcal conjunctivitis in the absence of appropriate prophylaxis [29]. Left untreated, gonorrheal ophthalmia neonatorum can progress to ulceration, endophthalmitis, perforation, or otherwise permanent vision loss within 24 h. Infants with gonorrheal ophthalmia neonatorum should be treated with frequent conjunctive lavage and intramuscular or intravenous ceftriaxone (25–50 mg/kg, up to 125 mg) and evaluated for disseminated gonococcal disease. The infant's mother and her sexual partners should also be treated. Infants born to mothers with known gonococcal infections should be treated with a single prophylactic dose of ceftriaxone or cefotaxime.

In sexually active individuals, autoinoculation of *N. gonorrhoeae* is the most common method of transmission, although transmission can also occur via direct ocular exposure to body fluids [34]. There is classically a concurrent genitourinary gonococcal infection, although this may not be symptomatic which can lead to delays in diagnosis. Treatment for gonococcal conjunctivitis depends on the presence or absence of corneal findings. In addition to saline lavage, gonococcal conjunctivitis requires a single dose of intramuscular ceftriaxone 1 g, a single dose of oral azithromycin 1 g, and a topical fluoroquinolone eyedrop or ointment. For gonococcal keratoconjunctivitis, admission to the hospital and the above therapies are required, but the ceftriaxone should instead be administered intravenously (instead of intramuscularly) 1 g every 12 h until significant clinical improvement is noted. Treatment for chlamydial coinfection is required, as well as treating their sexual contacts with oral antibiotics for both gonorrhea and chlamydia [35].

Meningococcal conjunctivitis can also be a rare cause of ophthalmia neonatorum, with a presentation similar to gonococcal conjunctivitis [33]. Patients treated with systemic antibiotics for primary meningococcal conjunctivitis (PMC) were less likely to develop invasive meningococcal disease (IMD), so topical antibiotics should not be used alone. Success was reported in treating PMC with 5 days of oral penicillin to 10 days of oral cefprozil, but no firm guidelines exist. If patients develop IMD, they require 7 days of intravenous ceftriaxone [33].

1.9 Complications

The severity of potential ophthalmic complications in hyperacute purulent conjunctivitis necessitates adequate treatment and monitoring. Due to the virulence of *Neisseria*, keratitis, corneal ulceration or perforation, and even endophthalmitis can occur in gonococcal and meningococcal conjunctivitis [33, 35–36]. In one study, limbal anterior stromal infiltrates were the most common corneal finding; these infiltrates were considered to be manifestations of hypersensitivity rather than a bacterial infiltrate [35].

Systemic morbidity is secondary to the often concurrent genitourinary gonococcal infections. Additionally, coinfection with *Chlamydia* and other sexually transmitted infections is common, so systemic therapy for patients and their sexual partners for gonorrhea and chlamydia is warranted to prevent potentially devastating sequelae such as pelvic inflammatory disease [37]. Work-up for other sexually transmitted infections should also be considered. *Neisseria meningitidis* conjunctivitis may also harbor a risk or developing invasive meningococcal disease. Because of the transmissibility through respiratory droplets, antibiotic chemoprophylaxis should also be instituted in close contacts of patients with positive cultures for *N. meningitidis* [33].

1.10   Chronic Bacterial Conjunctivitis

Conjunctivitis that has lasted for longer than 4 weeks is considered to be chronic conjunctivitis. Bacterial infections are relatively common causes of chronic conjunctivitis in the developed world, but they should nonetheless be considered in the differential diagnosis if appropriate.

1.10.1 Chlamydial Conjunctivitis

Chlamydia trachomatis can cause multiple distinct forms of conjunctivitis: trachoma, inclusion conjunctivitis, lymphogranuloma venereum, and ophthalmia neonatorum. The non-neonatal variations all cause a chronic follicular conjunctivitis with palpable or tender preauricular lymph nodes, but the variations are discrete for multiple reasons.

1.10.1.1   Trachoma

Although uncommon in the developed world, trachoma is the world's leading cause of infectious blindness [38]. Trachoma classically affects people in the developing world who are in relative poverty [38–39]. Additional risk factors, most of which correlate to socioeconomic status, include lack of access to water supply, facial cleanliness, and overcrowding.

In active or inflammatory trachoma, there is chronic inflammation of the conjunctiva caused by *Chlamydia trachomatis* serotypes A-C. Most commonly, this occurs in children less than 5 years of age. With aging, active trachoma decreases in incidence while cicatricial trachoma increases in incidence. Left untreated, up to 90% of patients will develop some degree of cicatricial trachoma over 25 years of age, though scarring itself will usually begin in late childhood and early adulthood. Women are more likely to develop cicatricial trachoma than men, likely due to their increased exposure to *C. trachomatis* while caring for young children [39].

Classic symptoms of active trachoma include irritation, foreign body sensation, discharge (which be mild), eyelid swelling, and photophobia. Signs of active trachoma, primarily seen on the everted upper lid, include follicular conjunctivitis and papillary hypertrophy. Active trachoma may be underdiagnosed due to the potential for children to be asymptomatic or with mild irritation that may be mistakenly considered "normal."

Cicatricial trachoma signs include scarring of the palpebral conjunctiva, scarring of limbal follicles (round, pigmented depressions known as Herbert's pits), entropion and lid distortion secondary to conjunctival scarring, and trichiasis. Palpebral conjunctival scarring can occur at any place in the palpebral conjunctiva; the formation of a horizontal, linear scar just superior to the eyelid margin is known as Arlt's line. Due to mechanical trauma to the cornea from trichiatic lashes and palpebral conjunctival scarring, corneal sequelae are common and potentially blinding in trachoma. Superficial pannus, diffuse punctate epithelial keratopathy, epithelial defects, ulceration, and scarring are all very realistic sequelae of cicatricial trachoma. Findings are often worse on the superior cornea due to the propensity of trachoma to affect the upper lid.

As a preventable cause of blindness, goals of trachoma management are preventative in nature. The SAFE (Surgery for trichiasis, Antibiotics, Facial cleanliness, Environmental improvement) effort is the World Health Organization's (WHO) primary strategy to eliminate blindness from trachoma worldwide. Surgery for trichiasis and entropion decrease the likelihood of corneal opacification and blindness; antibiotics have been shown to lower infection rates and can improve clinical signs; facial cleanliness and environmental improvements are aimed at improving the hygiene-related risk factors for trachoma in the community.

Surgery to prevent corneal opacification is dependent on each patient's particular needs. Epilation may be appropriate as a temporizing measure or in mild trachoma, while bilamellar tarsal rotation and posterior lamellar tarsal rotation procedures are recommended by the WHO. Primary limitations for surgical intervention in the SAFE strategy include awareness, fear, perceived costs, and access.

Antibiotic therapy can vary based on availability and of medications, but standard treatment includes either a single dose of azithromycin (20 mg/kg, up to 1 g) or topical tetracycline ointment twice daily for 6 weeks. Due to the difficulty of maintaining compliance with topical tetracycline ointment, a single dose of azithromycin is preferable if available.

For patients already with corneal opacification from trachoma, penetrating or lamellar keratoplasty are options to improve vision. Corneal transplantation is reserved for patients who have already optimized the ocular surface and addressed eyelid issues, as persistent entropion and trichiasis after keratoplasty would lead to poor graft survival. Availability and postoperative care limit the number of patients with trachoma-related corneal opacification who can receive corneal transplants, and penetrating keratoplasty in trachoma was considered to have a poor prognosis. However, a 2008 study of 127 eyes demonstrated 76.6% penetrating keratoplasty graft survival rate of 5 years for patients with trachomatous corneal scarring [40].

1.10.1.2 Inclusion Conjunctivitis

Non-neonatal inclusion conjunctivitis, sometimes known as adult inclusion conjunctivitis, is a chlamydial conjunctivitis that is considered a sexually transmitted infection [18]. Inclusion conjunctivitis is much more common in the developed world compared to trachoma, as *C. trachomatis* serotypes D-K are the most common cause of cervicitis in women and urethritis in men. The same serotypes D-K are responsible for neonatal chlamydial conjunctivitis. Similar to *N. gonorrhoeae* conjunctivitis, self-inoculation and genital-ocular contact are the primary modes of transmission for this conjunctivitis. Symptoms include redness, irritation, foreign body sensation, tearing, and mucopurulent discharge. Examination reveals a follicular conjunctivitis that may also be present on the superior palpebral conjunctiva. Subepithelial infiltrates can also be seen [18, 41].

Although patients may present in the acute stage of their illness, treatment with standard antibiotics used in acute bacterial conjunctivitis will often fail to treat inclusion conjunctivitis. This leads to the development of a chronic follicular conjunctivitis in many patients.

Inclusion conjunctivitis in sexually active individuals does not respond well to topical antibiotics. Multiple antibiotics have been shown to be effective in treating including conjunctivitis, though most common regimens are azithromycin 1 g (single dose or two doses given a week apart), doxycycline 100 mg twice daily for 7–10 days, or erythromycin 500 mg four times daily for 7–10 days.

1.10.1.3 Lymphogranuloma Venereum

Chlamydia trachomatis serotypes L1-L3 are causative agents of the sexually transmitted infection lymphogranuloma venereum (LGV) which typically results in a genital ulcer disease. Conjunctivitis appears to be the most common ocular manifestation of LGV, although ocular involvement appears to be very rare. Parinaud's oculoglandular syndrome with peripheral keratitis and perforation has been reported in one instance of ocular LGV, and another series reported conjunctivitis and keratitis in LGV [42–43]. Diagnosis of LGV can be made through serology.

Treatment for LGV usually consists of 21 days of oral doxycycline therapy, though other medications and regimens may work as well [44]. The patient with Parinaud's oculoglandular syndrome in LGV was treated successfully with 6 weeks of oral tetracycline [42].

1.10.2 Deep Fornix Syndrome

Deep fornix syndrome, also known as giant fornix syndrome, is a relatively underdiagnosed cause of recurrent and chronic mucopurulent conjunctivitis in the elderly. It is thought that dehiscence of the levator palpebrae superioris aponeurosis from the superior tarsus lengthens the fornices, as traction from the levator pulls the conjunctiva further back. Presentation usually occurs during or after the seventh decade of life. Women are more often affected than men. Unilateral pathology is more common, though bilateral cases have been seen. Some patients may have a history of chronic nasolacrimal duct obstruction or dacryocystitis as well [14].

Symptoms include redness, pain, tearing, foreign body sensation, and discharge. Examination will reveal upper lid ptosis, deep superior fornices, coagulum of mucopurulent material in the superior fornix, injection, and mucopurulent or purulent discharge. Pseudomembranes have also been reported. With chronic, undertreated conjunctivitis, punctate epitheliopathy, corneal neovascularization, scarring, epithelial defects, and ulceration are possible. Conjunctival cultures are most often positive for *Staphylococcus aureus*, and they should be routinely obtained in these patients due to the prevalence of methicillin-resistant *S. aureus* [14].

The management and course of deep fornix syndrome can often be difficult for clinicians and patients. First-line therapy includes frequent (every 1–2 h) topical steroids and topical antibiotics as well as systemic anti-staphylococcals [14]. Prednisolone acetate 1% is often used as the steroid, though fluorometholone and loteprednol may provide similar ocular surface benefits with a lower risk of steroid-induced ocular hypertension. Sweeping of the fornices with cotton tip applicators is recommended to debride the large coagulum from the fornices. Rinsing and sweeping the superior fornices with povidone-iodine has been reported to work in patients that did not improve with topical therapy [45]. Finally, surgical reconstruction of the fornix has also been successful in treating some patients that were refractive to more conservative measures [46].

1.10.3 Moraxella Conjunctivitis

Moraxella has been well known as a pathogen that causes angular and ulcerative blepharitis, but it should also be entertained in the differential for chronic follicular conjunctivitis. One study at a tertiary care center demonstrated 33 cases of *Moraxella* conjunctivitis over the course of a year [47]. Due to the potential for a follicular conjunctivitis, *Moraxella* has been misdiagnosed as adenovirus, herpesvirus, and *Chlamydia*. Performing Giemsa stains and obtaining conjunctival cultures prior to initiating treatment allows for quick rectification of a misdiagnosis that may have implications of a sexually transmitted infection from *Chlamydia*. Treatment can be guided by sensitivity results from microbiology.

1.11 Phlyctenular Keratoconjunctivitis

Phlyctenular keratoconjunctivitis is a type of inflammatory conjunctivitis from a hypersensitivity reaction. The triggering antigen is usually a bacterial protein usually from *Staphylococcus aureus*, but may also be from *Candida albicans*, virus, or nematode. Many patients have associated blepharitis. The diagnosis is mainly clinical. Patients have one or more small yellow-gray nodules (phlyctenules) that appear at the limbus, on the cornea, or on the bulbar conjunctiva and persist from few days to 2 weeks. The patients present with lacrimation, photophobia, and foreign body sensation when cornea is involved. Corneal lesions begin at the limbus and spread centrally, leaving no clear zone between the lesion and the limbus (Fig. 1.6).

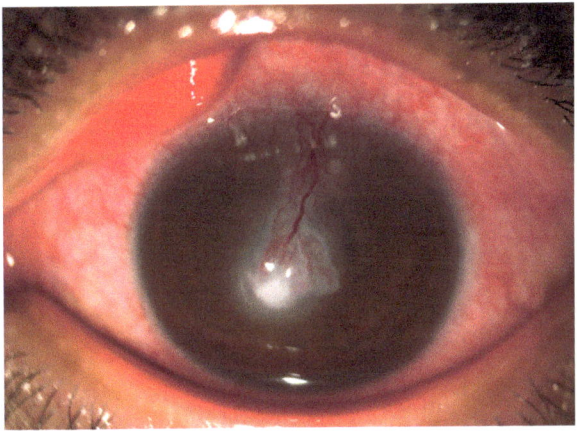

Fig. 1.6 Phlyctenular keratoconjunctivitis with leash of blood vessel. (Courtesy: Aravind Roy)

Conjunctival lesions are associated with mild symptoms, including tearing and foreign body sensation. Recurrence is known with associated blepharitis and may lead to corneal neovascularization and loss of visual acuity. Histopathologically, phlyctenules consist of subepithelial inflammatory nodules containing lymphocytes, histiocytes, neutrophils, and plasma cells.

Management requires both anti-inflammatory and antibacterial management, as well as management of chronic blepharitis. Aggressive lid hygiene with hot compresses, lid cleansers, and antibiotic drops is required to prevent disease recurrence. Topical corticosteroids should be tapered slowly to avoid recurrences. Systemic administration of tetracycline derivatives, such as doxycycline has been used to prevent recurrence. Tetracyclines should not be used in children under age 8 due to the risk of permanent tooth discoloration. It should be avoided in pregnant women and nursing mothers.

References

1. Høvding G. Acute bacterial conjunctivitis. Acta Ophthalmol. 2008;86(1):5–17.
2. McDonnell PJ. How do general practitioners manage eye disease in the community? Br J Ophthalmol. 1988;72(10):733–6.
3. Dart JK. Eye disease at a community health centre. Br Med J. 1986;293(6560):1477–80.
4. Everitt H, Little P. How do GPs diagnose and manage acute infective conjunctivitis? A GP survey. Fam Pract. 2002;19(6):658–60.
5. Kowalski RP, Nayyar SV, Romanowski EG, Shanks RMQ, Mammen A, Dhaliwal DK, Jhanji V. The prevalence of bacteria, fungi, viruses, and acanthamoeba from 3,004 cases of keratitis, endophthalmitis, and conjunctivitis. Eye Contact Lens. 2019; Online ahead of print.
6. Kowalski RP. Is antibiotic resistance a problem in the treatment of ophthalmic infections? J Expert Rev Ophthalmol. 2013;8(2):119–26.
7. Chandler JW, Gillette TE. Immunologic defense mechanisms of the ocular surface. Ophthalmology. 1983;90(6):585–91.
8. Dawson CR. How does the external eye resist infection. Investig Ophthalmol. 1976;15(12):971–4.
9. Stuchell RN, Farris RL, Mandel ID. Basal and reflex human tear analysis. II. Chemical analysis: lactoferrin and lysozyme. Ophthalmology. 1981;88(8):858–61.
10. Perkins RE, Kundsin RB, Pratt MV, Abrahamsen I, Leibowitz HM. Bacteriology of normal and infected conjunctiva. J Clin Microbiol. 1975;1(2):147–9.
11. Teweldemedhin M, Saravanan M, Gebreyesus A, Gebreegziabiher D. Ocular bacterial infections at Quiha Ophthalmic Hospital, Northern Ethiopia: an evaluation according to the risk factors and the antimicrobial susceptibility of bacterial isolates. BMC Infect Dis. 2017;17(1):207.
12. Høvding G. [Acute bacterial conjunctivitis]. Tidsskrift for den Norske Laegeforening: Tidsskrift for Praktisk Medicin, ny Raekke. 2004;124(11):1518–1520.
13. Schwartz B, Harrison LH, Motter JS, Motter RN, Hightower AW, Broome CV. Investigation of an outbreak of Moraxella conjunctivitis at a Navajo boarding school. Am J Ophthalmol. 1989;107(4):341–7.
14. Rose GE. The giant fornix syndrome: an unrecognized cause of chronic, relapsing, grossly purulent conjunctivitis. Ophthalmology. 2004;111(8):1539–45.
15. Patel PB, Diaz MCG, Bennett JE, Attia MW. Clinical features of bacterial conjunctivitis in children. Acad Emergency Med. 2007;14(1):1–5.
16. Rietveld RP, ter Riet G, Bindels PJ, Bink D, Sloos JH, van Weert HC. The treatment of acute infectious conjunctivitis with fusidic acid: a randomised controlled trial. Br J Gen Pract. 2005;55(521):924–30.

17. Duke-Elder S, Leigh AG. Inflammation of the conjunctiva and associated inflammation of the cornea. In: Duke-Elder S, editor. System of ophthalmology, Diseases of the outer eye, vol. VIII. St Louis: Mosby; 1961.
18. Katusic D, Petricek I, Mandic Z, Petric I, Salopek-Rabatic J, Kruzic V, Oreskovic K, Sikic J, Petricek G. Azithromycin vs doxycycline in the treatment of inclusion conjunctivitis. Am J Ophthalmol. 2003;135(4):447–51.
19. Lesser RL. Ocular manifestations of Lyme disease. Am J Med. 1995;98(4A):60S–2S.
20. Mombaerts IM, Maudgal PC, Knockaert DC. Bilateral follicular conjunctivitis as a manifestation of Lyme disease. Am J Ophthalmol. 1991;112(1):96–7.
21. Kivelä T, Tervo K, Ravila E, Tarkkanen A, Virtanen I, Tervo T. Pseudomembranous and membranous conjunctivitis. Immunohistochemical features. Acta Ophthalmol. 1992;70(4):534–42.
22. De Cock R. Membranous, pseudomembranous and ligneous conjunctivitis. Dev Ophthalmol. 1997;28:32–45.
23. Spektor FE, Eagle RC Jr, Nichols CW. Granulomatous conjunctivitis secondary to Treponema pallidum. Ophthalmology. 1981;88(8):863–5.
24. Faraj HG, Hoang-Xuan T. Chronic cicatrizing conjunctivitis. Curr Opin Ophthalmol. 2001;12(4):250–7.
25. Smith AF, Waycaster C. Estimate of the direct and indirect annual cost of bacterial conjunctivitis in the United States. BMC Ophthalmol. 2009;9:13.
26. Sheikh A, Hurwitz B, van Schayck CP, McLean S, Nurmatov U. Antibiotics versus placebo for acute bacterial conjunctivitis. Cochrane Database Syst Rev. 2012;9:CD001211.
27. Isenberg SJ, Apt L, Valenton M, Del Signore M, Cubillan L, Labrador MA, Chan P, Berman NG. A controlled trial of povidone-iodine to treat infectious conjunctivitis in children. Am J Ophthalmol. 2002;134(5):681–8.
28. Gigliotti F, Williams WT, Hayden FG, Hendley JO, Benjamin J, Dickens M, Gleason C, Perriello VA, Wood J. Etiology of acute conjunctivitis in children. J Pediatr. 1981;98(4):531–6.
29. Matejcek A, Goldman RD. Treatment and prevention of ophthalmia neonatorum. Can Fam Physician. 2013;59(11):1187–90.
30. Fitch CP, Rapoza PA, Owens S, Murillo-Lopez F, Johnson RA, Quinn TC, Pepose JS, Taylor HR. Epidemiology and diagnosis of acute conjunctivitis at an inner-city hospital. Ophthalmology. 1989;96(8):1215–20.
31. Margo CE, Hamed LM. Ocular syphilis. Surv Ophthalmol. 1992;37(3):203–20.
32. Belga S, Gratrix J, Smyczek P, Bertholet L, Read R, Roelofs K, Singh AE. Gonococcal conjunctivitis in adults: case report and retrospective review of cases in Alberta, Canada, 2000-2016. Sex Transm Dis. 2019;46(1):47–51.
33. Parikh SR, Campbell H, Mandal S, Ramsay ME, Ladhani SN. Primary meningococcal conjunctivitis: summary of evidence for the clinical and public health management of cases and close contacts. J Infect. 2019;79(6):490–4.
34. Bodurtha Smith AJ, Holzman SB, Manesh RS, Perl TM. Gonococcal conjunctivitis: a case report of an unusual mode of transmission. J Pediatr Adolesc Gynecol. 2017;30(4):501–2.
35. Ullman S, Roussel TJ, Culbertson WW, Forster RK, Alfonso E, Mendelsohn AD, Heidemann DG, Holland SP. Neisseria gonorrhoeae keratoconjunctivitis. Ophthalmology. 1987;94(5):525–31.
36. Lessing JN, Slingsby TJ, Betz M. Hyperacute gonococcal keratoconjunctivitis. J Gen Intern Med. 2019;34(3):477–8.
37. Lyss SB, Kamb ML, Peterman TA, Moran JS, Newman DR, Bolan G, Douglas JM Jr, Iatesta M, Malotte CK, Zenilman JM, Ehret J, Gaydos C, Newhall WJ, Project RESPECT Study Group. Chlamydia trachomatis among patients infected with and treated for Neisseria gonorrhoeae in sexually transmitted disease clinics in the United States. Ann Intern Med. 2003;139(3):178–85.
38. Lansingh VC. Trachoma. BMJ Clin Evid. 2016;2016:0706.
39. Taylor HR, Burton MJ, Haddad D, West S, Wright H. Trachoma. Lancet. 2014;384(9960):2142–52.
40. Al-Fawaz A, Wagoner MD, King Khaled Eye Specialist Hospital Corneal Transplant Study Group. Penetrating keratoplasty for trachomatous corneal scarring. Cornea. 2008;27(2):129–32.

41. Dawson CR, Juster R, Marx R, Daghfous MT, Ben Djerad A. Limbal disease in trachoma and other ocular chlamydial infections: risk factors for corneal vascularisation. Eye. 1989;3(Pt-2):204–9.
42. Buus DR, Pflugfelder SC, Schachter J, Miller D, Forster RK. Lymphogranuloma venereum conjunctivitis with a marginal corneal perforation. Ophthalmology. 1988;95(6):799–802.
43. Scheie HG, Crandall AS, et al. Keratitis associated with lymphogranuloma venereum. Am J Ophthalmol. 1947;30(5):624–7.
44. Workowski KA, Berman S, Centers for Disease Control and Prevention (CDC). Sexually transmitted diseases treatment guidelines, 2010. MMWR Recomm Rep. 2010;59(RR-12):1–110.
45. Karim R, Mandal N, Tuft S. Management of giant fornix syndrome with irrigation with povidone-iodine. BMJ Case Rep. 2018;2018:bcr2018225555.
46. Nabavi CB, Long JA, Compton CJ, Vicinanzo MG. A novel surgical technique for the treatment of giant fornix syndrome. Ophthalmic Plast Reconstr Surg. 2013;29(1):63–6.
47. Kowalski RP, Harwick JC. Incidence of Moraxella conjunctival infection. Am J Ophthalmol. 1986;101(4):437–40.

Lawson Ung, Jaya Rajaiya, and James Chodosh

2.1   Introduction

Viral conjunctivitis ("pink eye") is the most common form of conjunctival infection [1]. In the medical literature, viral conjunctivitis is widely regarded as a trivial disease, causing transient eye irritation, injection, chemosis, and increased lacrimation However, viral conjunctival infections are now understood to be caused by a rich and diverse consortium of viruses, many of which have distinct and variable patterns of disease presentation, unique epidemiologic features, and natural histories. While most cases will resolve spontaneously with no long-term complications, several viral infections have chronic manifestations that may result in visual impairment and disability. The viruses responsible for ocular infection also have wide-ranging tissue tropisms, and a significant proportion of affected patients will develop conjunctivitis as just one of the many clinical features associated with systemic disease. The social and economic burdens of viral conjunctivitis are compounded by the ease of transmission among its causative agents, which continue to be implicated in global and nosocomial outbreaks. In this chapter, we offer an overview of the etiologies and clinical syndromes associated with these infections, which remain an important but underappreciated cause of ocular morbidity.

2.2   The History of Viral Conjunctivitis

Historically, our understanding of viral conjunctivitis has been driven by clinical studies conducted in the wake of international and regional outbreaks. These research efforts led to the isolation of numerous pathogens and their

L. Ung · J. Rajaiya · J. Chodosh (✉)
Infectious Disease Institute and Department of Ophthalmology, Massachusetts Eye and Ear,
Harvard Medical School, Boston, MA, USA
e-mail: Lawson_Ung@meei.harvard.edu; Jaya_Rajaiya@meei.harvard.edu;
james_chodosh@meei.harvard.edu

© Springer Nature Singapore Pte Ltd. 2021   17
S. Das, V. Jhanji (eds.), *Infections of the Cornea and Conjunctiva*,
https://doi.org/10.1007/978-981-15-8811-2_2

conjunctivitis-associated types, including human adenovirus [2, 3] and human enteroviruses [4, 5]. However, references to epidemic conjunctivitis can be found in medical historiography dating back to at least the seventeenth and eighteenth centuries, and possibly earlier. In this early modern period, viral conjunctivitis was likely included among the many etiologies of "ophthalmia", a general term used to describe the red, inflamed, and/or blind eye [6, 7]. References to "ophthalmia" were dominated by descriptions of chronic, cicatrizing disease most consistent with *Chlamydia trachomatis* infection [8], which was itself erroneously believed to be caused by a viral pathogen originating from the Middle East [9]. However, other important outbreaks were described as having preferentially affected those in itinerant professions, including sailors, tradespeople, and the military [10]. The rapid and explosive nature of disease spread suggest that at least some outbreaks were viral or bacterial in nature [11]. Importantly, the physicians and historians who documented the spread of these epidemics were among the first to speculate that disease could be transmitted directly from individual to individual [12–14]. The circulation of this idea contributed to the gradual erosion of the prevailing miasmal theory of disease, which identified "bad air" as the source of all maladies. Therefore, early accounts of epidemic viral conjunctivitis likely had some role in the paradigm shift towards the germ-theory of disease, which would rise to prominence by the late nineteenth century [15].

2.3   Etiologies of Viral Conjunctivitis

Human adenoviruses, picornaviruses, and herpesviruses are the most common causes of viral conjunctivitis, accounting for up to 82% [16–19], 45% [20, 21], and 5% [16–20] of all cases, respectively. However, these figures should be treated as approximations because viral conjunctivitis remains a clinical diagnosis for the vast majority of patients, and laboratory confirmation is typically sought only in cases of diagnostic uncertainty and in particularly severe cases. Furthermore, it is intuitively obvious that the relative preponderance of these viral etiologies may differ in outbreak settings and/or with seasonal variation [22]. Nonetheless, the conjunctiva is a fertile tissue for many viral infections, which can be remembered with the mnemonic PHARAOH (Tables 2.1 and 2.2):

- **P**icornaviruses, e.g., enterovirus, and poxviruses, e.g., variola, vaccinia, molluscum contagiosum, and orf viruses
- **H**erpesviruses
- **A**denoviruses
- **R**ubella and rubeola (measles)
- **A**rboviruses (e.g., dengue, zika, and chikungunya)
- **O**ther (e.g., coronavirus, influenza virus, and Newcastle disease virus)
- **H**uman immunodeficiency virus (HIV)

Table 2.1 Etiologies of conjunctivitis (human DNA viruses)

Viral species	Family (size)	Subfamily	Genus	Nucleic acid	Genome size (kbp)	Envelope	Incubation period	Ocular tropisms
Adenoviruses								
Adenovirus	Adenoviridae (~75–90 nm)	No subfamily	Mastadenovirus	ds	30–37	No	Up to 14 days	Conjunctiva Cornea
Herpesviruses								
HHV-1 (HSV-1)	Herpesviridae (~120–260 nm)	Alphaherpesvirinae	Simplexvirus	ds	152.2	Yes	Primary infection: 1–28 days Reactivation: 2–3 days	Eyelids Conjunctiva Cornea Trabecular meshwork Uvea Retina Optic nerve
HHV-2 (HSV-2)		Alphaherpesvirinae	Simplexvirus	ds	154.7	Yes	Primary infection: 1–28 days Reactivation: 2–3 days	
HHV-3 (VZV)		Alphaherpesvirinae	Varicellovirus	ds	124.9	Yes	1–3 weeks	
HHV-4 (EBV)		Gammaherpesvirinae	Lymphocryptovirus	ds	71.8	Yes	6–7 weeks	Lacrimal gland
HHV-5 (HCMV)		Betaherpesvirinae	Cytomegalovirus	ds	235.6	Yes	3–12 weeks	Conjunctiva Cornea Uvea Retina Optic nerve
HHV-6A		Betaherpesvirinae	Roseolovirus	ds	160–162	Yes	1–2 weeks	Conjunctiva Uvea Retina
HHV-6B		Betaherpesvirinae	Roseolovirus	ds	160–162	Yes	1–2 weeks	Conjunctiva Uvea Retina
HHV-8 (KSHV)		Gammaherpesvirinae	Rhadinovirus	ds	137–138	Yes	Variable; may be up to years	Conjunctiva (Kaposi sarcoma)

(continued)

Table 2.1 (continued)

Viral species	Family (size)	Subfamily	Genus	Nucleic acid	Genome size (kbp)	Envelope	Incubation period	Ocular tropisms
Papillomaviruses								
HPV	Papillomaviridae (~55 nm)	Firstpapillomavirinae	Alphapapillomavirus	ds	7–8	No	2–3 months	Eyelid Conjunctiva
Poxviruses								
Variola virus	Poxviridae (up to 450 nm)	Chordopoxvirinae	Orthopoxvirus	ds	185.6	Yes	7–19 days	Eyelids Conjunctiva Cornea Uvea Retina Optic nerve
Vaccinia virus		Chordopoxvirinae	Orthopoxvirus	ds	194.7	Yes	5–7 days	Eyelids Conjunctiva Cornea Uvea
Molluscum contagiosum virus		Chordopoxvirinae	Molluscipoxvirus	ds	190.3	Yes	6–7 weeks	Eyelids Conjunctiva Cornea
Orf virus		Chordopoxvirinae	Parapoxvirus	ds	140.0	Yes	3–7 days	Eyelid Conjunctiva

Legend: *ds* double-stranded DNA; *kbp* kilobase pairs, as determined by reference to the NCBI Assembly

Adapted with permission from Chodosh J, Stroop WG. Introduction to Viruses in Ocular Disease. In: Tasman W, Jaeger EA, eds. Duane's Foundations of Clinical Ophthalmology. Philadelphia, USA: Lippincott Williams & Wilkins, 2005: Chapter 85

Table 2.2 Etiologies of conjunctivitis (human RNA viruses)

Viral species	Family (size)	Subfamily	Genus	Nucleic acid	Genome size (kbp)	Envelope	Incubation period	Ocular tropisms
Arboviruses								
Chikungunya virus	*Togaviridae* (~70 nm)	No subfamily	*Alphavirus*	ss (−)	11.8	Yes	1–12 days	Conjunctiva Cornea Uvea Retina Optic nerve
Dengue virus	*Flaviviridae* (~50 nm)	No subfamily	*Flavivirus*	ss (+)	10.7	Yes	3–10 days	Conjunctiva Cornea Uvea Retina Optic nerve
Rift Valley fever virus	*Bunyaviridae* (80–120 nm)	No subfamily	*Phlebovirus*	ss (−)	1.7	Yes	2–6 days	Conjunctiva Uvea Retina
Yellow fever virus	*Flaviviridae* (~50 nm)	No subfamily	*Flavivirus*	ss (+)	10.9	Yes	3–9 days	Conjunctiva Uvea Retina
Zika virus	*Flaviviridae* (~50 nm)	No subfamily	*Flavivirus*	ss (+)	10.8	Yes	3–14 days	Conjunctiva Cornea Uvea Retina Optic nerve
Coronaviruses								
Human coronaviruses[a]	*Coronaviridae* (120–160 nm)	*Coronavirinae*	*Alphacoronavirus* and *Betacoronavirus*	ss (+)	27–30	Yes	2–14 days	Conjunctiva

(continued)

Table 2.2 (continued)

Viral species	Family (size)	Subfamily	Genus	Nucleic acid	Genome size (kbp)	Envelope	Incubation period	Ocular tropisms
Orthomyxoviruses								
Influenza viruses[b]	Orthomyxoviridae (80–120 nm)	No subfamilies	Alphainfluenzaevirus Betainfluenzavirus Gammainfluenzavirus	ss (−)	10–14.6	Yes	1–4 days	Lacrimal gland Conjunctiva Cornea Uvea Retina Optic nerve
Paramyxoviruses								
Measles morbillivirus (measles, rubeola)	Paramyxoviridae (~150 nm)	Orthoparamyxovirinae	Morbillivirus	ss (−)	15.9	Yes	2–21 days	Conjunctiva Cornea Uvea Retina Optic nerve Cranial nerves
Mumps		Paramyxovirinae	Rubulavirus	ss (−)	15.4	Yes	12–25 days	Lacrimal gland Conjunctiva Sclera Cornea Uvea Retina Optic nerve Cranial nerves
Newcastle disease virus[c]		Paramyxovirinae	Avulavirus	ss (−)	15.2	Yes	1 day	Conjunctiva
Parainfluenza virus		Paramyxovirinae	Rubulavirus	ss (−)	15–17	Yes	2–7 days	Conjunctiva

Picornaviruses								
Enterovirus C and Enterovirus D[d]	*Picornaviridae* (30–32 nm)	No subfamily	*Enterovirus*	ss (+)	7–8	No	Up to 3 days	Conjunctiva Cornea
Rhinoviruses[e]		No subfamily	*Enterovirus*	ss (+)	7.1	No	<24 h	Conjunctiva
Retroviruses								
HIV-1 HIV-2	*Retroviridae* (80–100 nm)	*Orthoretrovirinae*	*Lentivirus*	ss (−)	9.2	Yes	3–12 weeks	Lacrimal gland Conjunctiva Cornea Uvea Retina Optic nerve
Togaviruses								
Rubella virus	*Togaviridae* (~70 nm)	No subfamily	*Rubivirus*	ss (−)	9.8	Yes	12–23 days	Conjunctiva Cornea Uvea Lens Retina

Legend: *ds* double-stranded DNA; *ss* single-stranded RNA; (+) positive sense; (−) negative sense; *kbp* kilobase pairs, as determined by reference to the NCBI Assembly

Adapted with permission from Chodosh J, Stroop WG. Introduction to Viruses in Ocular Disease. In: Tasman W, Jaeger EA, eds. Duane's Foundations of Clinical Ophthalmology. Philadelphia, USA: Lippincott Williams & Wilkins, 2005: Chapter 85

[a]Includes human coronaviruses 229E, NL63, OC43, HKU1, Middle-Eastern Respiratory Syndrome Coronavirus (MERS-CoV), Severe Acute Respiratory Syndrome coronavirus (SARS-CoV), and Severe Acute Respiratory Syndrome coronavirus 2 (SARS-CoV-2)

[b]Includes influenza A virus, influenza B virus, influenza C virus; influenza D virus is not known to cause disease in humans

[c]Also known as avian avulavirus 1

[d]Includes coxsackievirus A24 and enterovirus D70, respectively

[e]Includes species rhinovirus A, rhinovirus B, and rhinovirus C

The clinical presentations of viral conjunctivitis are mostly nonspecific, producing symptoms such as eye irritation, pain, pruritus, and foreign body sensation, and signs including conjunctival injection, discharge, edema, formation of follicles, papillae and/or membranes, and regional lymphadenopathy. Despite these common clinical findings, likely the result of convergent inflammatory pathways which are activated following viral infection, a weighted differential diagnosis can nonetheless be generated with an appreciation of certain patterns of ocular disease and their associated nonocular features. These may be pathognomonic or highly suggestive of certain viruses.

2.4   Adenoviral Conjunctivitis

2.4.1   The Human Adenoviruses

The human adenoviruses (HAdVs), belonging to the family *Adenoviridae* and genus *Mastadenovirus*, are a collection of nonenveloped, medium-sized (~70–90 nm), double-stranded DNA (dsDNA) viruses with a strong historical association with ocular infection [23, 24]. The first known clinical descriptions of adenoviral conjunctivitis were made by Austrian ophthalmologists Ernst Fuchs [25] and Karl Stellwag von Carion [26] during a large central European outbreak in the late nineteenth century. This disease was of a particularly severe form of adenoviral conjunctivitis subsequently termed as "epidemic keratoconjunctivitis" (EKC) [27], the only form of adenoviral conjunctivitis known to be accompanied by significant corneal infection. Particularly notable epidemics of EKC affecting thousands of patients were later reported in Madras in 1930 [28], and in the naval yards of Pearl Harbor in Hawaii and San Francisco in the early 1940s [29]. These latter outbreaks led to the popular designation of this mysterious affliction as "shipyard eye" [3, 30]. The causative agent of EKC would not come to light until the first adenovirus was serendipitously isolated in human adenoid tissue, by Rowe and colleagues in 1953 [31], amid efforts to identify the virus responsible for the common cold. The subsequent identification of HAdV type 8 (HAdV-D8) in conjunctival scrapings from an EKC patient [2] established the viral etiology of this disease. HAdVs are extremely contagious and resistant to environmental desiccation, and can be transmitted easily through contact with infected persons and their surroundings [32]. Currently, there are 103 HAdV types, across seven species (A to G), which have been formally recognized with whole genome sequencing (WGS) [23, 33]. In virology, WGS has succeeded serum neutralization and hemagglutination inhibition as the more accurate method of taxonomic classification. HAdV types are determined on the basis of unique nucleotide sequencing of major capsid proteins (penton, hexon, and/or fiber knob), or by unique patterns of genome recombination.

2.4.1.1   Clinical Syndromes Associated with Human Adenovirus
HAdV conjunctivitis is caused by species B (HAdV-B), D (HAdV-D), and E (HAdV-E) adenoviruses, which are classically associated with three distinct

syndromes: simple follicular conjunctivitis (types B3, E4, and B7), pharyngocon-junctival fever or PCF (types C2, B3, E4, B7, and B14), and EKC (types D8, D37, D53, D54, D56, D64, and D85). The incubation time for adenovirus ranges from 5 to 14 days. Simple follicular conjunctivitis, perhaps the most common form, is char-acterized by conjunctival injection, chemosis, edema, conjunctival follicle forma-tion, and serous discharge. Bilateral disease is common. PCF, as its name suggests, is a clinical syndrome characterized by febrile pharyngitis and follicular conjuncti-vitis. Although its name was coined following a nosocomial outbreak at the National Institutes of Health, Maryland, USA in 1954 [34], the first clinical descriptions of PCF were made by the French physician Beal during a Parisian epidemic in 1904 [35]. PCF is therefore also eponymously known as Beal's conjunctivitis [36]. These forms of HAdV conjunctivitis typically resolve spontaneously within 2 weeks of symptom onset, and usually do not require specific therapeutic intervention beyond symptomatic measures.

The most severe form of HAdV conjunctivitis is the aforementioned EKC, which may lead to chronic visual complications [32]. EKC is characterized by a classic constellation of signs including preauricular lymphadenopathy, hyperacute and sometimes membranous conjunctivitis, corneal epithelial keratitis, and the hallmark formation of delayed-onset subepithelial infiltrates (SEIs) (Fig. 2.1) [37]. Conjunctivitis seen in EKC is associated with the formation of exudative mem-branes which, if left untreated, may fibrose and lead to restriction of ocular motility [38]. The corneal manifestations of EKC distinguish this entity from other forms of HAdV conjunctivitis. In addition to a diffuse epithelial keratitis with punctate epi-thelial and/or macroepithelial erosions, SEIs develop in an estimated 20–30% of patients, leading to chronic, relapsing and remitting disease [39]. These SEIs, shown in animal models to involve aggregations of neutrophil-predominant leukocytes, are mediated by a complex inflammatory response within the corneal epithelium and stroma [40–42]. Their presence may result in reduced vision, photophobia, and glare. Despite decades of research in therapeutics, ranging from topical antiseptics [43–48], antivirals [49–51], and immunomodulators such as tacrolimus and

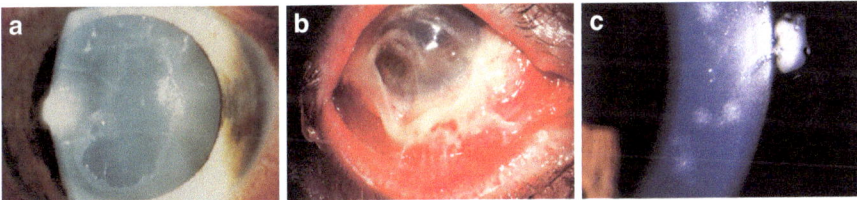

Fig. 2.1 Clinical Manifestations of Epidemic Keratoconjunctivitis (EKC): (**a**) geographic epithe-lial keratitis with a large epithelial defect; (**b**) severe, fulminant membranous conjunctivitis with symblepharon formation, which may lead to restriction of ocular motility; and (**c**) corneal subepi-thelial infiltrates (SEIs) as shown by slit lamp examination. Note the relatively uniform size of these SEIs, which tend to be <0.5 mm. SEIs seen in keratitis caused by other viruses (e.g. HSV and VZV) are often larger in diameter. [*Reproduced with permission from "Jonas RA, Ung L, Rajaiya J, Chodosh J. Mystery eye: Human adenovirus and the enigma of epidemic keratoconjunctivitis. Prog Retin Eye Res 2019: 100826" published by Elsevier*]

cyclosporin [52–56], topical corticosteroids remain the only treatment known to reliably alter the course of EKC. When expertly applied, topical corticosteroids may be administered to the eye following the removal of conjunctival membranes, and/ or to achieve remission in patients with chronic SEIs. However, tapering must be pursued slowly owing to the risk of rebound SEI formation.

2.5   Herpes Conjunctivitis

2.5.1   The Human Herpesviruses

The herpesviruses, belonging to order *Herpesvirales* and family *Herpesviridae*, are a collection of large (120–260 nm), spherical, dsDNA viruses composed of an icosahedral capsid, a protein-rich tegument, and an external lipid envelope [57–59]. Nine herpesvirus species are known to infect humans, and collectively they are known as the human herpesviruses 1 through 8 (HHV 1–8, with HHV-6 further subdivided into HHV-6A and HHV-6B). The viruses most strongly associated with conjunctivitis are the first five HHVs: HHV-1, otherwise known as herpes simplex virus type 1 (HSV-1); HHV-2 or herpes simplex virus type 2 (HSV-2); HHV-3 or varicella zoster virus (VZV); HHV-4 or Epstein-Barr virus (EBV); and HHV-5 or human cytomegalovirus (HCMV). Of the remaining HHVs, HHV-6 and HHV-8 (Kaposi sarcoma-associated herpesvirus, KSHV) also demonstrate ocular surface tropism [60–62] but have been more closely studied in other settings, including their potential role in oncogenesis [63–65]. All HHVs establish lifelong latent infections in a variety of cell types [66–69]. For example, the most common cause of ocular infection, HSV, remains nestled in sensory neurons within the trigeminal and dorsal root ganglia [70–74]. Persistence in extraneuronal tissues such as the cornea [75, 76] and ocular surface epithelium [77, 78] have also been reported. In general, the manifestations of herpetic eye disease occur as the result of primary infection, or the reactivation of latent virions within infected nerve ganglia.

2.5.2   Herpes Simplex Virus Conjunctivitis

HSV-1 and HSV-2, of the subfamily *Alphaherpesvirinae* and genus *Simplexvirus*, are indistinguishably associated with conjunctivitis. Conjunctival HSV infection typically manifests as an acute, unilateral, and diffuse follicular conjunctivitis resulting in increased lacrimation, foreign body sensation, and preauricular lymphadenopathy [79]. The application of fluorescein or rose bengal staining to the ocular surface may reveal characteristic bulbar geographic or dendritic ulcer(s) on slit lamp examination [80, 81]. The presence of blistering herpetic vesicles and/or ulcers found along the eyelid margin, periocular skin, lips, and oral cavity, in a nondermatomal distribution, is particularly suggestive of HSV. In these patients, it is critically important to carefully examine the cornea for evidence of epithelial, stromal, and/or endothelial keratitis. The presence of corneal disease mandates specific therapeutic interventions, including antiviral and/or topical corticosteroid therapy [82–84], along with considerations of oral antiviral prophylaxis. The involvement of any of these corneal layers, which may be the result of contiguous spread from adnexal lesions [85], represents a more severe form of infection which may lead to vision loss if not treated in a timely and appropriate manner. In the absence of corneal disease, HSV conjunctivitis typically follows a benign clinical course without specific intervention, and most cases will resolve within 2 weeks of onset [16], although rarely chronic blepharoconjunctivitis may last for months [79, 86]. An important caveat, however, is that viral reactivation may result in disease beyond the site of primary infection [84]. Patients with HSV conjunctivitis should therefore be counseled on the possibility of viral reactivation in both the ocular adnexa and cornea, which require prompt ophthalmological review.

2.5.3 Herpes Simplex Virus Conjunctivitis in Neonates

HSV is the most common viral cause of ophthalmia neonatorum, a form of neonatal conjunctivitis which develops in the first month after birth [87]. Although HSV may infect neonates in utero through transplacental transmission, most infections are caused by neonatal HSV exposure during delivery. This may occur either through contact with active genital lesions or silent shedding through the birth passage mucosa [88, 89]. Neonatal HSV affects up to 12 in 100,000 live births in the USA [90, 91], with over 60% of cases caused by HSV-2 [92]. Postpartum newborn checks are an opportune time to screen neonates for HSV infection, as lesions on the skin, eye, and mouth may arise between the first and third weeks of life [93]. Herpetic vesicles involving the periocular skin and lids are common, and may be associated with conjunctivitis [94]. The presence of findings consistent with HSV infection should prompt comprehensive examination of the anterior and posterior segments of the eye to assess for the presence of keratitis and/or chorioretinitis which, although rare, are sight-threatening and may result in cortical blindness in the developing infant. Also, and importantly, the presence of any indication for ocular HSV warrants immediate referral to a neonatologist or pediatrician, owing to the possibility of systemic HSV viremia. Suspicion for systemic HSV should prompt admission of the child for lumbar puncture, cultures and testing by polymerase chain reaction, and intravenous acyclovir. Neural and/or visceral HSV invasion may result in lifelong complications even with the timely administration of systemic antiviral therapy [95]. Unfortunately, despite advances in treatment, disseminated disease carries greater than 50% mortality rate [96].

2.5.4 Varicella Zoster Virus (VZV) Conjunctivitis

The varicella zoster virus (VZV) belongs to the *Alphaherpesvirinae* subfamily and genus *Varicellovirus* [59, 97]. Like its close relatives HSV-1 and HSV-2, VZV is a neurotrophic virus which establishes lifelong latency in neuronal ganglionic tissue, and is therefore capable of causing both primary and recurrent disease [98]. VZV is associated with two main clinical syndromes: primary varicella infection ("chickenpox") manifests as an intensely pruritic, vesicobullous rash during childhood; and herpes zoster, which is the result of viral reactivation, and estimated to affect 20–30% of the population over their lifetime [99, 100]. Primary VZV infection is occasionally associated with ocular manifestations [101, 102], most commonly bulbar conjunctival ulcers. Ocular VZV infection may also occur as the result of viral reactivation within the ophthalmic (V_1), and less commonly, the maxillary (V_2) divisions of the fifth cranial nerve [103], leading to a clinical syndrome known as herpes zoster ophthalmicus (HZO). HZO accounts for roughly one-fifth of all herpes zoster cases, and is characterized by the unilateral eruption of painful, crusty, maculopapular lesions in a classic dermatomal distribution. This clinical picture may be preceded by the formation of the same lesions at the nasal tip (Hutchinson's sign), representing involvement of the nasociliary branch of the ophthalmic nerve [104, 105]. The lesions associated with HZO are most apparent on the periorbital skin, eyelids, forehead, and nose, and may extend onto the conjunctiva and corneal limbus. Importantly, an insidious variant of HZO known as ophthalmic zoster sine herpete involves the *absence* of these characteristic skin lesions [106–108]. Conjunctivitis is the most common ocular manifestation of HZO [109, 110], is typically self-limiting, and does not require specific treatment. Very rarely, it may be associated with the formation of membranes and cicatricial disease [111]. As with HSV, it is critically important to carefully examine the cornea in HZO. Vision-threatening corneal involvement occurs in up to two-thirds of HZO patients [112], and may manifest as an epithelial, stromal, and/or endothelial keratitis. The presence of keratitis may warrant antiviral and/or corticosteroid therapy to salvage vision [113, 114]. Comprehensive reviews of HZO-associated corneal disease can be found elsewhere [112, 115].

2.5.5 Other Herpetic Etiologies of Conjunctivitis

HHV-4 (EBV) and HHV-5 (HCMV), both lymphotropic viruses, are now increasingly recognized as ocular surface pathogens. EBV, of the subfamily *Gammaherpesvirinae* and genus *Lymphocryptovirus*, has been mostly studied in the context of heterophile antibody-positive infectious mononucleosis (IM) [116], autoimmune conditions such as primary Sjogren's syndrome [117], and is now known to be an oncogenic virus owing to its close association with Burkitt's lymphoma [118] and epithelial cell neoplasia [119]. It has also been identified as an etiologic agent in ocular surface infections. CD21, the canonical EBV receptor, is found on B-lymphocytes as well as ocular surface epithelium [120–122]. EBV infection of B-lymphocytes, its site of viral latency, may encourage "transfer infection" to the basolateral surface of neighboring epithelial cells through the activation of B-lymphocyte-specific adhesion molecules [122]. This unique signaling biology may explain why conjunctivitis is seen in up to 40% [123] of patients with EBV-associated IM. EBV may manifest as a unilateral follicular conjunctivitis associated with lid edema, conjunctival hemorrhage, and palpable preauricular and/or cervical lymphadenopathy [124–127]. EBV is also a rare cause of Parinaud's oculoglandular syndrome, comprised of chronic granulomatous tarsal conjunctivitis and regional lymphadenopathy [125, 128]. Although less common, HCMV, belonging to the subfamily *Betaherpesvirinae* and genus *Cytomegalovirus*, has also been associated with viral conjunctivitis, specifically in the context of HIV infection [129–134]. Both EBV and HCMV conjunctivitis may be associated with potentially sight-threatening keratitis [135–140], uveitis [141–145], and retinitis [146–148], once again emphasizing the importance of thorough ophthalmic examination in conjunctivitis patients.

2.6   Picornavirus Conjunctivitis

The picornaviruses, belonging to the family *Picornaviridae*, are a collection of small (~30 nm), nonenveloped, icosahedral, positive-sense single-stranded RNA viruses [149]. Several members of the genus *Enterovirus* are associated with conjunctivitis, including four human enterovirus species (A–D) and three rhinovirus species (A–C). The most well-known clinical syndrome associated with the picornaviruses is acute hemorrhagic conjunctivitis (AHC), caused principally by human enterovirus species C (including coxsackievirus A24 variant, CA24v) and enterovirus species D (enterovirus type 70, EV70) [150, 151]. With an exceptionally short incubation time (≤24 h), AHC manifests as a rapid onset, painful, follicular conjunctivitis associated with eyelid swelling, epiphora, and serous or seromucoid discharge, initially arising in one eye but often quickly evolving into bilateral disease. The hallmark feature of AHC is the development of subconjunctival hemorrhages of varying severity, ranging from small petechial lesions to confluent areas of frank bleeding that are easily provoked by eye rubbing. Corneal punctate erosions and epithelial keratitis may occur in some patients, but subepithelial infiltrates are thought to be rare in enteroviral infection [152]. There is no specific therapy for AHC, and despite its striking clinical features, infection usually resolves within 1–2 weeks following symptom onset.

The emergence of AHC in the late 1960s, coinciding with the first successful lunar landing, led to this infection being named "Apollo 11 Disease" [153]. The first global pandemic of AHC occurred in 1969, with two main epicenters: Accra, Ghana [154, 155], and the Indonesian island of Java [153]. The disease spread rapidly throughout Africa, Asia, and continental Europe [4, 156], with 1.5 million people affected in the Indian cities of Mumbai and Calcutta alone [153, 157]. This emergent pathogen—later identified as EV70 from conjunctival scrapings of affected individuals [156]—was of significant global concern because of its neural tropism [158–160]. The neuroinvasive manifestations of EV70 include meningoencephalitis, myelitis, and cranial neuritis, and are clinically indistinguishable from infection caused by the feared poliovirus, which is also a member of the human enterovirus species C. Fortunately, the incidence of neurological disease caused by EV70 is not as high as that caused by polio. A large concurrent AHC outbreak arose in Singapore and Malaysia in 1971, leading to 60,000 cases [5]. Initially thought to be caused by the same virus that initiated the 1969 pandemic, the causative agent was later identified as CA24v [161]. EV70 and CA24v, both temperature-sensitive viruses [162, 163], continue to be implicated in periodic outbreaks [164–168], mostly affecting densely populated coastal cities in tropical climates. The largest outbreak since the 1970s occurred in South Korea in 2002, with CA24v-AHC affecting over one million individuals [169]. For reasons that are unclear, while EV70 has caused global pandemics, CA24v has remained mostly confined to Asia.

2.7 Poxvirus Conjunctivitis

2.7.1 Variola (Smallpox) Conjunctivitis

The *Poxviridae* family of viruses consists of large, ovoid, dsDNA viruses [170, 171]. Four are associated with ocular infection: variola, vaccinia, molluscum contagiosum, and orf viruses [172]. These viruses cause conjunctivitis principally through shedding of virions from adjacent infections on the periorbital skin and lid margins. The most lethal of all poxviruses is the variola or smallpox virus, belonging to the subfamily *Chordopoxvirinae* and genus *Orthopoxvirus*. Although smallpox was eradicated in 1977 [173], and no known natural reservoirs exist, smallpox and its close relatives remain of significant public health interest owing to their potential misuse as agents of bioterrorism and biological warfare [174, 175]. Smallpox, which has an incubation period of up to 19 days, is transmitted via respiratory droplets, direct contact, and fomites [176]. The clinical manifestations of smallpox include the generalized eruption of a disfiguring and painful pustular rash, often preceding overwhelming viremia and eventual death in 10–20% of all those infected [177]. The virus was also responsible for severe visual complications, occurring in up to 10% of all cases, and capable of affecting all structures in the eye [174]. The most common of these manifestations was the development of smallpox conjunctivitis of varying severity. While most cases were benign and characterized by subclinical conjunctivitis with mild watery discharge, more severe forms involved the formation of painful, weeping pustules on the eyelid, bulbar conjunctiva, and corneal limbus. These caused severe photophobia, profound injection, and chemosis. Active viral shedding in tears and from ocular surface pustules frequently led to corneal ulceration, the most common cause of smallpox-related blindness [178].

2.7.2 Vaccinia Conjunctivitis

The primary immunogenic ingredient in smallpox vaccines is a replication-competent vaccinia virus, a close relative of variola and also a member of the subfamily *Chordopoxvirinae* and genus *Orthopoxvirus*. Historically, vaccinia infections emerged as one of the unintended consequences of worldwide smallpox immunization programs [172, 179], with an estimated incidence of 1 in 40,000 primary vaccinations [180, 181]. Although the smallpox vaccine is no longer provided in most countries, it is still administered in selected populations. For example, the United States Department of Defense Smallpox Vaccination Program immunized nearly 500,000 military personnel in 2002 [182]. Smallpox immunization produces a distinct papule (up to 1 cm) at the site of injection, which harbors replicating vaccinia virus [183]. Vaccinia ocular infection is precipitated by accidental autoinoculation, from vaccination site to hand to eye [184]. The local papule left after vaccination is thought to shed virions for up to 3 weeks until the scab has fallen off [185]. Following an incubation period of 5–7 days, vaccinia infection of the eye typically results in the formation of white umbilicated pustules on the periorbital skin and eyelids [186, 187]. The same lesions may also arise on the conjunctiva, leading to an acute and diffuse papillary reaction, and serous or mucopurulent discharge [172]. Curiously, conjunctival follicles are not prominent. Vaccinia lesions on the conjunctiva may ulcerate [172], and in severe cases may be associated with the production of a thick, symblepharon-forming membrane. Corneal involvement is rare, occurring in ~1 of 1.2 million primary vaccination recipients [188]. Clinical signs can range from a mild epithelial keratitis to active stromal and endothelial disease, complicated by corneal ulceration. The Centers of Disease Control and Prevention recommends off-label application of topical antivirals (e.g., trifluridine) and consideration of vaccinia immune globulin in severe cases of vaccinia keratoconjunctivitis [183]. Importantly, acyclovir is reported to be ineffective in treating the ocular manifestations of vaccinia [172].

2.7.3 Other Poxvirus-Related Conjunctivitis

Infection with molluscum contagiosum virus, a member of the subfamily *Chordopoxvirinae* and genus *Molluscipoxvirus* [171], is characterized by the pathognomonic formation of multiple painless, discrete, dome-shaped papules with umbilicated centers on the skin. On occasion, molluscum contagiosum can also infect mucous membranes, including the conjunctiva [189]. Following an incubation period of 6–7 weeks, molluscum contagiosum may manifest as unilateral periocular and bulbar conjunctival papules associated with a secondary follicular conjunctivitis [190]. Although benign and not sight-threatening, chronic conjunctivitis has been reported in immunosuppressed patients and has been occasionally associated with cicatricial punctal occlusion [191]. Corneal signs, if present, may include corneal micropannus formation and punctate epithelial keratitis [192]. Anecdotal evidence suggests that oral acyclovir might be effective in treating this disease [193], but elimination of the molluscum lesion on the eyelid margin by incision, excision, or curettage eliminates the source of viral replication and is generally curative in immune competent individuals [191]. The last of the poxviruses capable of infecting humans is the orf virus, belonging to the subfamily *Chordopoxvirinae* and genus *Parapoxvirus*. Orf virus is trophic to sheep and goats, causing pustular dermatitis of the mouth, nose, and teats [194]. However, zoonotic transmission of orf virus has been reported in humans following close contact with livestock, with case reports of maculopapular lesions arising along the canthal folds and conjunctiva, associated with a self-limited mild to moderate conjunctivitis [194].

2.8   Other Important Causes of Viral Conjunctivitis

2.8.1   Arbovirus Conjunctivitis

The arboviruses, an informal acronym for "arthropod-borne" viruses, are transmitted through arthropod vectors including mosquitoes and ticks [195]. The arboviruses, which are single-stranded RNA viruses, have gained international notoriety in recent years owing to their rapid global dissemination. In the last decade alone, outbreaks have swept through the Americas, Africa, and Asia, driven primarily by the tropical and subtropical spread of the mosquito species *Aedes aegypti* and *Aedes albopictus*. The most prominent of these include dengue and zika viruses, both of the family *Flaviviridae* and genus *Flavivirus*; and chikungunya virus, of the family *Togaviridae* and genus *Alphavirus*. Others include Rift Valley fever [196] and yellow fever viruses [197]. The presenting features of arboviral infection vary widely, ranging from asymptomatic disease to an acute febrile illness characterized by constitutional malaise, myalgia, polyarticular arthralgia, headache, and a generalized morbilliform exanthem [198]. Ocular infection may occur as a self-limiting, nonpurulent conjunctivitis with retro-orbital pain [199–201], seen most commonly as the presenting features of zika and chikungunya infection, to potentially sight-threatening uveitis [202, 203], chorioretinitis [204, 205], and optic neuritis [206, 207]. Arboviral infections should be considered part of a weighted differential diagnosis for patients seen in endemic countries and returned travellers, particularly important in resource-constrained settings with limited access to laboratory testing [208]. No specific treatments exist for arbovirus-associated conjunctivitis.

2.8.2   Measles, Mumps, and Rubella Conjunctivitis

The worldwide availability of vaccines against measles, mumps, and rubella (MMR) viruses has led to significant decreases in their overall incidence. However, recent worldwide measles epidemics in 2019 reflect alarming declines in vaccination rates owing to vaccine skepticism and/or hesitancy, as well as waning immunity from childhood immunization [209–211]. The MMR viruses are transmitted through respiratory droplets, direct contact, and fomites. Affected individuals typically develop a prodrome of fever, generalized malaise, and arthralgia, followed by the eruption of a generalized morbilliform exanthem. Conjunctivitis features in 60–70% of all acute presentations of rubella [212] and measles [213], but is less common in mumps [214]. The follicular conjunctivitis caused by these viruses is clinically indistinguishable from other viral causes, although a range of associated ocular and extra-ocular signs may provide diagnostic clues to etiology. For example, acute mumps infection is traditionally associated with parotitis and dacryoadenitis, while measles is associated with pathognomonic Koplik spots— small, raised lesions on an erythematous base—along mucosal surfaces, most commonly on the buccal mucosa but also occasionally found on the conjunctiva [215, 216]. The conjunctivitis seen in measles can be accompanied by corneal ulceration, which occurs within 2 weeks of the viral exanthem [217]. The combination of conjunctivitis, rash, and respiratory symptoms in unvaccinated patients, particularly young children, should always prompt suspicion of MMR infection and referral for urgent medical evaluation.

2.8.3 Conjunctivitis Associated with Human Immunodeficiency Virus

The human immunodeficiency virus (HIV) is associated with either primary or secondary infections of nearly all ocular structures [218]. HIV-associated conjunctivitis may arise through several mechanisms. In acute seroconversion illness, which usually occurs in the first few weeks following HIV infection as the immune system generates detectable levels of HIV antibody, a mild and self-limiting conjunctivitis may develop as part of a flu-like syndrome characterized by malaise, coryza, sore throat, and generalized lymphadenopathy [219, 220]. Progressive immune destruction in HIV-infected patients is associated with an increased risk of reactivation of HSV [221, 222] and HZO [223]. The association between HIV infection and risk of recurrent HZO is particularly strong [224]. HZO occurs in up to 15% of all HIV-infected persons [225], and the relative incident risk of recurrent disease is estimated to be approximately six times that of HIV-negative individuals [226]. HZO in HIV-infected patients is more likely to involve the cornea [227], and more likely to result in chronic pseudodendritiform keratitis, with lesions that lack the characteristic terminal bulbs and central staining seen in HSV epithelial keratitis [228]. HZO in young patients should warrant consideration of HIV testing, particularly in those who may disclose a history of high-risk sexual activity and/or intravenous drug use.

HIV is also associated with increased severity of other ocular infections. In immunocompromised persons, lesions caused by molluscum contagiosum are usually of greater size and number, and secondary chronic conjunctivitis is common [229]. Additionally, opportunistic pathogens which are not usually associated with conjunctival disease may more commonly manifest on the ocular surface of HIV-infected persons, including *Mycobacterium tuberculosis* [230], *Pneumocystis carinii* [231], and microsporidia [232, 233]. A third mechanism by which HIV may result in conjunctivitis is through immune reconstitution inflammatory syndrome (IRIS), which occurs in the months immediately following the initiation of highly active antiretroviral therapy. This condition is characterized by the paradoxical worsening of the inflammatory manifestations of preexisting infections, some of which may have escaped detection at a prior stage [234]. IRIS may unmask previously subclinical HZO [235], microsporidial keratoconjunctivitis [236], and molluscum contagiosum [237]. Finally, HIV is associated with conjunctival microangiopathic changes in up to 80% of patients, mirroring those also found in the retina [238, 239]. Considered to be benign, vascular changes including microaneurysm formation and segmental vessel tortuosity are usually best appreciated at the corneal limbus. However, the pathogenesis of these changes, and their possible relation to HIV infection, remain unclear.

2.8.4   Other Causes of Conjunctivitis

The viruses described above are not an exhaustive list of those capable of causing ocular surface infection. The human papilloma virus (HPV), belonging to the family *Papillomaviridae*, subfamily *Firstpapillomavirinae*, and genus *Alphapapillomavirus* [240], is a ubiquitous epitheliotrophic virus which is acquired through close contact with infected body surfaces. Neonatal peripartum transmission occurs through the birth passage, while adult transmission occurs through intimate contact with infected persons [241]. Importantly, several HPV subtypes have oncogenic properties and are now considered causative agents of squamous cell neoplasia [242, 243]. Although these causal associations are strongest in the setting of cervical cancer, HPV has also been implicated in the pathogenesis of conjunctival tumors. HPV subtypes 6 and 11 are classically associated with the formation of benign conjunctival papillomas, which are composed of pinkish-red fibrous bands of tissue and pathognomonic frond-like vascular loops [244–246]. In contrast, HPV subtypes 16 and 18 are associated with ocular surface squamous neoplasia (OSSN), which encompasses premalignant conjunctival intraepithelial neoplasia (CIN) [247, 248] and malignant squamous cell carcinoma [249, 250]. Chronic immune suppression is a strong risk factor for the development of HPV-associated OSSN, the incidence of which increased dramatically with the emergence of HIV/AIDS in the 1980s [251].

A range of respiratory viruses, including coronavirus [252], influenza virus [253], parainfluenza virus [254], are also known to cause conjunctivitis. Early studies of the 2019–2020 coronavirus disease (COVID-19) pandemic, caused by the Severe Acute Respiratory Syndrome coronavirus (SARS-CoV-2), have now analyzed a cumulative volume of over 55,000 laboratory-confirmed cases [255, 256]. "Conjunctival congestion", most likely representing viral conjunctivitis, has been reported to be a presenting feature in approximately 0.8% of all infected patients. It is likely, therefore, that conjunctivitis will continue to feature as part of case-finding matrices used in further epidemiologic studies as the global outbreak unfolds. Another family of viruses which have caused multiple pandemics in the last century, the influenza viruses, are also important causes of conjunctivitis. It is known that certain types (e.g., human and avian influenza A, H7 subtype [257, 258]) have an unusual affinity for the ocular surface, possibly through preferential binding to terminal sialic acids on the surface of conjunctival epithelium [259]. The eye is not often thought of as a portal of entry for respiratory viral infections, or a site of viral replication, but recent findings suggest that the ocular surface may serve as an important conduit to subsequent nasopharyngeal and respiratory infection by these viruses.

Newcastle disease is caused by avian avulavirus 1 of the family *Paramyxoviridae* and genus *Avulavirus*, which occasionally causes outbreaks in poultry workers and veterinarians who may come into contact with poultry secretions and droppings [260–262]. The first known case was described in a poultry worker inadvertently exposed to fluid from a fertilized chicken egg [263]. The patient later developed generalized malaise, fever, headache, and mucopurulent conjunctivitis, with a clinical course lasting a week before an uneventful recovery. This form of conjunctivitis produces a follicular or papillary reaction associated with hyperemic and edematous changes. The future emergence of novel viruses, particularly those capable of zoonotic transmission, will continue to expand the list of pathogens capable of causing ocular surface infection.

2.9   Diagnostic Evaluation of Viral Conjunctivitis

2.9.1   Traditional Methods of Diagnosis

In most cases of viral conjunctivitis, the diagnosis is made on the basis of clinical findings, and identification of the precise causative agent is unnecessary. However, all patients with viral conjunctivitis should undergo a thorough anterior and posterior segment examination at the slit lamp, as there may be signs which can significantly alter the differential diagnosis. Conjunctivitis associated with corneal findings, anterior chamber inflammation or posterior pole changes, and/or relevant extraocular features, should warrant consideration of alternative and possibly more severe diagnoses. It is vitally important, for instance, to establish whether HSV or VZV infection is confined to the conjunctiva, or if there is corneal involvement. As emphasized earlier, the presence of keratitis can alter how the patient should be treated. Unusual or atypical findings may also warrant laboratory testing. Viral culture has long been considered the gold standard of virus detection, but is limited by its relatively poor sensitivity [264] and protracted turnaround time. Tzanck smears, which are prepared by using hematoxylin-eosin, Giemsa, or Papanicolaou stains on material collected from deroofed vesicular lesions, may be used to identify multinucleated giant (Tzanck) cells and acidophilic nuclear inclusion bodies that are strongly suggestive of herpetic infection. However, these smears alone are poorly sensitive and cannot distinguish between HSV and VZV [114]. Paired acute and convalescent serology is rarely helpful because several weeks must elapse before a demonstrable rise in antibody titers, after which the therapeutic window may have closed.

2.9.2   Molecular Diagnosis of Viral Infections

It is now possible to diagnose a variety of viral infections with diagnostic molecular assays. For instance, polymerase chain reaction (PCR) assays have been used to diagnose HSV from conjunctival swabs and/or tears, with reported sensitivities of up to 92% [265]. However, because viral shedding may occur in otherwise asymptomatic individuals [266], PCR is prone to false-positive results and unable to differentiate active from latent infection. Molecular assays have also been used for adenoviral conjunctivitis. Point-of-care tools such as the RPS Adeno Detector and its later model, the AdenoPlus (Rapid Pathogen Screening, Fl) are both US Food and Drug Administration-approved devices which detect adenovirus in tear samples based on an enzyme-linked immunosorbent assay (ELISA) specific to the highly conserved HAdV hexon protein, with results available within 10 min. While company-sponsored trials have reported sensitivities and specificities of over 85% for the RPS Adeno Detector [267] and AdenoPlus [268], their application in real clinical scenarios has yielded less encouraging results, with sensitivities and specificities ranging from 39.5–50% and 92–95.5%, respectively [269, 270]. PCR is regarded as a more accurate molecular test for HAdV conjunctivitis, and its use continues to shed new light on pathogens that may cause ocular disease that is indistinguishable from that caused by HAdV. For instance, an international, multicenter randomized clinical trial investigating the use of auriclosene in participants clinically diagnosed with EKC showed that 22% of those recruited were PCR-negative for HAdV [271]. A substantial proportion of these patients developed SEIs, suggesting that there are other viruses—yet to be identified—which are capable of causing EKC or EKC-like syndromes.

2.9.3 Whole Genome Sequencing

The advent of whole genome sequencing (WGS) has changed how epidemiologic investigations are conducted in emerging outbreaks. The procurement of data in real time as an epidemic evolves is particularly helpful in identifying the causative agent, its origins, and modes of transmission. In one recent example, WGS was used to guide infection control procedures during a nosocomial outbreak of systemic and ocular HAdV-B3 in a neonatal intensive care unit, which led to a total of 23 infections and four newborn deaths [272]. During this event, WGS was performed on nasopharyngeal aspirates of affected patients and their surrounding environment, quickly identifying HAdV-B3 as the culprit pathogen. These data showed that the outbreak had been driven primarily through the repeated use of ophthalmic instruments used to screen newborns for retinopathy of prematurity [272, 273], and this knowledge allowed for immediate modifications to be made to isolation procedures and clinical workflows. WGS may also provide unprecedented insights into the molecular epidemiology of implicated pathogens, allowing for spatial and/or geographic mapping in a variety of community and healthcare settings [22]. With a deeper understanding of viral transmission dynamics, it is possible to implement interventions that may mitigate risk of exposure in large populations. As costs decline and sequencing efficiency improves, WGS may also one day be optimized as a diagnostic tool for individualized clinical care.

2.10   Management of Viral Conjunctivitis

Despite years of research in potential therapies, few, if any, agents have been found to fundamentally alter the course of viral conjunctivitis. Where pertinent, specific treatments have been described in the text above. For the most common etiologies, supportive therapies including cool compresses, artificial tears, and topical nonsteroidal anti-inflammatory drugs [274] may offer symptomatic relief to some patients. Conjunctival membranes, which occur most frequently in EKC, can be gently removed and treated with a topical corticosteroid. In the absence of effective medications, prevention of disease transmission is even more critical. Patients with pink eye should be counseled regarding the importance of hand hygiene and self-quarantine, minimizing close contact with others and their personal articles. As a general rule, patients should be advised that viral shedding should be expected to occur for at least 10 days following symptom onset [32, 275]. This may warrant a brief furlough from work or school until symptoms have subsided, which is particularly important for healthcare workers who may come into contact with immunocompromised patients, the elderly, and neonates. For eye care providers, it is important to ensure ophthalmic instruments are cleaned thoroughly with hospital-grade disinfectants (e.g., chlorine-based agents [276]) after every patient encounter, and to avoid repeated use of common bottled ophthalmic medications (e.g., topical cycloplegic and anesthetic eye drops) across different patients. Follow-up should be initiated on an as-needed basis, and patients should be informed that any changes to their vision should prompt urgent ophthalmology review.

2.11   Conclusions and Future Directions

Despite its burden of disease and costs to society, viral conjunctivitis remains an underappreciated cause of ocular morbidity. Although many of the etiologies of viral conjunctivitis produce stereotypical symptoms and clinical findings, these infections should not be considered a homogenous disorder. Rather, the virosphere is replete with agents that infect the eye, either as a localized process or as a part of systemic infection. Eliciting a thorough patient history and comprehensive physical examination is important for all patients, and the presence of other ocular and/or systemic findings should prompt consideration of less common etiologies and definitive diagnostic testing. The history of viral conjunctivitis outbreaks in the last century strongly suggests that new and emerging viruses will cause wide-scale disease outbreaks in the future. Indeed, the viruses discussed in this chapter do not form an exhaustive list of all viral agents capable of infecting the ocular surface. Further research in molecular diagnostics may bring us closer to a more complete understanding of the pathogenesis, epidemiology, and disease associations of viruses, in ways that may inform future inquiries into urgently needed novel therapeutics for this age-old disease.

References

1. Azari AA, Barney NP. Conjunctivitis: a systematic review of diagnosis and treatment. JAMA. 2013;310(16):1721–9.
2. Jawetz E, Kimura SJ, Hanna L, Coleman VR, Thygeson P, Nicholas A. Studies on the etiology of epidemic keratoconjunctivitis. Am J Ophthalmol. 1955;40(5 Pt-2):200–9; discussion, 209–11.
3. Jawetz E. The story of shipyard eye. Br Med J. 1959;1(5126):873–6.
4. Mirkovic RR, Kono R, Yin-Murphy M, Sohier R, Schmidt NJ, Melnick JL. Enterovirus type 70: the etiologic agent of pandemic acute haemorrhagic conjunctivitis. Bull World Health Organ. 1973;49(4):341–6.
5. Mirkovic RR, Schmidt NJ, Yin-Murphy M, Melnick JL. Enterovirus etiology of the 1970 Singapore epidemic of acute conjunctivitis. Intervirology. 1974;4(2):119–27.
6. Sichel J. On the treatment of ophthalmia in general. Boston Med Surg J. 1838;18(22):347–52.
7. Friedenwald H. Paths of progress of ophthalmology. Arch Ophthalmol. 1942;27(6):1047–96.
8. Law FW. Egyptian ophthalmia. Br J Ophthalmol. 1939;23(2):81–95.
9. Thygeson P. Present status of the viral keratoconjunctivitis problem. Am J Ophthalmol. 1957;43(4 Part-2):3–10.
10. De Laey JJ. Military ophthalmia and the Napoleonic campaign in Egypt. Acta Ophthalmol. 2015;93(S255).
11. Wilson RP. Ophthalmia Ægyptiaca. Am J Ophthalmol. 1932;15(5):405–6.
12. Meyerhof M. A short history of ophthalmia during the Egyptian campaigns of 1798-1807. Br J Ophthalmol. 1932;16(3):129–52.
13. Maccallan AF. The history of ophthalmology in Egypt. Br J Ophthalmol. 1927;11(12):602–9.
14. No author listed. Egyptian ophthalmia. Can Med Assoc J. 1915;5(10):918–20.
15. Lederberg J. Infectious history. Science. 2000;288(5464):287–93.
16. Uchio E, Takeuchi S, Itoh N, Matsuura N, Ohno S, Aoki K. Clinical and epidemiological features of acute follicular conjunctivitis with special reference to that caused by herpes simplex virus type 1. Br J Ophthalmol. 2000;84(9):968–72.
17. Stenson S, Newman R, Fedukowicz H. Laboratory studies in acute conjunctivitis. Arch Ophthalmol. 1982;100(8):1275–7.
18. Harding SP, Mallinson H, Smith JL, Clearkin LG. Adult follicular conjunctivitis and neonatal ophthalmia in a Liverpool eye hospital, 1980-1984. Eye. 1987;1(P-4):512–21.
19. Woodland RM, Darougar S, Thaker U, Cornell L, Siddique M, Wania J, Shahet M. Causes of conjunctivitis and keratoconjunctivitis in Karachi, Pakistan. Trans R Soc Trop Med Hyg. 1992;86(3):317–20.
20. Akcay E, Carhan A, Höndur G, Tufan ZK, Duru N, Kiliç S, Ensari EN, Uğurlu N, Çağıl N. Molecular identification of viral agents associated with acute conjunctivitis: a prospective controlled study. Braz J Infect Dis. 2017;21(4):391–5.
21. Chang CH, Lin KH, Sheu MM, Huang WL, Wang HZ, Chen CW. The change of etiological agents and clinical signs of epidemic viral conjunctivitis over an 18-year period in southern Taiwan. Graefes Arch Clin Exp Ophthalmol. 2003;241(7):554–60.
22. Zhang L, Zhao N, Huang X, Jin X, Geng X, Chan TC, Liu S. Molecular epidemiology of acute hemorrhagic conjunctivitis caused by coxsackie A type 24 variant in China, 2004–2014. Sci Rep. 2017;7:45202.
23. Seto D, Chodosh J, Brister JR, Jones MS, Members of the Adenovirus Research C. Using the whole-genome sequence to characterize and name human adenoviruses. J Virol. 2011;85(11):5701–2.
24. International Committee on Taxonomy of Viruses (ICTV). Adenoviridae. Secondary Adenoviridae; 2011. https://talk.ictvonline.org/ictv-reports/ictv_9th_report/dsdna-viruses-2011/w/dsdna_viruses/93/adenoviridae. Accessed 4 Jan 2020.
25. Fuchs E. Keratitis punctata superficialis. Alfred Hölder; 1889.

26. von Carion SK. A peculiar form of corneal inflammation. Wien Klin Wochenschr. 1889;2:613–4.
27. Hogan MJ, Crawford JW. Epidemic Keratoconjunctivitis: (Superficial Punctate Keratitis, Keratitis Subepithelialis, Keratitis Maculosa, Keratitis Nummularis) with a review of the literature and a report of 125 cases. Am J Ophthalmol. 1942;25(9):1059–78.
28. Wright RE. Superficial Punctate Keratitis. Br J Ophthalmol. 1930;14(11):595–601.
29. Hogan MJ, Crawford JW. Epidemic Keratoconjunctivitis: (Superficial Punctate Keratitis, Keratitis Subepithelialis, Keratitis Maculosa, Keratitis Nummularis) with a review of the literature and a report of 125 cases. Am J Ophthalmol. 2018;190:xxix–xlii.
30. Kuh C. Epidemic keratoconjunctivitis: "shipyard eye". Cal West Med. 1943;58(1):18–9.
31. Rowe WP, Huebner RJ, Gilmore LK, Parrott RH, Ward TG. Isolation of a cytopathogenic agent from human adenoids undergoing spontaneous degeneration in tissue culture. Proc Soc Exp Biol Med. 1953;84(3):570–3.
32. Jonas RA, Ung L, Rajaiya J, Chodosh J. Mystery eye: human adenovirus and the enigma of epidemic keratoconjunctivitis. Prog Retin Eye Res. 2019;100826
33. Ismail AM, Lee JS, Lee JY, Singh G, Dyer DW, Seto D, Chodosh J, Rajaiya J. Adenoviromics: mining the human adenovirus species D Genome. Front Microbiol. 2018;9:2178.
34. Parrott RH, Rowe WP, Huebner RJ, Bernton HW, McCullough N. Outbreak of febrile pharyngitis and conjunctivitis associated with type 3 adenoidal-pharyngeal-conjunctival virus infection. N Engl J Med. 1954;251(27):1087–90.
35. Béal R. Sur une forme particulière de conjonctivite aiguë avec follicules. Ann d'ocul. 1907;87:1.
36. Thygeson P. Etiology and differential diagnosis of non-trachomatous follicular conjunctivitis. Bull World Health Organ. 1957;16(5):995–1011.
37. Chodosh J, Miller D, Stroop WG, Pflugfelder SC. Adenovirus epithelial keratitis. Cornea. 1995;14(2):167–74.
38. Chintakuntlawar AV, Chodosh J. Cellular and tissue architecture of conjunctival membranes in epidemic keratoconjunctivitis. Ocul Immunol Inflamm. 2010;18(5):341–5.
39. Butt AL, Chodosh J. Adenoviral keratoconjunctivitis in a tertiary care eye clinic. Cornea. 2006;25(2):199–202.
40. Rajaiya J, Zhou X, Barequet I, Gilmore MS, Chodosh J. Novel model of innate immunity in corneal infection. In Vitro Cell Dev Biol Anim. 2015;51(8):827–34.
41. Chodosh J. Human adenovirus type 37 and the BALB/c mouse: progress toward a restricted adenovirus keratitis model (an American Ophthalmological Society thesis). Trans Am Ophthalmol Soc. 2006;104:346–65.
42. Chintakuntlawar AV, Astley R, Chodosh J. Adenovirus type 37 keratitis in the C57BL/6J mouse. Invest Ophthalmol Vis Sci. 2007;48(2):781–8.
43. Monnerat N, Bossart W, Thiel MA. Povidone-iodine for treatment of adenoviral conjunctivitis: an in vitro study. Klin Monatsbl Augenheilkd. 2006;223(5):349–52.
44. Pelletier JS, Stewart K, Trattler W, Ritterband DC, Braverman S, Samson CM, Liang B, Capriotti JA. A combination povidone-iodine 0.4%/dexamethasone 0.1% ophthalmic suspension in the treatment of adenoviral conjunctivitis. Adv Ther. 2009;26(8):776–83.
45. Özen Tunay Z, Ozdemir O, Petricli IS. Povidone iodine in the treatment of adenoviral conjunctivitis in infants. Cutan Ocul Toxicol. 2015;34(1):12–5.
46. Yazar H, Yarbag A, Balci M, Teker B, Tanyeri P. The effects of povidone iodine (pH 4.2) on patients with adenoviral conjunctivitis. J Pak Med Assoc. 2016;66(8):968–70.
47. Kovalyuk N, Kaiserman I, Mimouni M, Cohen O, Levartovsky S, Sherbany H, Mandelboim M. Treatment of adenoviral keratoconjunctivitis with a combination of povidone-iodine 1.0% and dexamethasone 0.1% drops: a clinical prospective controlled randomized study. Acta Ophthalmol. 2017;95(8):e686–92.
48. Pepose JS, Ahuja A, Liu W, Narvekar A, Haque R. Randomized, controlled, phase 2 trial of povidone-iodine/dexamethasone ophthalmic suspension for treatment of adenoviral conjunctivitis. Am J Ophthalmol. 2018;194:7–15.

49. de Oliveira CB, Stevenson D, LaBree L, McDonnell PJ, Trousdale MD. Evaluation of Cidofovir (HPMPC, GS-504) against adenovirus type 5 infection in vitro and in a New Zealand rabbit ocular model. Antivir Res. 1996;31(3):165–72.

50. Hillenkamp J, Reinhard T, Ross RS, Böhringer D, Cartsburg O, Roggendorf M, De Clercq E, Godehardt E, Sundmacher R. Topical treatment of acute adenoviral keratoconjunctivitis with 0.2% cidofovir and 1% cyclosporine: a controlled clinical pilot study. Arch Ophthalmol. 2001;119(10):1487–91.

51. Hillenkamp J, Reinhard T, Ross RS, Böhringer D, Cartsburg O, Roggendorf M, De Clercq E, Godehardt E, Sundmacher R. The effects of cidofovir 1% with and without cyclosporin a 1% as a topical treatment of acute adenoviral keratoconjunctivitis: a controlled clinical pilot study. Ophthalmology. 2002;109(5):845–50.

52. Levinger E, Trivizki O, Shachar Y, Levinger S, Verssano D. Topical 0.03% tacrolimus for subepithelial infiltrates secondary to adenoviral keratoconjunctivitis. Graefes Arch Clin Exp Ophthalmol. 2014;252(5):811–6.

53. Ghanem RC, Vargas JF, Ghanem VC. Tacrolimus for the treatment of subepithelial infiltrates resistant to topical steroids after adenoviral keratoconjunctivitis. Cornea. 2014;33(11):1210–3.

54. Berisa Prado S, Riestra Ayora AC, Lisa Fernández C, Chacón Rodríguez M, Merayo-Lloves J, Alfonso Sánchez JF. Topical tacrolimus for corneal subepithelial infiltrates secondary to adenoviral keratoconjunctivitis. Cornea. 2017;36(9):1102–5.

55. Levinger E, Slomovic A, Sansanayudh W, Bahar I, Slomovic AR. Topical treatment with 1% cyclosporine for subepithelial infiltrates secondary to adenoviral keratoconjunctivitis. Cornea. 2010;29(6):638–40.

56. Jeng BH, Holsclaw DS. Cyclosporine A 1% eye drops for the treatment of subepithelial infiltrates after adenoviral keratoconjunctivitis. Cornea. 2011;30(9):958–61.

57. Cohen JI. Introduction to herpesviridae. In: Mandell GL, Bennett JE, Dolin R, editors. Mandell, Douglas and Bennett's principles and practice of infectious diseases. Philadelphia: Churchill Livingstone Elsevier; 2010. p. 1937–42.

58. Schiffer JT, Corey L. Herpes simplex virus. In: Mandell GL, Bennett JE, Dolin R, editors. Mandell, Douglas and Benett's principles and practice of infectious diseases. Philadelphia: Churchill Livingstone Elsevier; 2010. p. 1943–62.

59. Davison AJ. Herpesvirus systematics. Vet Microbiol. 2010;143(1):52–69.

60. Okuno T, Hooper LC, Ursea R, Smith J, Nussenblatt R, Hooks JJ, Hayashi K. Role of human herpes virus 6 in corneal inflammation alone or with human herpesviruses. Cornea. 2011;30(2):204–7.

61. Boto-de-los-Bueis A, Romero Gómez MP, del Hierro ZA, Sanchez EG, Mediero S, Noval S. Recurrent ocular surface inflammation associated with human herpesvirus 6 infection. Eye Contact Lens. 2015;41(3):e11–3.

62. Reiser BJ, Mok A, Kukes G, Kim JW. Non–AIDS-related Kaposi Sarcoma involving the tarsal conjunctiva and eyelid margin. Arch Ophthalmol. 2007;125(6):838–40.

63. Shuler JD, Holland GN, Miles SA, Miller BJ, Grossman I. Kaposi Sarcoma of the conjunctiva and eyelids associated with the acquired immunodeficiency syndrome. Arch Ophthalmol. 1989;107(6):858–62.

64. Razzaque A. Oncogenic potential of human herpesvirus-6 DNA. Oncogene. 1990;5(9):1365–70.

65. Daibata M, Taguchi T, Taguchi H, Miyoshi I. Integration of human herpesvirus 6 in a Burkitt's lymphoma cell line. Br J Haematol. 1998;102(5):1307–13.

66. Johnson DC, Baines JD. Herpesviruses remodel host membranes for virus egress. Nat Rev Microbiol. 2011;9(5):382–94.

67. Stevens JG. Human herpesviruses: a consideration of the latent state. Microbiol Rev. 1989;53(3):318–32.

68. Pepose JS, Keadle TL, Morrison LA. Ocular herpes simplex: changing epidemiology, emerging disease patterns, and the potential of vaccine prevention and therapy. Am J Ophthalmol. 2006;141(3):547–57.

69. Burnet FM, Williams SW. Herpes simplex: a new point of view. Med J Aust. 1939;1:637–42.

70. Margolis TP, Dawson CR, LaVail JH. Herpes simplex viral infection of the mouse trigeminal ganglion. Immunohistochemical analysis of cell populations. Invest Ophthalmol Vis Sci. 1992;33(2):259–67.
71. Wilson AC, Mohr I. A cultured affair: HSV latency and reactivation in neurons. Trends Microbiol. 2012;20(12):604–11.
72. Roizman B, Whitley RJ. An inquiry into the molecular basis of HSV latency and reactivation. Annu Rev Microbiol. 2013;67:355–74.
73. Tullo AB, Shimeld C, Blyth WA, Hill TJ, Easty DL. Spread of virus and distribution of latent infection following ocular herpes simplex in the non-immune and immune mouse. J Gen Virol. 1982;63(Pt-1):95–101.
74. Asbell PA, Centifanto-Fitzgerald YM, Chandler JW, Kaufman HE. Analysis of viral DNA in isolates from patients with recurrent herpetic keratitis. Invest Ophthalmol Vis Sci. 1984;25(8):951–4.
75. Scriba M. Extraneural localisation of herpes simplex virus in latently infected guinea pigs. Nature. 1977;267(5611):529–31.
76. Pavan-Langston D, Rong BL, Dunkel EC. Extraneuronal herpetic latency: animal and human corneal studies. Acta Ophthalmol Suppl. 1989;192:135–41.
77. Maggs DJ, Chang E, Nasisse MP, Mitchell WJ. Persistence of herpes simplex virus type 1 DNA in chronic conjunctival and eyelid lesions of mice. J Virol. 1998;72(11):9166–72.
78. Doller E, Aucker J, Weissbach A. Persistence of herpes simplex virus type 1 in rat neurotumor cells. J Virol. 1979;29(1):43–50.
79. Darougar S, Wishart MS, Viswalingam ND. Epidemiological and clinical features of primary herpes simplex virus ocular infection. Br J Ophthalmol. 1985;69(1):2–6.
80. Sridhar U, Bansal Y, Choudhury S, Gupta AK. Conjunctival dendrite in a case of primary herpes simplex infection. Br J Ophthalmol. 2004;88(4):590–1.
81. Laibson PR. Current therapy of herpes simplex virus infection of the cornea. Int Ophthalmol Clin. 1973;13(4):39–52.
82. White ML, Chodosh J. Herpes simplex virus keratitis: a treatment guideline [Hoskins Center for Quality Eye Care and American Academy of Ophthalmology website]. Secondary Herpes simplex virus keratitis: a treatment guideline [Hoskins Center for Quality Eye Care and American Academy of Ophthalmology website]. 2014. https://www.aao.org/clinical-statement/herpes-simplex-virus-keratitis-treatment-guideline. Accessed 4 Jan 2020.
83. Wilhelmus KR, Gee L, Hauck WW, Kurinij N, Dawson CR, Jones DB, Barron BA, Kaufman HE, Sugar J, Hyndiuk RA, et al. Herpetic eye disease study. A controlled trial of topical corticosteroids for herpes simplex stromal keratitis. Ophthalmology. 1994;101(12):1883–95; discussion 1895–6.
84. Herpetic Eye Disease Study Group. Acyclovir for the prevention of recurrent herpes simplex virus eye disease. N Engl J Med. 1998;339(5):300–6.
85. Chodosh J, Stroop WG. Introduction to viruses in ocular disease. In: Tasman W, Jaeger EA, editors. Duane's foundations of clinical ophthalmology. Philadelphia: Lippincott Williams & Wilkins; 2005; Chapter 85.
86. Wishart MS, Darougar S, Viswalingam ND. Recurrent herpes simplex virus ocular infection: epidemiological and clinical features. Br J Ophthalmol. 1987;71(9):669–72.
87. Isenberg SJ, Apt L, Wood M. A controlled trial of povidone-iodine as prophylaxis against ophthalmia neonatorum. N Engl J Med. 1995;332(9):562–6.
88. Prober CG, Corey L, Brown ZA, Hensleigh PA, Frenkel LM, Bryson YJ, Whitley RJ, Arvin AM. The management of pregnancies complicated by genital infections with herpes simplex virus. Clin Infect Dis. 1992;15(6):1031–8.
89. Brown ZA, Benedetti J, Ashley R, Burchett S, Selke S, Berry S, Vontver LA, Corey L. Neonatal herpes simplex virus infection in relation to asymptomatic maternal infection at the time of labor. N Engl J Med. 1991;324(18):1247–52.
90. Sullivan-Bolyai J, Hull HF, Wilson C, Corey L. Neonatal herpes simplex virus infection in King County, Washington: increasing incidence and epidemiologic correlates. JAMA. 1983;250(22):3059–62.

91. Stone KM, Brooks CA, Guinan ME, Alexander ER. National surveillance for neonatal herpes simplex virus infections. Sex Transm Dis. 1989;16(3):152–6.
92. Whitley RJ, Corey L, Arvin A, Lakeman FD, Sumaya CV, Wright PF, Dunkle LM, Steele RW, Soong SJ, Nahmias AJ, et al. Changing presentation of herpes simplex virus infection in neonates. J Infect Dis. 1988;158(1):109–16.
93. Csonka GW, Coufalik ED. Chlamydial, gonococcal, and herpes virus infections in neonates. Postgrad Med J. 1977;53(624):592–4.
94. Nahmias AJ, Visintine AM, Caldwell DR, Wilson LA. Eye infections with herpes simplex viruses in neonates. Surv Ophthalmol. 1976;21(2):100–5.
95. Kohl S. Neonatal herpes simplex virus infection. Clin Perinatol. 1997;24(1):129–50.
96. Whitley R, Arvin A, Prober C, Corey L, Burchett S, Plotkin S, Starr S, Jacobs R, Powell D, Nahmias A, et al. Predictors of morbidity and mortality in neonates with herpes simplex virus infections. N Engl J Med. 1991;324(7):450–4.
97. Davison AJ, Eberle R, Ehlers B, Hayward GS, McGeoch DJ, Minson AC, Pellett PE, Roizman B, Studdert MJ, Thiry E. The order herpesvirales. Arch Virol. 2009;154(1):171–7.
98. Liesegang TJ. Varicella-zoster virus eye disease. In: Tasman W, Jaeger EA, editors. Duane's foundations of clinical ophthalmology. Philadelphia: Lippincott Williams & Wilkins; 2005; Chapter 94.
99. Opstelten W, Zaal MJW. Managing ophthalmic herpes zoster in primary care. BMJ. 2005;331(7509):147–51.
100. Liesegang TJ. Herpes zoster ophthalmicus natural history, risk factors, clinical presentation, and morbidity. Ophthalmology. 2008;115(2-Suppl):S3–12.
101. Matsuo T, Koyama M, Matsuo N. Acute retinal necrosis as a novel complication of chickenpox in adults. Br J Ophthalmol. 1990;74(7):443–4.
102. Poonyathalang A, Sukavatcharin S, Sujirakul T. Ischemic retinal vasculitis in an 18-year-old man with chickenpox infection. Clin Ophthalmol. 2014;8:441–3.
103. Esiri MM, Tomlinson AH. Herpes Zoster. Demonstration of virus in trigeminal nerve and ganglion by immunofluorescence and electron microscopy. J Neurol Sci. 1972;15(1):35–48.
104. Zaal MJ, Volker-Dieben HJ, D'Amaro J. Prognostic value of Hutchinson's sign in acute herpes zoster ophthalmicus. Graefes Arch Clin Exp Ophthalmol. 2003;241(3):187–91.
105. Hutchinson J. Clinical report on herpes zoster frontalis ophthalmicus (shingles affecting the forehead and nose). R Lond Ophthalmic Hosp Rep. 1864;3(72):865–6.
106. Goon P, Wright M, Fink C. Ophthalmic zoster sine herpete. J R Soc Med. 2000;93(4):191–2.
107. Sigireddi RR, Lyons LJ, Beaver HA, Lee AG. Herpes zoster ophthalmicus: pre-eruption phase sine herpete. Am J Ophthalmol Case Rep. 2018;10:201–2.
108. Lewis GW. Zoster sine herpete. Br Med J. 1958;2(5093):418–21.
109. Szeto SK, Chan TC, Wong RL, Ng AL, Li EY, Jhanji V. Prevalence of ocular manifestations and visual outcomes in patients with herpes zoster ophthalmicus. Cornea. 2017;36(3):338–42.
110. Tran KD, Falcone MM, Choi DS, Goldhardt R, Karp CL, Davis JL, Galor A. Epidemiology of herpes zoster ophthalmicus: recurrence and chronicity. Ophthalmology. 2016;123(7):1469–75.
111. Ryan-Graham MA, Durand M, Pavan-Langston D. AIDS and the anterior segment. Int Ophthalmol Clin. 1998;38(1):241–63.
112. Liesegang TJ. Corneal complications from herpes zoster ophthalmicus. Ophthalmology. 1985;92(3):316–24.
113. Jeng BH. Herpes zoster eye disease: new ways to combat an old foe? Ophthalmology. 2018;125(11):1671–4.
114. Liesegang TJ. Diagnosis and therapy of herpes zoster ophthalmicus. Ophthalmology. 1991;98(8):1216–29.
115. Wenkel H, Rummelt V, Fleckenstein B, Naumann GO. Detection of varicella zoster virus DNA and viral antigen in human eyes after herpes zoster ophthalmicus. Ophthalmology. 1998;105(7):1323–30.
116. Epstein MA, Achong BG, Barr YM. Virus particles in cultured lymphoblasts from Burkitt's lymphoma. Lancet. 1964;1(7335):702–3.

117. Fox RI, Pearson G, Vaughan JH. Detection of Epstein-Barr virus-associated antigens and DNA in salivary gland biopsies from patients with Sjogren's syndrome. J Immunol. 1986;137(10):3162–8.
118. Henle G, Henle W, Diehl V. Relation of Burkitt's tumor-associated herpes-type virus to infectious mononucleosis. Proc Natl Acad Sci U S A. 1968;59(1):94–101.
119. Lo AK, Lo KW, Tsao SW, Wong HL, Hui JWY, To KF, Hayward DS, Chui YL, Lau YL, Takada K, Huang DP. Epstein-Barr virus infection alters cellular signal cascades in human nasopharyngeal epithelial cells. Neoplasia. 2006;8(3):173–80.
120. Levine J, Pflugfelder SC, Yen M, Crouse CA, Atherton SS. Detection of the complement (CD21)/Epstein-Barr virus receptor in human lacrimal gland and ocular surface epithelia. Reg Immunol. 1990;3(4):164–70.
121. Roberts ML, Luxembourg AT, Cooper NR. Epstein-Barr virus binding to CD21, the virus receptor, activates resting B cells via an intracellular pathway that is linked to B cell infection. J Gen Virol. 1996;77(Pt-12):3077–85.
122. Shannon-Lowe C, Rowe M. Epstein-Barr virus infection of polarized epithelial cells via the basolateral surface by memory B cell-mediated transfer infection. PLoS Pathog. 2011;7(5):e1001338.
123. Librach IM. Ocular symptoms in glandular fever. Br J Ophthalmol. 1956;40(10):619–21.
124. Tanner OR. Ocular manifestations of infectious mononucleosis. AMA Arch Ophthalmol. 1954;51(2):229–41.
125. Meisler DM, Bosworth DE, Krachmer JH. Ocular infectious mononucleosis manifested as Parinaud's Oculoglandular syndrome. Am J Ophthalmol. 1981;92(5):722–6.
126. Wilhelmus KR. Ocular involvement in infectious mononucleosis. Am J Ophthalmol. 1981;91(1):117–8.
127. Matoba AY. Ocular disease associated with Epstein-Barr virus infection. Surv Ophthalmol. 1990;35(2):145–50.
128. Charbel Issa P, Eis-Hübinger AM, Klatt K, Holz FG, Loeffler KU. Oculoglandular syndrome associated with reactivated Epstein-Barr-virus infection. Br J Ophthalmol. 2008;92(6):740–855.
129. Garau J, Kabins S, DeNosaquo S, Lee G, Keller R. Spontaneous cytomegalovirus mononucleosis with conjunctivitis. Arch Intern Med. 1977;137(11):1631–2.
130. Khadem M, Kalish SB, Goldsmith J, Fetkenhour C, O'Grady RB, Phair JP, Chrobak M. Ophthalmologic findings in Acquired Immune Deficiency Syndrome (AIDS). Arch Ophthalmol. 1984;102(2):201–6.
131. Lee-Wing MW, Hodge WG, Diaz-Mitoma F. The prevalence of herpes family virus DNA in the conjunctiva of patients positive and negative for human immunodeficiency virus using the polymerase chain reaction. Ophthalmology. 1999;106(2):350–4.
132. Pathanapitoon K, Ausayakhun S, Kunavisarut P, Pungrasame A, Sirirungsi W. Detection of cytomegalovirus in vitreous, aqueous and conjunctiva by polymerase chain reaction (PCR). J Med Assoc Thail. 2005;88(2):228–32.
133. Wilhelmus KR, Font RL, Lehmann RP, Cernoch PL. Cytomegalovirus keratitis in acquired immunodeficiency syndrome. Arch Ophthalmol. 1996;114(7):869–72.
134. Holland GN, Pepose JS, Pettit TH, Gottlieb MS, Yee RD, Foos RY. Acquired immune deficiency syndrome: ocular manifestations. Ophthalmology. 1983;90(8):859–73.
135. Matoba AY, Wilhelmus KR, Jones DB. Epstein-Barr viral stromal keratitis. Ophthalmology. 1986;93(6):746–51.
136. Pinnolis M, McCulley JP, Urman JD. Nummular keratitis associated with infectious mononucleosis. Am J Ophthalmol. 1980;89(6):791–4.
137. Matoba AY, Jones DB. Corneal subepithelial infiltrates associated with systemic Epstein-Barr viral infection. Ophthalmology. 1987;94(12):1669–71.
138. Koizumi N, Inatomi T, Suzuki T, Shiraishi A, Ohashi Y, Kandori M, Miyazaki D, Inoue Y, Soma T, Nishida K, Takase H, Sugita S, Mochizuki M, Kinoshita S, Japan Corneal Endotheliitis Study Group. Clinical features and management of cytomegalovirus corneal

endotheliitis: analysis of 106 cases from the Japan corneal endotheliitis study. Br J Ophthalmol. 2015;99(1):54–8.

139. Koizumi N, Yamasaki K, Kawasaki S, Sotozono C, Inatomi T, Mochida C, Kinoshita S. Cytomegalovirus in aqueous humor from an eye with corneal endotheliitis. Am J Ophthalmol. 2006;141(3):564–5.

140. Kandori M, Inoue T, Takamatsu F, Kojima Y, Hori Y, Maeda N, Tano Y. Prevalence and features of keratitis with quantitative polymerase chain reaction positive for cytomegalovirus. Ophthalmology. 2010;117(2):216–22.

141. Morishima N, Miyakawa S, Akazawa Y, Takagi S. A case of uveitis associated with chronic active Epstein-Barr virus infection. Ophthalmologica. 1996;210(3):186–8.

142. Touge C, Agawa H, Sairenji T, Inoue Y. High incidence of elevated antibody titers to Epstein-Barr virus in patients with uveitis. Arch Virol. 2006;151(5):895–903.

143. Usui M, Sakai J. Three cases of EB virus-associated uveitis. Int Ophthalmol. 1990;14(5–6):371–6.

144. Chee SP, Jap A. Presumed fuchs heterochromic iridocyclitis and Posner-Schlossman syndrome: comparison of cytomegalovirus-positive and negative eyes. Am J Ophthalmol. 2008;146(6):883–9.e1.

145. Chee SP, Bacsal K, Jap A, Se-Thoe SY, Cheng CL, Tan BH. Clinical features of cytomegalovirus anterior uveitis in immunocompetent patients. Am J Ophthalmol. 2008;145(5):834–40.

146. Jacobson MA, Zegans M, Pavan PR, O'Donnell JJ, Sattler F, Rao N, Owens S, Pollard R. Cytomegalovirus retinitis after initiation of highly active antiretroviral therapy. Lancet. 1997;349(9063):1443–5.

147. Pertel P, Hirschtick R, Phair J, Chmiel J, Poggensee L, Murphy R. Risk of developing cytomegalovirus retinitis in persons infected with the human immunodeficiency virus. J Acquir Immune Defic Syndr. 1992;5(11):1069–74.

148. Schaal S, Kagan A, Wang Y, Chan CC, Kaplan HJ. Acute retinal necrosis associated with Epstein-Barr virus: immunohistopathologic confirmation. JAMA Ophthalmol. 2014;132(7):881–2.

149. Zell R, Delwart E, Gorbalenya AE, Hovi T, King AMQ, Knowles NJ, Lindberg AM, Pallansch MA, Palmenberg AC, Reuter G, Simmonds P, Skern T, Stanway G, Yamashita T. ICTV report consortium. ICTV virus taxonomy profile: picornaviridae. J Gen Virol. 2017;98(10):2421–2.

150. Supanaranond K, Takeda N, Yamazaki S. The complete nucleotide sequence of a variant of coxsackievirus A24, an agent causing acute hemorrhagic conjunctivitis. Virus Genes. 1992;6(2):149–58.

151. Hierholzer JC, Hilliard KA, Esposito JJ. Serosurvey for "Acute Hemorrhagic Conjunctivitis" Virus (Enterovirus 70) antibodies in the Southeastern United States, with review of the literature and some epidemiologic implications. Am J Epidemiol. 1975;102(6):533–44.

152. Sklar VEF, Patriarca PA, Onorato IM, Langford MP, Clark SW, Culbertson WW, Forster RK. Clinical findings and results of treatment in an outbreak of acute hemorrhagic conjunctivitis in Southern Florida. Am J Ophthalmol. 1983;95(1):45–54.

153. Kono R. Apollo 11 disease or acute hemorrhagic conjunctivitis: a pandemic of a new enterovirus infection of the eyes. Am J Epidemiol. 1975;101(5):383–90.

154. Chatterjee S, Quarcoopome CO, Apenteno A. An epidemic of acute conjunctivitis in Ghana. Ghana Med J. 1970;9(1):9–11.

155. Chatterjee S, Quarcoopome CO, Apenteng A. Unusual type of epidemic conjunctivitis in Ghana. Br J Ophthalmol. 1970;54(9):628–30.

156. Kono R, Sasagawa A, Ishii K, Sugiura S, Ochi M. Pandemic of new type of conjunctivitis. Lancet. 1972;1(7762):1191–4.

157. Ray I, Chakravarty MS, Mukherjee MK, Chakravarty SK, Roy IS, Mitra BK, Sen AK, Sen GC, Sarkar JK. Laboratory investigations of an epidemic of conjunctivitis in Calcutta—a preliminary report. Bull Calcutta Sch Trop Med. 1972;20(1):1–2.

158. Wadia NH, Wadia PN, Katrak SM, Misra VP. A study of the neurological disorder associated with acute haemorrhagic conjunctivitis due to enterovirus 70. J Neurol Neurosurg Psychiatry. 1983;46(7):599–610.

159. Kono R, Miyamura K, Tajiri E, Sasagawa A, Phuapradit P. Virological and serological studies of neurological complications of acute hemorrhagic conjunctivitis in Thailand. J Infect Dis. 1977;135(5):706–13.

160. Hung TP, Sung SM, Liang HC, Landsborough D, Green IJ. Radiculomyelitis following acute haemorrhagic conjunctivitis. Brain. 1976;99(4):771–90.

161. Yin-Murphy M, Lim KH. Picornavirus epidemic conjunctivitis in Singapore. Lancet. 1972;2(7782):857–8.

162. Stanton GJ, Langford MP, Baron S. Effect of interferon, elevated temperature, and cell type on replication of acute hemorrhagic conjunctivitis viruses. Infect Immun. 1977;18(2):370–6.

163. Miyamura K, Takeda N, Yamazaki S. Characterization of a temperature-sensitive defect of enterovirus 70: effect of elevated temperature on in vitro transcription. J Virol. 1984;51(1):192–8.

164. Shulman LM, Manor Y, Azar R, Handsher R, Vonsover A, Mendelson E, Rothman S, Hassin D, Halmut T, Abramovitz B, Varsano N. Identification of a new strain of fastidious enterovirus 70 as the causative agent of an outbreak of hemorrhagic conjunctivitis. J Clin Microbiol. 1997;35(8):2145–9.

165. Goh KT, Ooi PL, Miyamura K, Ogino T, Yamazaki S. Acute haemorrhagic conjunctivitis: seroepidemiology of coxsackievirus A24 variant and enterovirus 70 in Singapore. J Med Virol. 1990;31(3):245–7.

166. Maitreyi RS, Dar L, Muthukumar A, Vajpayee M, Xess I, Vajpayee RB, Seth P, Broor S. Acute hemorrhagic conjunctivitis due to enterovirus 70 in India. Emerg Infect Dis. 1999;5(2):267–9.

167. Uchio E, Yamazaki K, Ishikawa H, Matsunaga I, Asato Y, Aoki K, Ohno S. An epidemic of acute haemorrhagic conjunctivitis caused by enterovirus 70 in Okinawa, Japan, in 1994. Graefes Arch Clin Exp Ophthalmol. 1999;237(7):568–72.

168. Christopher S, John TJ, Charles V, Ray S. Coxsackievirus A24 variant EH 24/70 and enterovirus type 70 in an epidemic of acute haemorrhagic conjunctivitis-a preliminary report. Indian J Med Res. 1977;65(5):593–5.

169. Oh MD, Park S, Choi Y, Kim H, Lee K, Park W, Yoo Y, Kim EC, Choe K. Acute hemorrhagic conjunctivitis caused by coxsackievirus A24 variant, South Korea, 2002. Emerg Infect Dis. 2003;9(8):1010–2.

170. Lefkowitz EJ, Wang C, Upton C. Poxviruses: past, present and future. Virus Res. 2006;117(1):105–18.

171. International Committee on Taxonomy of Viruses (ICTV). Poxviridae. Secondary Poxviridae. 2011. https://talk.ictvonline.org/ictv-reports/ictv_9th_report/dsdna-viruses-2011/w/dsdna_viruses/74/poxviridae. Accessed 2 Feb 2020.

172. Pepose JS, Margolis TP, LaRussa P, Pavan-Langston D. Ocular complications of smallpox vaccination. Am J Ophthalmol. 2003;136(2):343–52.

173. Breman JG, Arita I, Smallpox Eradication Unit, World Health Organization. The confirmation and maintenance of smallpox eradication. Geneva, Switzerland: World Health Organization; 1980.

174. Semba RD. The ocular complications of smallpox and smallpox immunization. Arch Ophthalmol. 2003;121(5):715–9.

175. McFadden G. Poxvirus tropism. Nat Rev Microbiol. 2005;3(3):201–13.

176. Breman JG, Henderson DA. Diagnosis and management of smallpox. N Engl J Med. 2002;346(17):1300–8.

177. Foege WH, Millar JD, Henderson DA. Smallpox eradication in West and Central Africa. Bull World Health Organ. 1975;52(2):209–22.

178. Baker AR. Eye complications of smallpox. Some observations during the recent epidemic in Cleveland. JAMA. 1903;XLI(11):645–8.

179. Sinaiko AA. Keratitis postvaccinolosa. Arch Ophthalmol. 1931;5(1):91–2.

180. Lane JM, Ruben FL, Neff JM, Millar JD. Complications of smallpox vaccination, 1968. N Engl J Med. 1969;281(22):1201–8.

181. Ruben FL, Lane JM. Ocular vaccinia: an epidemiologic analysis of 348 cases. Arch Ophthalmol. 1970;84(1):45–8.
182. Grabenstein JD, Winkenwerder J, William. US military smallpox vaccination program experience. JAMA. 2003;289(24):3278–82.
183. Cono J, Casey CG, Bell DM, Centers for Disease Control and Prevention. Smallpox vaccination and adverse reactions. Guidance for clinicians. MMWR Recomm Rep. 2003;52(RR-4):1–28.
184. Neff JM, Lane JM, Fulginiti VA, Henderson DA. Contact vaccinia—transmission of vaccinia from smallpox vaccination. JAMA. 2002;288(15):1901–5.
185. Koplan JP, Marton KI. Smallpox vaccination revisited. Some observations on the biology of vaccinia. Am J Trop Med Hyg. 1975;24(4):656–63.
186. Cramblett HG, Szwed CF, Utz JP, Kasel JA, McCullough NB. Accidental infection with vaccinia virus; a case report illustrating laboratory studies and problems of vaccination. Pediatrics. 1957;20(6):1020–32.
187. Moffatt AB. Vaccinia of the conjunctival sac. Br J Ophthalmol. 1952;36(4):211–3.
188. Ellis PP, Winograd LA. Current concepts of ocular vaccinia. Trans Pac Coast Otoophthalmol Soc Annu Meet. 1963;44:141–8.
189. Robinson MR, Udell IJ, Garber PF, Perry HD, Streeten BW. Molluscum contagiosum of the eyelids in patients with acquired immune deficiency syndrome. Ophthalmology. 1992;99(11):1745–7.
190. Ringeisen AL, Raven ML, Barney NP. Bulbar conjunctival molluscum contagiosum. Ophthalmology. 2016;123(2):294.
191. Gonnering RS, Kronish JW. Treatment of periorbital Molluscum contagiosum by incision and curettage. Ophthalmic Surg. 1988;19(5):325–7.
192. Charteris DG, Bonshek RE, Tullo AB. Ophthalmic molluscum contagiosum: clinical and immunopathological features. Br J Ophthalmol. 1995;79(5):476–81.
193. Mutalik SD, Rasal YD. Successful use of oral acyclovir in ophthalmic molluscum contagiosum. Indian Dermatol Online J. 2019;10(4):456–9.
194. Freeman G, Bron AJ, Juel-Jensen B. Ocular infection with orf virus. Am J Ophthalmol. 1984;97(5):601–4.
195. Cleton N, Koopmans M, Reimerink J, Godeke GJ, Reusken C. Come fly with me: review of clinically important arboviruses for global travelers. J Clin Virol. 2012;55(3):191–203.
196. Deutman AF, Klomp HJ. Rift valley fever retinitis. Am J Ophthalmol. 1981;92(1):38–42.
197. Grobbelaar AA, Weyer J, Moolla N, Jansen van Vuren P, Moises F, Paweska JT. Resurgence of yellow fever in Angola, 2015-2016. Emerg Infect Dis. 2016;22(10):1854–5.
198. Chadwick D, Arch B, Wilder-Smith A, Paton N. Distinguishing dengue fever from other infections on the basis of simple clinical and laboratory features: application of logistic regression analysis. J Clin Virol. 2006;35(2):147–53.
199. Petersen LR, Jamieson DJ, Powers AM, Honein MA. Zika virus. N Engl J Med. 2016;374(16):1552–63.
200. Manangeeswaran M, Kielczewski JL, Sen HN, Xu BC, Ireland DDC, McWilliams IL, Chan CC, Caspi RR, Verthelyi D. Zika virus infection causes persistent chorioretinal lesions. Emerg Microbes Infect. 2018;7(1):96.
201. Wikan N, Smith DR. Zika virus: history of a newly emerging arbovirus. Lancet Infect Dis. 2016;16(7):e119–26.
202. Furtado JM, Esposito DL, Klein TM, Teixeira-Pinto T, da Fonseca BA. Uveitis associated with Zika virus infection. N Engl J Med. 2016;375(4):394–6.
203. Kodati S, Palmore TN, Spellman FA, Cunningham D, Weistrop B, Sen HN. Bilateral posterior uveitis associated with Zika virus infection. Lancet. 2017;389(10064):125–6.
204. Mahendradas P, Ranganna SK, Shetty R, Balu R, Narayana KM, Babu RB, Shetty BK. Ocular manifestations associated with chikungunya. Ophthalmology. 2008;115(2):287–91.
205. Ng AW, Teoh SC. Dengue eye disease. Surv Ophthalmol. 2015;60(2):106–14.
206. Karesh JW, Mazzoli RA, Heintz SK. Ocular manifestations of mosquito-transmitted diseases. Mil Med. 2018;183(Suppl-1):450–8.

207. Zaidi MB, De Moraes CG, Petitto M, Yepez JB, Sakuntabhai A, Simon-Loriere E, Prot M, Ruffie C, Kim SS, Allikmets R, Terwilliger JD, Lee JH, Maestre GE. Non-congenital severe ocular complications of Zika virus infection. JMM Case Rep. 2018;5(6):e005152.
208. Rodriguez-Morales AJ, Villamil-Gomez WE, Franco-Paredes C. The arboviral burden of disease caused by co-circulation and co-infection of dengue, chikungunya and Zika in the Americas. Travel Med Infect Dis. 2016;14(3):177–9.
209. Clemmons NS, Redd SB, Gastanaduy PA, Marin M, Patel M, Fiebelkorn AP. Characteristics of large mumps outbreaks in the United States, July 2010-December 2015. Clin Infect Dis. 2019;68(10):1684–90.
210. Hahne S, Macey J, van Binnendijk R, Kohl R, Dolman S, van der Veen Y, Tipples G, Ruijs H, Mazzulli T, Timen A, van Loon A, de Melkeret H. Rubella outbreak in the Netherlands, 2004-2005: high burden of congenital infection and spread to Canada. Pediatr Infect Dis J. 2009;28(9):795–800.
211. Mahase E. Measles cases rise 300% globally in first few months of 2019. BMJ 2019; 365: l1810.
212. Hara J, Fujimoto F, Ishibashi T, Seguchi T, Nishimura K. Ocular manifestations of the 1976 rubella epidemic in Japan. Am J Ophthalmol. 1979;87(5):642–5.
213. Kayikçioglu Ö, Kir E, Söyler M, Güler C, Irkeç M. Ocular findings in a measles epidemic among young adults. Ocul Immunol Inflamm. 2000;8(1):59–62.
214. Meyer RF, Sullivan JH, Oh JO. Mumps conjunctivitis. Am J Ophthalmol. 1974;78(6):1022–4.
215. Lefebvre N, Camuset G, Bui E, Christmann D, Hansmann Y. Koplik spots: a clinical sign with epidemiological implications for measles control. Dermatology. 2010;220(3):280–1.
216. Xavier S, Forgie SED. Koplik spots revisited. CMAJ. 2015;187(8):600.
217. Foster A, Sommer A. Corneal ulceration, measles, and childhood blindness in Tanzania. Br J Ophthalmol. 1987;71(5):331.
218. Jabs DA. Ocular manifestations of HIV infection. Trans Am Ophthalmol Soc. 1995;93:623–83.
219. Aggarwal M, Rein J. Acute human immunodeficiency virus syndrome in an adolescent. Pediatrics. 2003;112(4):e323.
220. Gaines H, von Sydow M, Pehrson PO, Lundbegh P. Clinical picture of primary HIV infection presenting as a glandular-fever-like illness. BMJ. 1988;297(6660):1363–8.
221. Liesegang TJ. Herpes simplex virus epidemiology and ocular importance. Cornea. 2001;20(1):1–13.
222. Hodge WG, Margolis TP. Herpes simplex virus keratitis among patients who are positive or negative for human immunodeficiency virus: an epidemiologic study. Ophthalmology. 1997;104(1):120–4.
223. Ayena KD, Amedome KM, Agbo AR, Kpetessou-Ayivon AL, Dzidzinyo BK, Djagnikpo PA, Banla M, Baloet KP. [Ocular manifestations in HIV/AIDS patients undergoing highly active antiretroviral treatment (HAART) in Togo]. Med Trop (Mars). 2010;70(2):137–140.
224. Liesegang TJ. Herpes zoster virus infection. Curr Opin Ophthalmol. 2004;15(6):531–6.
225. Cunningham ET Jr, Margolis TP. Ocular manifestations of HIV infection. N Engl J Med. 1998;339(4):236–44.
226. Hodge WG, Seiff SR, Margolis TP. Ocular opportunistic infection incidences among patients who are HIV positive compared to patients who are HIV negative. Ophthalmology. 1998;105(5):895–900.
227. Ali R, Kim JY, Henderson BA. Adnexal and anterior segment manifestations of HIV/AIDS. Int Ophthalmol Clin. 2007;47(2):15–32.
228. Engstrom RE, Holland GN. Chronic herpes zoster virus keratitis associated with the acquired immunodeficiency syndrome. Am J Ophthalmol. 1988;105(5):556–8.
229. Schulz D, Sarra GM, Koerner UB, Garweg JG. Evolution of HIV-1-related conjunctival molluscum contagiosum under HAART: report of a bilaterally manifesting case and literature review. Graefes Arch Clin Exp Ophthalmol. 2004;242(11):951–5.
230. Babu RB, Sudharshan S, Kumarasamy N, Therese L, Biswas J. Ocular tuberculosis in acquired immunodeficiency syndrome. Am J Ophthalmol. 2006;142(3):413–8.

231. Ruggli GM, Weber R, Messmer EP, Font RL, Moll C, Bernauer W. Pneumocystis carinii infection of the conjunctiva in a patient with acquired immune deficiency syndrome. Ophthalmology. 1997;104(11):1853–6.
232. Lowder CY, McMahon JT, Meisler DM, Dodds EM, Calabrese LH, Didier ES, Cali A. Microsporidial keratoconjunctivitis caused by Septata intestinalis in a patient with acquired immunodeficiency syndrome. Am J Ophthalmol. 1996;121(6):715–7.
233. Weber R, Kuster H, Visvesvara GS, Bryan RT, Schwartz DA, Lüthy R. Disseminated microsporidiosis due to encephalitozoon hellem: pulmonary colonization, microhematuria, and mild conjunctivitis in a patient with AIDS. Clin Infect Dis. 1993;17(3):415–9.
234. Meintjes G, Lawn SD, Scano F, Maartens G, French MA, Worodria W, Elliott JH, Murdoch D, Wilkinson RJ, Seyler C, John L, van der Loeff MS, Reiss P, Lynen L, Janoff EN, Gilks C, Colebunders R, International Network for the Study of HIV-associated IRIS. Tuberculosis-associated immune reconstitution inflammatory syndrome: case definitions for use in resource-limited settings. Lancet Infect Dis. 2008;8(8):516–23.
235. Pagani JM, Duan JQ. Highly active antiretroviral therapy-induced immune recovery in an HIV-positive patient with a history of herpes zoster ophthalmicus. Optometry. 2011;82(2):77–82.
236. Gajdatsy AD, Tay-Kearney M-L. Microsporidial keratoconjunctivitis after HAART. Clin Exp Ophthalmol. 2001;29(5):327–9.
237. Ratnam I, Chiu C, Kandala N-B, Easterbrook PJ. Incidence and risk factors for immune reconstitution inflammatory syndrome in an ethnically diverse HIV type 1–infected cohort. Clin Infect Dis. 2006;42(3):418–27.
238. Teich SA. Conjunctival vascular changes in AIDS and AIDS-related complex. Am J Ophthalmol. 1987;103(3 Pt-1):332–3.
239. Engstrom RE Jr, Holland GN, Hardy WD, Meiselman HJ. Hemorheologic abnormalities in patients with human immunodeficiency virus infection and ophthalmic microvasculopathy. Am J Ophthalmol. 1990;109(2):153–61.
240. Bernard HU. The clinical importance of the nomenclature, evolution and taxonomy of human papillomaviruses. J Clin Virol. 2005;32(Suppl-1):S1–6.
241. Burd EM. Human papillomavirus and cervical cancer. Clin Microbiol Rev. 2003;16(1):1–17.
242. Shields CL, Shields JA. Tumors of the conjunctiva and cornea. Surv Ophthalmol. 2004;49(1):3–24.
243. Sjö NC, Heegaard S, Prause JU, von Buchwald C, Lindeberg H. Human papillomavirus in conjunctival papilloma. Br J Ophthalmol. 2001;85(7):785–7.
244. McDonnell PJ, McDonnell JM, Kessis T, Green WR, Shah KV. Detection of human papillomavirus type 6/11 DNA in conjunctival papillomas by in situ hybridization with radioactive probes. Hum Pathol. 1987;18(11):1115–9.
245. Shields CL, Shields JA. Conjunctival tumors in children. Curr Opin Ophthalmol. 2007;18(5):351–60.
246. Sjö NC, von Buchwald C, Cassonnet P, Norrild B, Prause JU, Vinding T, Heegaard S. Human papillomavirus in normal conjunctival tissue and in conjunctival papilloma: types and frequencies in a large series. Br J Ophthalmol. 2007;91(8):1014–5.
247. Scott IU, Karp CL, Nuovo GJ. Human papillomavirus 16 and 18 expression in conjunctival intraepithelial neoplasia. Ophthalmology. 2002;109(3):542–7.
248. Lauer SA, Malter JS, Meier JR. Human papillomavirus type 18 in conjunctival intraepithelial neoplasia. Am J Ophthalmol. 1990;110(1):23–7.
249. Odrich MG, Jakobiec FA, Lancaster WD, Kenyon KR, Kelly LD, Kornmehl EW, Steinert RF, Grove AS Jr, Shore JW, Gregoire L, et al. A spectrum of bilateral squamous conjunctival tumors associated with human papillomavirus type 16. Ophthalmology. 1991;98(5):628–35.
250. McDonnell JM, Mayr AJ, Martin WJ. DNA of human papillomavirus type 16 in dysplastic and malignant lesions of the conjunctiva and cornea. N Engl J Med. 1989;320(22):1442–6.
251. Gichuhi S, Sagoo MS, Weiss HA, Burton MJ. Epidemiology of ocular surface squamous neoplasia in Africa. Tropical Med Int Health. 2013;18(12):1424–43.

252. van der Hoek L, Pyrc K, Jebbink MF, Vermeulen-Oost W, Berkhout RJ, Wolthers KC, Wertheim-van Dillen PM, Kaandorp J, Spaargaren J, Berkhout B. Identification of a new human coronavirus. Nat Med. 2004;10(4):368–73.

253. Fouchier RA, Schneeberger PM, Rozendaal FW, Broekman JM, Kemink SAG, Munster V, Kuiken T, Rimmelzwaan GF, Schutten M, van Doornum GJJ, Kock G, Bosman A, Koopmans M, Osterhaus ADME. Avian influenza A virus (H7N7) associated with human conjunctivitis and a fatal case of acute respiratory distress syndrome. Proc Natl Acad Sci U S A. 2004;101(5):1356–61.

254. Yang TY, Lu CY, Kao CL, Chen RT, Ho YH, Yang SC, Lee PI, Chen JM, Lee CY, Huang LM. Clinical manifestations of parainfluenza infection in children. J Microbiol Immunol Infect. 2003;36(4):270–4.

255. Guan W-J, Ni Z-y, Hu Y, Liang WH, Ou CQ, He JX, Liu L, Shan H, Lei CL, Hui DSC, Du B, Li LJ, Zeng G, Yuen KY, Chen RC, Tang CL, Wang T, Chen PY, Xiang J, Li SY, Wang JL, Liang ZJ, Peng YX, Wei L, Liu Y, Hu YH, Peng P, Wang JM, Liu JY, Chen Z, Li G, Zheng ZJ, Qiu SQ, Luo J, Ye CJ, Zhu SY, Zhong NS; China Medical Treatment Expert Group for Covid-19. Clinical characteristics of coronavirus disease 2019 in China. N Engl J Med. 2020; [Online ahead of print].

256. World Health Organization. Report of the WHO-China Joint Mission on Coronavirus Disease 2019 (COVID-19). WHO; 2020.

257. Belser JA, Lash RR, Garg S, Tumpey TM, Maines TR. The eyes have it: influenza virus infection beyond the respiratory tract. Lancet Infect Dis. 2018;18(7):e220–7.

258. Koopmans M, Wilbrink B, Conyn M, Natrop G, van der Nat H, Vennema H, Meijer A, van Steenbergen J, Fouchier R, Osterhaus A, Bosman A. Transmission of H/N7 avian influenza A virus to human beings during a large outbreak in commercial poultry farms in the Netherlands. Lancet. 2004;363(9409):587–93.

259. Belser JA, Zeng H, Katz JM, Tumpey TM. Ocular tropism of influenza A viruses: identification of H7 subtype-specific host responses in human respiratory and ocular cells. J Virol. 2011;85(19):10117–25.

260. Nelson CB, Pomeroy BS, Schrall K, Park WE, Lindeman RJ. An outbreak of conjunctivitis due to Newcastle disease virus (NDV) occurring in poultry workers. Am J Public Health Nations Health. 1952;42(6):672–8.

261. Trott DG, Pilsworth R. Outbreaks of conjunctivitis due to the Newcastle disease virus among workers in chicken-broiler factories. Br Med J. 1965;2(5477):1514–7.

262. Lippmann O. Human conjunctivitis due to the Newcastle-disease virus of fowls. Am J Ophthalmol. 1952;35(7):1021–8.

263. Burnet FM. Human infection with the virus of Newcastle disease of fowls. Med J Aust. 1943;2(16):313–4.

264. Wilson DA, Yen-Lieberman B, Schindler S, Asamoto K, Schold JD, Procop GW. Should varicella-zoster virus culture be eliminated? A comparison of direct immunofluorescence antigen detection, culture, and PCR, with a historical review. J Clin Microbiol. 2012;50(12):4120–2.

265. Elnifro EM, Cooper RJ, Klapper PE, Yeo AC, Tullo AB. Multiplex polymerase chain reaction for diagnosis of viral and chlamydial keratoconjunctivitis. Invest Ophthalmol Vis Sci. 2000;41(7):1818–22.

266. Kaufman HE, Azcuy AM, Varnell ED, Sloop GD, Thompson HW, Hill JM. HSV-1 DNA in tears and saliva of normal adults. Invest Ophthalmol Vis Sci. 2005;46(1):241–7.

267. Sambursky R, Tauber S, Schirra F, Kozich K, Davidson R, Cohen EJ. The RPS Adeno detector for diagnosing adenoviral conjunctivitis. Ophthalmology. 2006;113(10):1758–64.

268. Sambursky R, Trattler W, Tauber S, Starr C, Friedberg M, Boland T, McDonald M, DellaVecchia M, Luchs J. Sensitivity and specificity of the AdenoPlus test for diagnosing adenoviral conjunctivitis. JAMA Ophthalmol. 2013;131(1):17–22.

269. Holtz KK, Townsend KR, Furst JW, Myers JF, Binnicker MJ, Quigg SM, Maxson JA, Espy MJ. An assessment of the AdenoPlus point-of-care test for diagnosing adenoviral

conjunctivitis and its effect on antibiotic stewardship. Mayo Clin Proc Innov Qual Outcomes. 2017;1(2):170–5.

270. Kam KY, Ong HS, Bunce C, Ogunbowale L, Verma S. Sensitivity and specificity of the AdenoPlus point-of-care system in detecting adenovirus in conjunctivitis patients at an ophthalmic emergency department: a diagnostic accuracy study. Br J Ophthalmol. 2015;99(9):1186–9.

271. Lee CS, Lee AY, Akileswaran L, Stroman D, Najafi-Tagol K, Kleiboeker S, Chodosh J, Magaret A, Wald A, Van Gelder RN, BAYnovation Study Group. Determinants of outcomes of adenoviral keratoconjunctivitis. Ophthalmology. 2018;125(9):1344–53.

272. Sammons JS, Graf EH, Townsend S, Hoegg CL, Smathers SA, Coffin SE, Williams K, Mitchell SL, Nawab U, Munson D, Quinn G, Binenbaum G. Outbreak of adenovirus in a neonatal intensive care unit: critical importance of equipment cleaning during inpatient ophthalmologic examinations. Ophthalmology. 2019;126(1):137–43.

273. Chodosh J. Neonatal intensive care eye. Ophthalmology. 2019;126(1):144–5.

274. Gordon YJ, Araullo-Cruz T, Romanowski EG. The effects of topical nonsteroidal anti-inflammatory drugs on adenoviral replication. Arch Ophthalmol. 1998;116(7):900–5.

275. Chodosh J. Epidemic keratoconjunctivitis. In: Melki S, Fava MA, editors. Cornea and refractive atlas of clinical wisdom. 1st ed. Thorofare, NJ: Slack; 2011. p. 91–6.

276. Rutala WA, Peacock JE, Gergen MF, Sobsey MD, Weber DJ. Efficacy of hospital germicides against adenovirus 8, a common cause of epidemic keratoconjunctivitis in health care facilities. Antimicrob Agents Chemother. 2006;50(4):1419–24.

Chlamydia Conjunctivitis

3

Darby D. Miller

3.1 Introduction

Chlamydial infections are the most common cause of infectious blindness in the world [1]. Each of the three species, *C. trachomatis, C. pneumoniae*, and *C. psittaci*, has clinical manifestations in humans. *C. pneumoniae* causes systemic disease without ocular manifestations whereas *C. psittaci*, specifically the avian strain, has been known to cause conjunctivitis [2]. *C. trachomatis* causes the majority of ocular disease in humans including trachoma, neonatal and adult inclusion conjunctivitis, and lymphogranuloma venereum. This chapter will focus on the different species of *Chlamydia* that cause ocular disease, namely *C. trachomatis* and, to a lesser extent, *C. psittaci*.

3.2 Pathophysiology

Chlamydia is an obligate intracellular, gram-negative bacterium that exists in two distinct forms during its biphasic life cycle: the replicative reticulate body (RB) and the infectious elementary body (EB). The small and metabolically inactive EBs invade the host cell by endocytosis and then differentiate into larger, metabolically active RBs. The RB is the intracellular form and replicates in a membrane-bound inclusion compartment. They produce energy by utilizing the host cell metabolic activity. RBs transform back into EBs that can disseminate by lysis of the host cell or by infecting adjacent cells [3–5].

When considering Chlamydial infections in humans, specific serovars result in specific clinical manifestations. Serovars A-C are associated with trachoma. The vast majority of ocular disease is caused by *C. trachomatis*, and trachoma accounts

D. D. Miller (✉)
Mayo Clinic, Jacksonville, FL, USA
e-mail: Miller.Darby@mayo.edu

© Springer Nature Singapore Pte Ltd. 2021
S. Das, V. Jhanji (eds.), *Infections of the Cornea and Conjunctiva*,
https://doi.org/10.1007/978-981-15-8811-2_3

for 3% of the causes of blindness worldwide [1]. Serovars D-K are associated with neonatal and adult conjunctivitis. Serovars L1-3 are associated with lymphogranuloma venereum [5].

3.3 Trachoma

3.3.1 Epidemiology

According to the World Health Organization (WHO), an estimated 232 million people living in trachoma-endemic districts are at risk, more than 21 million have active trachoma, and approximately 7.3 million require surgery for trachomatous trichiasis. An estimated 2.2 million people are visually impaired as a result of trachoma, 1.2 million of whom are blind. Trachoma is endemic in more than 50 countries in Africa, Asia, Central and South America, Australia, and the Middle East (Fig. 3.1). Africa has the largest burden of trachoma with an estimated 18 million cases of active trachoma (85% of all cases globally) and 3.2 million cases of trichiasis (44% of all cases globally) [6].

Children younger than 5 years old are most susceptible to infection and have the highest prevalence of active disease. The prevalence of active trachoma and conjunctival scarring are inversely related: active trachoma decreases with age while the rates of conjunctival scarring increase [7–10]. Although rates of active trachoma

Distribution of trachoma, worldwide, 2012

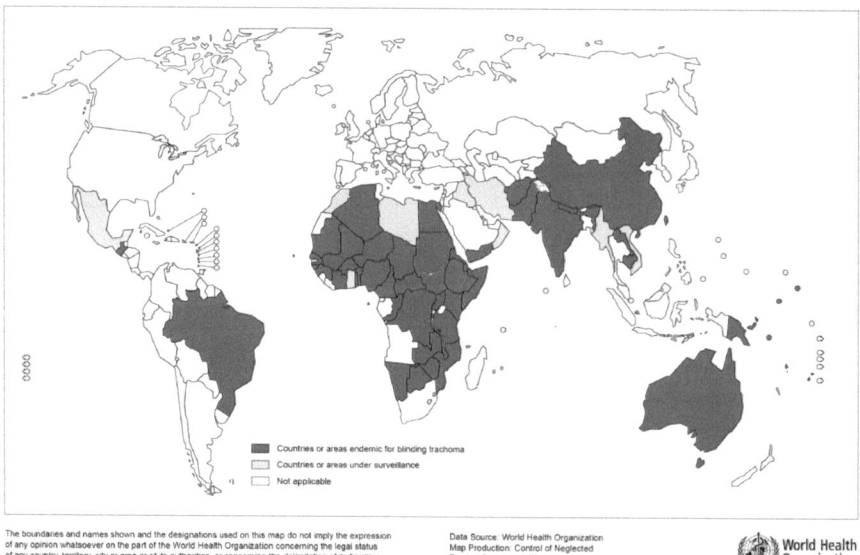

Fig. 3.1 Distribution of trachoma. According to the World Health Organization in 2012. (Source: WHO Alliance for the Global Elimination of Blinding Trachoma by the year 2020. Progress report on elimination of trachoma, 2013. Wkly Epidemiol Rec 2014;89(39):421–8)

are similar in males and females at young ages, trichiasis and visual impairment are more common in women than men in adulthood [8]. Endemic areas typically have populations with poor personal and community hygiene. Risk factors for developing trachoma include low socioeconomic status, crowding, insufficient sanitation facilities, and inadequate water supply [11].

3.3.2   Pathogenesis

The most common mode of *C. trachomatis* transmission is direct contact with ocular and nasal discharges from infected individuals. *C. trachomatis* can also be spread by eye-seeking flies such as *Musca sorbens* and by contact with fomites [12].

Persistent and recurrent infections result in the conjunctival and corneal scarring seen with trachoma. To better assess the stages of the disease, the WHO developed Detailed and Simplified Grading Systems. The simplified classification of trachomatous disease is the most widely accepted and used by health care personnel [13]. It is straightforward and provides a grading system which follows the natural history of trachoma (Fig 3.2) [14, 15]. The five stages of this classification system are:

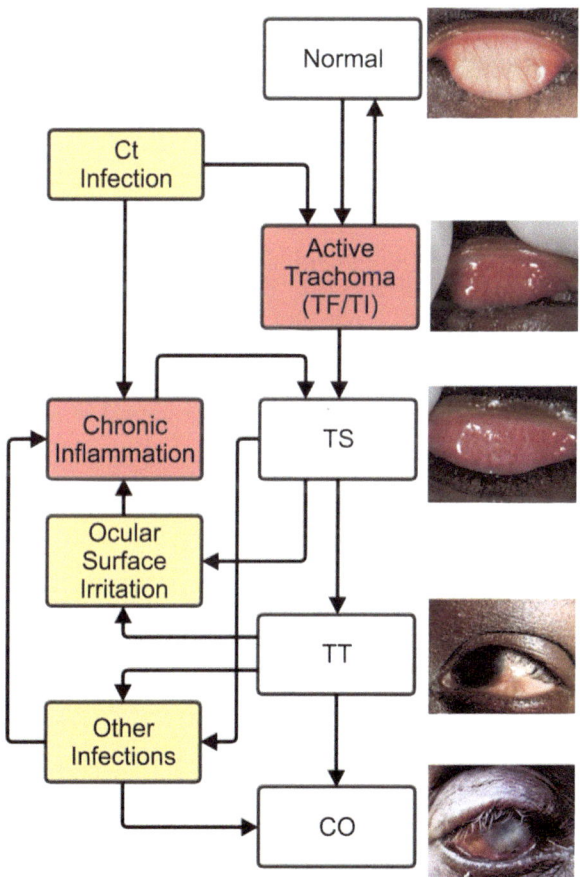

Fig. 3.2 Stages of Trachoma. *TF* trachomatous inflammation, follicular; *TI* trachomatous inflammation, intense; *TS* trachomatous scarring; *TT* Trachomatous trichiasis; *CO* Corneal opacification. (Source: Ramadhani AM, Derrick T, Holland MJ, Burton MJ. Blinding Trachoma: Systematic Review of Rates and Risk Factors for Progressive Disease. PLoS Negl Trop Dis 2016;10(8):e0004859)

1. Trachomatous inflammation—follicular (TF): the presence of five or more follicles in the superior tarsal conjunctiva. The follicles must be at least 0.5 mm in diameter.
2. Trachomatous inflammation—intense (TI): pronounced inflammatory thickening of the tarsal conjunctiva that obscures more than half of the normal deep tarsal vessels.
3. Trachomatous scarring (TS): the presence of scarring in the tarsal conjunctiva.
4. Trachomatous trichiasis (TT): at least one eyelash rubs on the eyeball. Evidence of recent removal of inturned eyelashes should also be graded as trichiasis.
5. Corneal opacity (CO): easily visible corneal opacity over the pupil. Such corneal opacities cause significant visual impairment, and visual acuity should be measured if possible.

Clinically, trachoma infection initially presents with a follicular conjunctivitis. Symptoms include irritation, hyperemia, discharge, and blurry vision. Active disease is characterized by TF and TI and is mostly seen in children. The blinding effects of the infection typically present later in life. Thus TS, TT, and CO are more common in adulthood [16]. Additional ocular exam findings include Herbert's pits, limbal scarring secondary to the necrosis of follicles, and Arlt's line, linear scarring on the upper tarsus [17]. As scarring progresses, cicatricial lid abnormalities along with trichiasis eventually lead to corneal pannus, scarring, and opacification [16].

There is no solitary accepted gold standard for laboratory testing of *C. trachomatis*. Signs of active infection in patients can be present long after the infection has resolved, and DNA or RNA is undetectable at that time [18]. Thus trachoma primarily remains a clinical diagnosis.

On histopathology, TF of the conjunctiva is characterized by a mixed inflammatory response of lymphocytes, neutrophils, macrophages, and plasma cells (particularly IgA). The diffuse infiltration is also marked by interspersed follicles of B cells surrounded by T cells [19]. Inflammatory changes close to the conjunctival surface indicate that the epithelium has an integral role in the pathogenesis of trachoma [20]. Changes in type I and type V collagen are characteristic of TS and natural killer cells have been implicated in scar formation [21]. In vivo confocal microscopy can now be used to quantitate inflammation and connective tissue scarring [20, 22].

3.3.3 Management

To better address the public health need, the WHO-led Global Alliance for the Elimination of Trachoma by 2020 (GET 2020) was established in 1997. The WHO recommends the implementation of the SAFE strategy which addresses the disease at four different stages [16]. The SAFE strategy acronym stands for:

- Surgery to correct trichiasis
- Antibiotics to treat chlamydial infection

- Facial cleanliness to reduce transmission of ocular infection
- Environmental improvements to suppress transmission of infection including access to water and sanitation

When implemented, the SAFE strategy results in substantial reductions in the transmission of *Chlamydia* as well as a decline in active trachoma [23].

3.3.4 Surgery

Trachomatous trichiasis and entropion can cause corneal scarring and opacification and ultimately vision loss which can be permanent. Surgical correction of the eyelid and eyelashes aims to stop the detrimental effect of trichiasis and entropion. Although eyelash epilation is a temporary, short-term treatment option, it has been shown to decrease the risk of corneal opacification [24]. For patients with mild TT who decline surgery or do not have access to surgical treatment, self-epilation and regular follow-up has shown to have comparable change in vision and corneal opacity when compared to surgical patients [25]. Eyelid surgery, however, is preferred over epilation and is a long-term solution.

Although different surgical options are available, bilamellar tarsal rotation and posterior lamellar rotation procedures are recommended by the WHO [26, 27]. In 2018, over 146,000 people with trachomatous trichiasis were provided with corrective eyelid surgery [28]. Postoperative antibiotics, specifically azithromycin, have been shown to improve surgical outcomes [29]. Unfortunately, tarsoconjunctival scarring in trachoma can still progress even after tarsal rotational procedures, which can result in recurrence of trichiasis [30]. Surgical outcomes can be improved by addressing inadequate peripheral dissection, asymmetric suture positioning and tension, irregular incision, and lash location [31].

3.3.5 Antibiotics

The goal of antibiotic treatment is to reduce the burden of active infection. By lowering the prevalence of *C. trachomatis*, transmission of infection within endemic communities is interrupted and ultimately prevents the ocular sequelae of trachoma. Systemic treatment with macrolide or tetracycline antibiotics is effective in the TF and TI stages of acute infection. Azithromycin 1 g given as a single-dose oral therapy is preferred if the medication is available and affordable [32]. It is well tolerated when given as a single dose and avoids the risk of noncompliance that is associated with a prolonged course of antibiotics. Single-dose azithromycin has also been shown to be as effective as a 2 week course of an oral tetracycline. An alternative to azithromycin is a 2 week course of oral doxycycline 100 mg twice daily. In addition to oral therapy, topical erythromycin or tetracycline ointment twice daily for 6 weeks is an effective treatment in helping to eliminate the acute infection [33]. Regardless of the regimen, antibiotic treatment should also be administered to the patient's sexual partner(s). For pregnant women or children under the age of 8 years, oral erythromycin is preferred.

The WHO guidelines recommend mass distribution of antibiotics according to the prevalence of TF. In 2018, according to the WHO, over 89 million people were treated with antibiotics to eliminate trachoma [28]. Single-dose azithromycin remains the preferred antibiotic regimen as it reduces the prevalence of active trachoma and ocular infection in communities. Antibiotic resistance is a concern and has been documented in certain communities [34, 35].

3.3.6 Facial Cleanliness and Environmental Improvements

Facial cleanliness and environmental improvements address the principal cause of trachoma and are primary prevention components of the WHO's SAFE strategy for trachoma elimination. Although mass distribution of antibiotics can reduce the burden of disease, personal and community hygiene play an essential role in controlling the spread of trachoma. Maximizing facial cleanliness and environmental improvements involves not only information dissemination but also behavior change techniques [36].

Facial cleanliness has been linked to a lower risk of trachoma as well as decreasing the severity of active disease [37]. When facial cleanliness is implemented in concert with mass distribution of antibiotics, there is a clear and positive impact on trachoma [38]. The addition of environmental improvements, such as the use of a household pit latrine, is independently associated with lessening active trachoma [39]. The goal of safe disposal of excreta is to reduce fly populations. Access to water and sanitation are also crucially important in achieving the goal of facial cleanliness and environmental improvements.

Each component of the SAFE strategy plays an integral role in combating trachoma. Simultaneous implementation of antibiotics, facial cleanliness, and environmental improvements, along with SAFE evaluations within 6–12 months after mass distribution of azithromycin, are crucial to the reduction of trachoma [40]. As of January 2020, 13 countries had reported achieving trachoma elimination goals. Trachoma remains hyperendemic, however, in 24 countries spread across Africa, Central and South America, Asia, Australia, and the Middle East [28].

3.4   Inclusion Conjunctivitis

3.4.1   Neonatal Inclusion Conjunctivitis

Neonatal inclusion conjunctivitis (NIC), also known as ophthalmia neonatorum (ON), occurs within the first 30 days of life. The three most common etiologies include chemical, viral, and bacterial. Bacterial causes consist of *Neisseria gonorrhoeae, Pseudomonas aeruginosa*, as well as *Staphylococcus, Streptococcus*, and *Haemophilus* species. *C. trachomatis*, however, accounts for approximately 40% of

ON cases and is thus the most common cause of infectious neonatal conjunctivitis worldwide [41, 42].

C. trachomatis neonatal conjunctivitis is associated with serovars D-K, which cause urogenital disease, and is acquired from the birth canal during delivery. Clinically, it is characterized by bilateral hyperemia, mucopurulent discharge, eyelid edema, pseudomembranes, and a papillary reaction. The acute infection typically occurs within 5–14 days after birth. While the incidence of chlamydial infections in pregnant women in the United States is approximately 8%, between 30 to 50% of infants born to a mother with an active chlamydial infection will develop NIC [43]. Prompt diagnosis and treatment are essential to preventing progression and long-term sequelae such as scarring of the cornea and conjunctiva.

In addition to clinical findings, laboratory studies are valuable in the diagnosis of NIC. Importantly, the studies allow *C. trachomatis* to be differentiated from other organisms such as *N. gonorrhoeae* and *Pseudomonas*, both of which have sight-threatening potential that can be rapid and severe. When obtaining a conjunctival specimen, scrapings of the tarsal conjunctiva must contain epithelial cells since *C. trachomatis* is an obligate intracellular organism. Exudate cultures and routine conjunctival swabs are inadequate for testing. Historically, laboratory diagnosis was made by direct detection of inclusion bodies with the Giemsa stain. Although pathognomonic for chlamydial infection, sensitivity of this test is less than 40% [44]. Other methods of laboratory diagnosis include culture with McCoy cells, fluorescein-labeled monoclonal tests, and polymerase chain reaction (PCR) testing [45]. Due to its high specificity, cell culture remains the preferred method for legal cases and epidemiological studies [46]. Culture with McCoy cells reportedly has >95% specificity and approximately 60% sensitivity. Highly sensitive nucleic acid amplification tests (NAATs), such as PCR-based testing, are used to routinely diagnose chlamydial infection and have a specificity of 95% and sensitivity of >90% [47]. When compared with PCR-based testing, fluorescein-labeled monoclonal tests achieve a similar level of specificity and sensitivity [48]. Although *C. trachomatis* isolation by cell culture is still frequently used worldwide, PCR-based testing is becoming the gold standard.

Prophylaxis of neonatal chlamydial conjunctivitis has historically consisted of topical silver nitrate, erythromycin, or tetracycline drops. However, chemical conjunctivitis occurs in 50–90% of infants treated with silver nitrate and its use has been suspended in several countries [49]. Currently, in the United States, prophylaxis with erythromycin ophthalmic ointment immediately after birth is mandated in most states [50]. Confirmed cases should be treated immediately with systemic erythromycin or azithromycin. Erythromycin is recommended for 14 days at a dose of 50 mg/kg body weight per day. Azithromycin can be given at 20 mg/kg per day as a 3-day course. A recent study suggests that erythromycin at 50 mg/kg per day for 14 days results in higher numbers of cure than does azithromycin [51]. If confirmed by culture, the mother and her sexual partners must also be treated with systemic doxycycline 100 mg twice daily for seven days if neither pregnant nor breast-feeding. If pregnant or breast-feeding, erythromycin 250 to 500 mg four times daily for seven days is effective. Several countries, however, have halted ocular prophylaxis of newborns and replaced it with prenatal prevention and care [52]. Prenatal screening, along with diagnosis and management of chlamydial disease during pregnancy, is the preferred approach to preventing NIC.

3.4.2 Adult Inclusion Conjunctivitis

Chlamydia is the most common notifiable disease in the United States and typically affects sexually active young adults. Since 1994, it has comprised the largest proportion of all sexually transmitted diseases reported to the Centers for Disease Control and Prevention (CDC) [53]. Untreated infections can result in pelvic inflammatory disease (PID), ectopic pregnancy, and conjunctivitis. Pregnant women can pass the infection to their infants during delivery, potentially resulting in NIC. Adult inclusion conjunctivitis (AIC), similar to NIC, is caused by *Chlamydia trachomatis* serotypes D-K. It is spread via direct inoculation from the genitalia. A sizeable percentage of patients with AIC will have a concomitant genital infection [54]. Thus, AIC should be thought of as a systemic disease. Systemic therapy of the patient and their sexual partner is required [55].

The initial presentation of AIC is an acute, unilateral follicular conjunctivitis with an enlarged, preauricular lymph node on the ipsilateral side (Fig. 3.3). Similar to NIC, ocular manifestations of AIC begin 5–14 after inoculation. The follicular conjunctivitis eventually becomes chronic and bilateral. Follicles are most prominent in the lower palpebral conjunctiva and inferior fornix [56]. AIC can also be characterized by hyperemia, mucopurulent discharge, tearing, chemosis, subepithelial corneal infiltrates, and pseudomembranes [57].

Laboratory diagnosis of AIC is comparable to NIC. Conjunctival scrapings can be evaluated using Giemsa stains and cultured with McCoy cells. Similar to NIC, PCR is becoming the gold standard for diagnosis in most countries due to its superior specificity and sensitivity. AIC patients and their partners must be treated

Fig. 3.3 Follicular conjunctivitis of the inferior palpebral conjunctiva. (Courtesy: Jason Calhoun, Mayo Clinic)

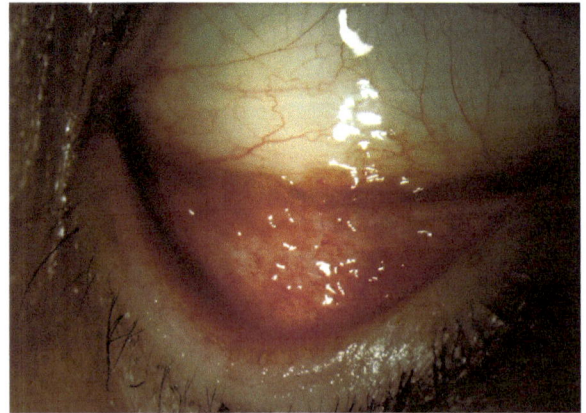

systemically and single-dose azithromycin 1 g is preferred. Alternative medication regimens include doxycycline 100 mg twice daily or erythromycin 500 mg four times per day. Both are given for 7 days but doxycycline should be avoided in pregnancy. Adjunct topical therapy includes erythromycin or tetracycline ointment twice daily for 2–3 weeks [58, 59].

3.5 Lymphogranuloma Venereum

Lymphogranuloma venereum (LGV) is a sexually transmitted disease and is caused by *C. trachomatis* serotypes L1-3. It is most frequently seen in sexually active young adults and affects both sexes equally. LGV can cause potentially severe infections with irreversible consequences if treatment is not initiated promptly. Early and accurate diagnosis is necessary. The initial clinical manifestations of LGV can include tender inguinal lymphadenopathy, a self-limited and painless genital ulcer or papule, and/or proctitis [60].

Ocular involvement secondary to LGV is unusual but can present as Parinaud's oculoglandular syndrome. Clinically, it is characterized by a bilateral papillary and/or follicular conjunctivitis in addition to prominent and tender preauricular and cervical lymphadenopathy [61]. Peripheral corneal infiltrates, episcleritis, iridocyclitis, and optic neuritis have also been reported [62].

Diagnosis is based on clinical suspicion and the exclusion of other etiologies, in addition to laboratory studies. Genital lesions, rectal specimens, and lymph node specimens can be tested for *C. trachomatis* by culture, direct immunofluorescence, or nucleic acid detection [63]. The recommended systemic therapy cures the infection and prevents further damage to tissues. Treatment consists of doxycycline 100 mg twice daily for 21 days, erythromycin 500 mg four times per day for 21 days, or azithromycin 1 g once per week for 3 weeks. Pregnant and lactating women should be treated with erythromycin [64]. The patient and partner should be screened for concomitant sexually transmitted diseases.

3.6 Chlamydia Psittaci

Psittacosis is an infection caused by *Chlamydia psittaci* and is an uncommon cause of conjunctivitis. The natural host of *C. psittaci* is birds and mammals. Individuals with exposure to birds such as poultry industry employees are at the greatest risk of infection. Inhalation of the aerosolized organism causes an atypical pneumonia. Other clinical manifestations can include severe headache, myalgias, and mental status changes. Ocular involvement is rare but is characterized by a bilateral follicular conjunctivitis involving the superior and inferior palpebral, and occasionally bulbar, conjunctiva (Fig. 3.4) [65].

Fig. 3.4 Follicular
conjunctivitis of the
superior tarsal conjunctiva.
(Courtesy: Jason Calhoun,
Mayo Clinic)

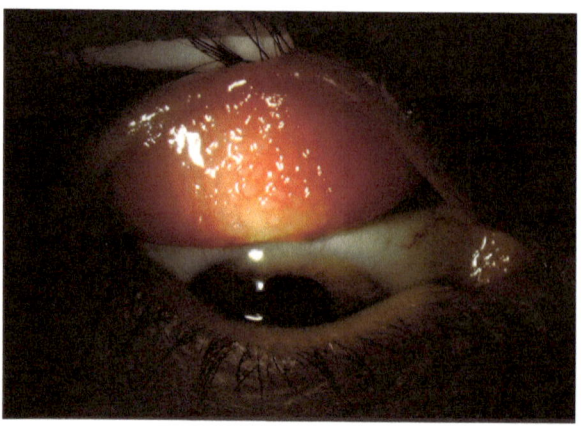

Infection should be suspected in patients with exposure history and relevant clinical indicators. Complement fixation titers can be beneficial in diagnosis but PCR remains the most effective method when differentiating *C. psittaci* from other organisms [66]. Treatment consists of oral tetracycline 500 mg four times per day or doxycycline 100 mg twice daily for at least 2 weeks. With prompt recognition and treatment, the prognosis is excellent.

3.7   Summary

Chlamydial infections are the most common cause of infectious blindness in the world. Each of the three species, C. trachomatis, C. pneumoniae, and C. psittaci, has clinical manifestations in humans. C. trachomatis causes the vast majority of ocular disease in humans.

References

1. Pascolini D, Mariotti SP. Global estimates of visual impairment: 2010. Br J Ophthalmol. 2012;96(5):614–8.
2. Center for Disease Control and Prevention. Compendium of measures to control Chlamydia psittaci infection among humans (psittacosis) and pet birds (avian chlamydiosis), 1998. MMWR Recomm Rep. 1998;47(RR-10):1–14.
3. Fischer A, Rudel T. Safe haven under constant attack—the Chlamydia-containing vacuole. Cell Microbiol. 2018;20(10):e12940.
4. Clarke IN. Evolution of Chlamydia trachomatis. Ann N Y Acad Sci. 2011;1230:E11–8.
5. Peeling RW, Brunham RC. Chlamydiae as pathogens: new species and new issues. Emerg Infect Dis. 1996;2(4):307–19.
6. WHO Alliance for the Global Elimination of Blinding Trachoma by the year 2020. Progress report on elimination of trachoma, 2013. Wkly Epidemiol Rec. 2014;89(39):421–8.
7. Ngondi J, Onsarigo A, Adamu L, Matende I, Baba S, Reacher M, Emerson P, Zingeser J. The epidemiology of trachoma in Eastern Equatoria and Upper Nile States, southern Sudan. Bull World Health Organ. 2005;83(12):904–12.

8. West SK, Munoz B, Turner VM, Mmbaga BB, Taylor HR. The epidemiology of trachoma in central Tanzania. Int J Epidemiol. 1991;20(4):1088–92.
9. Grassly NC, Ward ME, Ferris S, Mabey DC, Bailey RL. The natural history of trachoma infection and disease in a Gambian cohort with frequent follow-up. PLoS Negl Trop Dis. 2008;2(12):e341.
10. Courtright P, Sheppard J, Schachter J, Said ME, Dawson CR. Trachoma and blindness in the Nile Delta: current patterns and projections for the future in the rural Egyptian population. Br J Ophthalmol. 1989;73(7):536–40.
11. Wright HR, Turner A, Taylor HR. Trachoma. Lancet. 2008;371(9628):1945–54.
12. Witkin SS, Minis E, Athanasiou A, Leizer J, Linhares IM. Chlamydia trachomatis: the persistent pathogen. Clin Vaccine Immunol. 2017;24(10):e00203–17.
13. Thylefors B, Dawson CR, Jones BR, West SK, Taylor HR. A simple system for the assessment of trachoma and its complications. Bull World Health Organ. 1987;65(4):477–83.
14. Ramadhani AM, Derrick T, Holland MJ, Burton MJ. Blinding trachoma: systematic review of rates and risk factors for progressive disease. PLoS Negl Trop Dis. 2016;10(8):e0004859.
15. Bowman RJ, Jatta B, Cham B, Bailey RL, Faal H, Myatt M, Foster A, Johnson GJ. Natural history of trachomatous scarring in the Gambia: results of a 12-year longitudinal follow-up. Ophthalmology. 2001;108(12):2219–24.
16. Taylor HR, Burton MJ, Haddad D, West S, Wright H. Trachoma. Lancet. 2014;384(9960):2142–52.
17. Dawson CR, Juster R, Marx R, Daghfous MT, Ben Djerad A. Limbal disease in trachoma and other ocular chlamydial infections. risk factors for corneal vascularisation. Eye. 1989;3(Pt-2):204–9.
18. Keenan JD, Lakew T, Alemayehu W, Melese M, House JI, Acharya NR, Porco TC, Gaynor BD, Lietman TM. Slow resolution of clinically active trachoma following successful mass antibiotic treatments. Arch Ophthalmol. 2011;129(4):512–3.
19. el-Asrar AM, Van den Oord JJ, Geboes K, Missotten L, Emarah MH, Desmet V. Immunopathology of trachomatous conjunctivitis. Br J Ophthalmol. 1989;73(4):276–82.
20. Hu VH, Weiss HA, Massae P, Courtright P, Makupa W, Mabey DC, Bailey RL, Burton MJ. In vivo confocal microscopy in scarring trachoma. Ophthalmology. 2011;118(11):2138–46.
21. Hu VH, Luthert PJ, Derrick T, Pullin J, Weiss HA, Massae P, Mtuy T, Makupa W, Essex D, Mabey DC, Bailey RL, Holland MJ, Burton MJ. Immunohistochemical analysis of scarring trachoma indicates infiltration by natural killer and undefined CD45 negative cells. PLoS Negl Trop Dis. 2016;10(5):e0004734.
22. Hu VH, Holland MJ, Cree IA, Pullin J, Weiss HA, Massae P, Makupa W, Mabey DC, Bailey RL, Burton MJ, Luthert P. In vivo confocal microscopy and histopathology of the conjunctiva in trachomatous scarring and normal tissue: a systematic comparison. Br J Ophthalmol. 2013;97(10):1333–7.
23. Ngondi J, Gebre T, Shargie EB, Adamu L, Ejigsemahu Y, Teferi T, Zerihun M, Ayele B, Cevallos V, King J, Emerson PM. Evaluation of three years of the SAFE strategy (surgery, antibiotics, facial cleanliness and environmental improvement) for trachoma control in five districts of Ethiopia hyperendemic for trachoma. Trans R Soc Trop Med Hyg. 2009;103(10):1001–10.
24. Rajak SN, Habtamu E, Weiss HA, Bedri A, Gebre T, Genet A, Khaw PT, Bailey RL, Mabey DC, Gilbert CE, Emerson PM, Burton MJ. Epilation for trachomatous trichiasis and the risk of corneal opacification. Ophthalmology. 2012;119(1):84–9.
25. Habtamu E, Rajak SN, Tadesse Z, Wondie T, Zerihun M, Guadie B, Gebre T, Kello AB, Callahan K, Mabey DC, Khaw PT, Gilbert CE, Weiss HA, Emerson PM, Burton MJ. Epilation for minor trachomatous trichiasis: four-year results of a randomised controlled trial. PLoS Negl Trop Dis. 2015;9(3):e0003558.
26. Reacher MH, Muñoz B, Alghassany A, Daar AS, Elbualy M, Taylor HR. A controlled trial of surgery for trachomatous trichiasis of the upper lid. Arch Ophthalmol. 1992;110(5):667–74.
27. Reacher M, Foster A, Huber J. Trichiasis surgery for trachoma. In: The bilamellar tarsal rotation procedure. Geneva: World Health Organization; 1993. WHO/PBL/93.29; 2011.

28. World Health Organization. Trachoma. https://www.who.int/news-room/fact-sheets/detail/trachoma. Accessed 20 July 2020.
29. Burton M, Habtamu E, Ho D, Gower EW. Interventions for trachoma trichiasis. Cochrane Database Syst Rev. 2015;2015(11):CD004008.
30. Diab MM, Allen RC, Gawdat TI, Saif AS. Trachoma elimination, approaching 2020. Curr Opin Ophthalmol. 2018;29(5):451–7.
31. Habtamu E, Wondie T, Aweke S, Tadesse Z, Zerihun M, Gashaw B, Wondimagegn GS, Mengistie HD, Rajak SN, Callahan K, Weiss HA, Burton MJ. Predictors of trachomatous trichiasis surgery outcome. Ophthalmology. 2017;124(8):1143–55.
32. Bailey RL, Arullendran P, Whittle HC, Mabey DC. Randomised controlled trial of single-dose azithromycin in treatment of trachoma. Lancet. 1993;342(8869):453–6.
33. World Health Organization. Report of the first meeting of the WHO alliance for the global elimination of trachoma. Geneva: World Health Organization; 2000.
34. Evans JR, Solomon AW, Kumar R, Perez Á, Singh BP, Srivastava RM, Harding-Esch E. Antibiotics for trachoma. Cochrane Database Syst Rev. 2019;(9, 9):CD001860.
35. Fry AM, Jha HC, Lietman TM, Chaudhary JS, Bhatta RC, Elliott J, Hyde T, Schuchat A, Gaynor B, Dowell SF. Adverse and beneficial secondary effects of mass treatment with azithromycin to eliminate blindness due to trachoma in Nepal. Clin Infect Dis. 2002;35(4):395–402.
36. Delea MG, Solomon H, Solomon AW, Freeman MC. Interventions to maximize facial cleanliness and achieve environmental improvement for trachoma elimination: a review of the grey literature. PLoS Negl Trop Dis. 2018;12(1):e0006178.
37. West S, Muñoz B, Lynch M, Kayongoya A, Chilangwa Z, Mmbaga BB, Taylor HR. Impact of face-washing on trachoma in Kongwa, Tanzania. Lancet. 1995;345(8943):155–8.
38. Ngondi J, Onsarigo A, Matthews F, Reacher M, Brayne C, Baba S, Solomon AW, Zingeser J, Emerson PM. Effect of 3 years of SAFE (surgery, antibiotics, facial cleanliness, and environmental change) strategy for trachoma control in southern Sudan: a cross-sectional study. Lancet. 2006;368(9535):589–95.
39. Ngondi J, Matthews F, Reacher M, Baba S, Brayne C, Emerson P. Associations between active trachoma and community intervention with Antibiotics, Facial cleanliness, and Environmental improvement (A,F,E). PLoS Negl Trop Dis. 2008;2(4):e229.
40. Ngondi J, Gebre T, Shargie EB, Adamu L, Teferi T, Zerihun M, Ayele B, King JD, Cromwell EA, Emerson PM. Estimation of effects of community intervention with antibiotics, facial cleanliness, and environmental improvement (A,F,E) in five districts of Ethiopia hyperendemic for trachoma. Br J Ophthalmol. 2010;94(3):278–81.
41. Hammerschlag MR, Roblin PM, Gelling M, Tsumura N, Jule JE, Kutlin A. Use of polymerase chain reaction for the detection of Chlamydia trachomatis in ocular and nasopharyngeal specimens from infants with conjunctivitis. Pediatr Infect Dis J. 1997;16(3):293–7.
42. Zloto O, Gharaibeh A, Mezer E, Stankovic B, Isenberg S, Wygnanski-Jaffe T. Ophthalmia neonatorum treatment and prophylaxis: IPOSC global study. Graefes Arch Clin Exp Ophthalmol. 2016;254(3):577–82.
43. Hammerschlag MR. Chlamydial and gonococcal infections in infants and children. Clin Infect Dis. 2011;53(Suppl-3):S99–102.
44. Madhavan HN, Rao SK, Natarajan K, Sitalakshmi G, Jayanthi I, Roy S. Evaluation of laboratory tests for diagnosis of chlamydial infections in conjunctival specimens. Indian J Med Res. 1994;100:5–9.
45. Solomon AW, Peeling RW, Foster A, Mabey DC. Diagnosis and assessment of trachoma. Clin Microbiol Rev. 2004;17(4):982–1011.
46. Shao L, Guo Y, Jiang Y, Liu Y, Wang M, You C, Liu Q. Sensitivity of the standard Chlamydia trachomatis culture method is improved after one additional in vitro passage. J Clin Lab Anal. 2016;30(5):697–701.
47. Quinn TC. DNA amplification assays: a new standard for diagnosis of Chlamydia trachomatis infections. Ann Acad Med Singap. 1995;24(4):627–33.

48. Yip PP, Chan WH, Yip KT, Que TL, Kwong NS, Ho CK. The use of polymerase chain reaction assay versus conventional methods in detecting neonatal chlamydial conjunctivitis. J Pediatr Ophthalmol Strabismus. 2008;45(4):234–9.
49. Nishida H, Risemberg HM. Silver nitrate ophthalmic solution and chemical conjunctivitis. Pediatrics. 1975;56(3):368–73.
50. US Preventive Services Task, Force CSJ, Krist AH, Owens DK, Barry MJ, Caughey AB, Davidson KW, Doubeni CA, Epling JW Jr, Kemper AR, Kubik M, Landefeld CS, Mangione CM, Silverstein M, Simon MA, Tseng CW, Wong JB. Ocular prophylaxis for gonococcal ophthalmia neonatorum: US Preventive Services Task Force reaffirmation recommendation statement. JAMA. 2019;321(4):394–8.
51. Zikic A, Schünemann H, Wi T, Lincetto O, Broutet N, Santesso N. Treatment of neonatal chlamydial conjunctivitis: a systematic review and meta-analysis. J Pediatr Infect Dis Soc. 2018;7(3):e107–15.
52. Darling EK, McDonald H. A meta-analysis of the efficacy of ocular prophylactic agents used for the prevention of gonococcal and chlamydial ophthalmia neonatorum. J Midwifery Womens Health. 2010;55(4):319–27.
53. Centers for Disease Control and Prevention. Chlamydia. https://www.cdc.gov/std/stats18/chlamydia.htm.
54. Postema EJ, Remeijer L, van der Meijden WI. Epidemiology of genital chlamydial infections in patients with chlamydial conjunctivitis; a retrospective study. Genitourin Med. 1996;72(3):203 5.
55. Garland SM, Malatt A, Tabrizi S, Grando D, Lees MI, Andrew JH, Taylor HR. Chlamydia trachomatis conjunctivitis. Prevalence and association with genital tract infection. Med J Aust. 1995;162(7):363–6.
56. Coppens I, Abu el-Asrar AM, Maudgal PC, Missotten L. Incidence and clinical presentation of chlamydial keratoconjunctivitis: a preliminary study. Int Ophthalmol. 1988;12(4):201–5.
57. Stenson S. Adult inclusion conjunctivitis. Clinical characteristics and corneal changes. Arch Ophthalmol. 1981;99(4):605–8.
58. O'Connell CM, Ferone ME. Chlamydia trachomatis genital infections. Microb Cell. 2016;3(9):390–403.
59. Keegan MB, Diedrich JT, Peipert JF. Chlamydia trachomatis infection: screening and management. J Clin Outcomes Manag. 2014;21(1):30–8.
60. Ceovic R, Gulin SJ. Lymphogranuloma venereum: diagnostic and treatment challenges. Infect Drug Resist. 2015;8:39–47.
61. Buus DR, Pflugfelder SC, Schachter J, Miller D, Forster RK. Lymphogranuloma venereum conjunctivitis with a marginal corneal perforation. Ophthalmology. 1988;95(6):799–802.
62. Albert D, Miller J, Azar D, Blodi B, editors. Albert & Jakobiec's principles & practice of ophthalmology. 3rd ed. Philadelphia: Saunders Elsevier; 2008. p. 4796–7; Chapter 345.
63. Stoner BP, Cohen SE. Lymphogranuloma venereum 2015: clinical presentation, diagnosis, and treatment. Clin Infect Dis. 2015;61(Suppl-8):S865–73.
64. O'Byrne P, MacPherson P, DeLaplante S, Metz G, Bourgault A. Approach to lymphogranuloma venereum. Can Fam Physician. 2016;62(7):554–8.
65. Vandendriessche S, Rybarczyk J, Schauwvlieghe PP, Accou G, Van den Abeele AM, Vanrompay D. A bird's-eye view of chronic unilateral conjunctivitis: remember about Chlamydia psittaci. Microorganisms. 2019;7(5):118.
66. Lietman T, Brooks D, Moncada J, Schachter J, Dawson C, Dean D. Chronic follicular conjunctivitis associated with Chlamydia psittaci or Chlamydia pneumoniae. Clin Infect Dis. 1998;26(6):1335–40.

Ophthalmia Neonatorum

Jamila G. Hiasat and Ken K. Nischal

4.1 Introduction

Ophthalmia (*Latin*: inflammation of the membranes or coats of the eye) Neonatorum (*Latin*: of the newborn), is also known as neonatal conjunctivitis. Ophthalmia Neonatorum (ON) is defined as an acute, mucopurulent conjunctivitis, presenting in the first 4 weeks of life [1, 2]. Initially ON was used only for cases due to *Neisseria gonorrhoeae* [3], but it now encompasses any inflammation due to any entity (e.g., chlamydia trachomatis, chemical, etc.) [4].

ON is a clinical diagnosis and may involve the eyelids, conjunctiva, cornea, and/ or lacrimal apparatus. Therefore, dacryocystitis cases which usually present with purulent recurrent conjunctivitis should also technically fall within the definition of ON. Both conditions can be coded under the term "neonatal conjunctivitis and dacryocystitis" [5]. Therefore, any infant presenting with signs of external eye infection within the first 4 weeks of life should be treated as ON unless proven otherwise [6].

4.2 Incidence

The incidence of ON varies between 1.6 and 24% according to different studies from varying geographical locations, and depends on the socioeconomic character of the area. Under-notification of infectious diseases [6] and limitations in reporting suggest numbers are an underestimate; nearly 85% of combined chlamydial and gonococcal cases in infants less than 1 year do not report the specimen source so are not counted among cases [7]. With a broader definition including cases with unknown, other, or missing specimen sources, the prevalence of gonococcal ON, for

J. G. Hiasat · K. K. Nischal (✉)
Division of Pediatric Ophthalmology, Strabismus, and Adult Motility, UPMC Children's Hospital of Pittsburgh, University of Pittsburgh School of Medicine, Pittsburgh, PA, USA
e-mail: hiasatjg@upmc.edu; nischalkk@upmc.edu

© Springer Nature Singapore Pte Ltd. 2021
S. Das, V. Jhanji (eds.), *Infections of the Cornea and Conjunctiva*,
https://doi.org/10.1007/978-981-15-8811-2_4

example, may possibly be as high as 1.1–1.6 cases per 100,000 live births from 2010 to 2015 [7].

Neisseria gonorrhoeae and *Chlamydia trachomatis* were major causes of microbial neonatal conjunctivitis before the twenty-first century. The prevalence [8] and incidence of neonatal conjunctivitis has decreased because of the development of antibiotics, more widespread use of prepartum examination, and increased number of cesarean section [9].

Since the institution of neonatal ocular prophylaxis, the incidence of gonococcal conjunctivitis, for example, has decreased dramatically in the Western world [10, 11] with a reduction from 10 to 0.3% [11]. In the United States, ON caused by *N. gonorrhoeae* has an incidence of 0.3 per 1000 live births, while *Chlamydia trachomatis* represents 8.2 of 1000 cases [12]. In another study, when defined as gonorrhea in infants less than 1 year with a specimen source of "eye" or "conjunctiva," there were an estimated 0.4 cases or fewer per 100,000 live births per year during 2013–2017 [13].

The geographic variation is illustrated by the fact that rates in New Zealand are 145.9 per 100,000 births per year for Chlamydial infections and 3.79 per 100,000 births per year for Gonorrhea infections [14], while in Pakistan 17% of 1010 babies developed neonatal conjunctivitis with Staphylococcus aureus (65% of all positive cultures) which was the most causative agent [15].

A global study investigating the incidence of ON cases presenting to members of the American Association of Pediatric Ophthalmology and Strabismus (AAPOS) found that ophthalmologists encountered 0–5 cases per year per practitioner, with *Chlamydia trachomatis* being the most common reported organism (35%) [4].

4.3   Etiology

The specific cause of neonatal conjunctivitis can be correlated to the onset of conjunctivitis [10, 11, 16, 17].

- First 24 h of life: Chemical causes (silver nitrate drops or from prophylactic eye drops like erythromycin drops, gentamicin drops).
- 24–48 h of life: Bacterial causes are most likely (*Neisseria gonorrhoeae*, *Staphylococcus aureus*).
- 5–14 days of life: *Chlamydia trachomatis*.
- 6–14 days of life: Herpes keratoconjunctivitis.
- 5–18 days: *Pseudomonas aerugi*nosa.

Etiology can also be classified as either sexually transmitted or non-sexually transmitted. An association between neonates with purulent conjunctivitis and mothers with vaginal discharge was first described in 1750 [1]. Sexually transmitted causes tend to include *N. gonorrhoeae* and *Chlamydia trachomatis*. *N. gonorrhoeae*

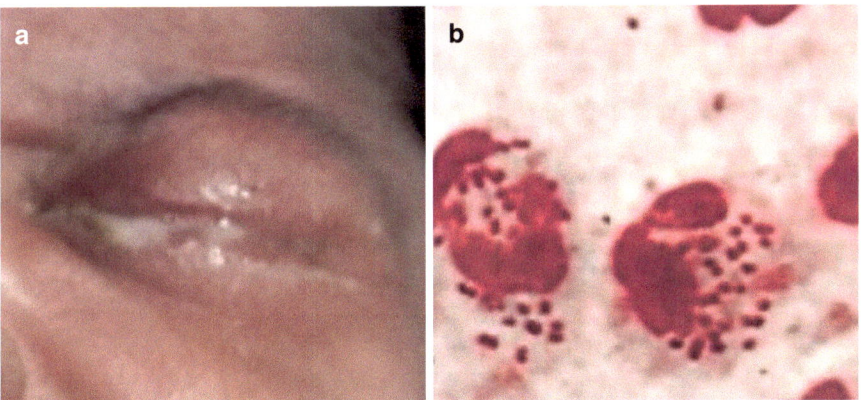

Fig. 4.1 Composite figure showing a neonate with purulent discharge and swollen lids (**a**). The gram stain shows gram-negative intracellular diplococci, suggesting *N. gonorrhea* as the causative organism (**b**)

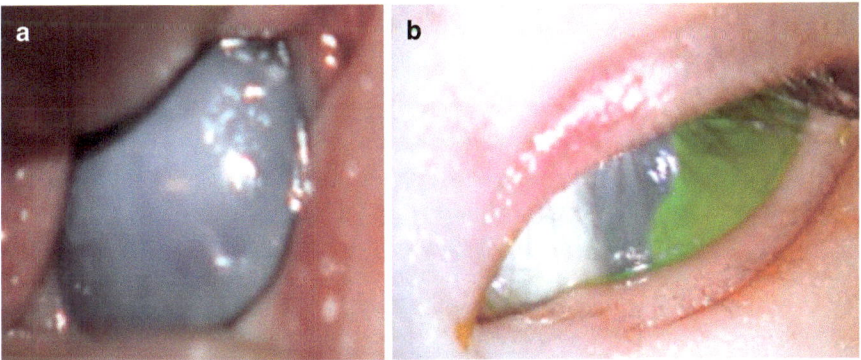

Fig. 4.2 Infant with geographic ulcer due to HSV, prior to (**a**) and after staining with topical fluorescein (**b**)

accounts for less than 1% of ophthalmia cases worldwide; however, of the babies born to mothers infected with *N. gonorrhoeae,* up to 48% develop ophthalmia neonatorum (Fig. 4.1). While *Chlamydia trachomatis* accounts for 2–40% of ophthalmia neonatorum cases [18]. Non-sexually transmitted bacteria, like *Staphylococcus aureus*, *Streptococcal* species, gram-negative bacteria (*Haemophilus spp.*, *Escherichia coli*, *Pseudomonas aeruginosa*), and *Haemophilus*, account for 30–50% of ON cases [19, 20]. Much less commonly, neonatal conjunctivitis is caused by viral infections (herpes simplex, adenovirus, enteroviruses) (Fig. 4.2). Unusual organisms causing neonatal conjunctivitis like *Serratia marcescens* (*S. marcescens*) are usually seen as nosocomial infections associated with significant morbidity and mortality in the neonatal intensive care units (NICU) [21]. Chemical conjunctivitis can be seen after silver nitrate prophylactic treatment.

4.4 Clinical Symptoms

ON caused by *N. gonorrhoeae* typically presents in the first 3–4 days of life. The neonate may present with mild conjunctival hyperemia and discharge. In severe cases, there is marked chemosis, copious discharge, and potentially rapid corneal ulceration and perforation of the eye. Systemic infection can cause sepsis, meningitis, and arthritis.

Chlamydia trachomatis is an obligate intracellular bacterium that causes neonatal inclusion conjunctivitis. The onset of conjunctivitis usually occurs around 1 week of age [22], although onset may be earlier, especially in cases with premature rupture of membranes. ON due to *Chlamydia* can have a delayed peak at around the age of 2-week-old. This is explained by the fact that the first-line empirical therapy with topical eye drops is not sufficiently effective against chlamydia and may not eradicate the infection, hence delaying the onset of symptoms and diagnosis [22]. Eye infection is characterized by minimal to moderate discharge, mild swelling of the eyelids, and hyperemia with a papillary reaction of the conjunctiva. Severe cases may be accompanied by more copious discharge and pseudomembrane formation. *Chlamydial* infection in infants differs from that in adults in several ways: in infants, there is little to no follicular response, membrane formation may occur, and there is greater mucopurulent discharge.

Herpes simplex virus (HSV) infection is usually secondary to HSV type 2 and typically presents later than infection with *N. gonorrhoeae* or *C. trachomatis*, frequently in the second week of life. Any child diagnosed with HSV ON must have a full systemic evaluation to exclude pneumonitis, hepatitis, and encephalitis.

Chemical conjunctivitis refers to a mild, self-limited irritation and redness of the conjunctiva occurring in the first 24 h after instillation of silver nitrate, a preparation used for prophylaxis against ophthalmia neonatorum. This condition improves spontaneously by the second day of life.

4.5 Pathophysiology

The causative organism usually infects the infant through direct contact during passage through the birth canal. Infection can ascend to the uterus, especially if there is prolonged rupture of membranes, so even infants delivered by a cesarean section can be infected.

4.6 Diagnosis and Investigation

Diagnosis of ON is a clinical diagnosis supported by appropriate laboratory investigations. This should include immediate conjunctival scraping with Gram stain to look for gram-negative intracellular diplococci to exclude or confirm a presumptive diagnosis of *N. gonorrhoeae* infection, since this organism can cause rapid corneal ulceration if left undiagnosed and therefore untreated (Fig. 4.1).

Culture on chocolate agar or Thayer Martin for *N. gonorrhoeae* and culture on blood agar for other bacteria are performed. Additionally, a conjunctival scraping should be done to rule out chlamydial infection by using antigen immunodetection and polymerase chain reaction. If the corneal epithelium is involved, a culture and polymerase chain reaction for herpes simplex virus is indicated.

In *Chlamydia trachomatis* infection, polymerase chain reaction (PCR) [23], direct fluorescent antibody staining, and Giemsa-stained epithelial cells from conjunctival scraping can be useful and essential in some cases to make the diagnosis [12]. Serology is not informative in these local epithelial infections [24]. Attempts at DNA sequencing of *Chlamydia* positive samples were successful and the results revealed multiple genotypes with a clear 48% dominance of genotype E contributing to both neonatal and adult conjunctivitis. The dominance of genotype E may be due to the different tissue tropism of these strains for the conjunctival mucosa of neonates or is a reflection of the actual dominance of circulating urogenital strains among humans [25].

The standard diagnostic tests for the isolation of the virus in herpetic conjunctivitis are virus culture and viral DNA detection by PCR. Patients with signs of systemic infection that look unwell may have spread disease manifesting as meningitis, bacteremia, arthritis, or sepsis; on those cases, additional investigation including blood culture, cerebrospinal fluid for gram stain or joint are warranted [26]. Evaluation of meningitis, bronchitis, and hepatitis with systemic disease is mandatory in cases of neonatal herpetic conjunctivitis.

4.7 Prophylaxis

The concept of ON prophylaxis is the best method adapted ever since Credes introduced it in 1884 to control ON disease burden and complications [19, 27]. Prevention of ophthalmia neonatorum can be effectively practiced through antenatal care by treating sexually transmitted infections in pregnant women, newborn screening, and ocular prophylaxis. A combination of these three will reduce the ocular morbidity and blindness in the pediatric population, particularly in underdeveloped nations [1].

In the absence of ocular prophylaxis, studies have estimated transmission rates of gonococcal infections of 30–50% from the mother to the newborn [4]. Neonatal ocular prophylaxis is mandated in most states and is considered most effective when administered up to 1 h after birth.

A 2.5% povidone-iodine has been used immediately after birth [28]. A clinical trial for ophthalmia neonatorum conducted in Kenya showed that a 2.5% solution of povidone-iodine was more effective and less toxic than erythromycin or silver nitrate ointment. Povidone-iodine is particularly useful in developing countries because of its low cost and ease of application [29]. Chemical conjunctivitis has been reported with use of silver nitrate but not 2.5% povidone-iodine solution.

Erythromycin ophthalmic ointment is currently the only FDA-approved prophylactic agent available in the United States [30]. Failure of prophylaxis may be due to either poor compliance of protocols or reinfection.

4.8   Management

ON is an acute emergency and requires immediate treatment and referral because of the significant risk of corneal perforation and intraocular infection that can very quickly lead to blindness, if the cause is *N. gonorrhoeae* [1]. Since a mother may have multiple sexually transmitted diseases, infants with one type of ON should be screened for other such diseases. Public health authorities should be contacted to initiate evaluation and treatment of other maternal contacts in cases of sexually transmitted diseases.

Ideally, a swab of the discharge should be obtained in order to determine which organism is responsible. In the absence of easy access to laboratory diagnosis, the World Health Organization recommends that babies should be treated for both gonococcal and chlamydial infections.

World Health Organization (WHO) treatment recommendations for ON due to *C. trachomatis* include oral erythromycin, while topical erythromycin is recommended as an adjunct therapy. The purpose of the systemic therapy is to decrease the risk for pneumonitis and also prevent the relapse of conjunctivitis.

For gonococcal ON, the recommended treatment is a single dose of intramuscular ceftriaxone injection (50 mg/kg of body weight, maximum 125 mg). An alternative regimen is cefotaxime 100 mg/kg in a single dose [14] others are kanamycin and spectinomycin [2].

For chlamydial ON, the recommendation is 50 mg/kg of erythromycin syrup per day, divided into 4 doses, for 14 days. Topical erythromycin can be used as adjunct therapy as well. Conjunctivitis secondary to *Staphylococcal* species and pseudomonas requires treatment with systemic antibiotics. On the other hand, patients with herpes simplex conjunctivitis should have treatment with systemic antiviral therapy, along with topical ophthalmic drugs, including 0.15% ganciclovir or 1% trifluridine for 14 days [3, 4, 30].

Recommendations about management in asymptomatic babies born to mothers infected with *Chlamydia trachomatis* infection exist; these babies require close monitoring for the appearance of clinical symptoms suggestive of chlamydia ocular or respiratory infections [31, 32].

4.9   Complications

These may be immediate, long term, or treatment related. Immediate ones are usually seen in cases of gonococcal ON which is associated with a high risk of corneal perforation [33] and untreated gonococcal ophthalmia neonatorum can result in corneal scarring, ocular perforation, and blindness as early as 24 h after birth [34, 35, 36].

Late ones include corneal opacity which contributes to a significant proportion of blinding eye diseases in Asia and Africa [37]. Sixty percent of blindness that occurs in children under 12 years is due to corneal opacity mostly from infections resulting in huge social and economic burden to the family and society in India [38]. There are no published contemporary estimates of gonococcal ON-related blindness in the US; it is considered rare in industrialized countries [39]. Even historical information about gonococcal ON-related blindness is limited. In the late nineteenth century, prior to Crede's prophylaxis with silver nitrate, ON, primarily caused by gonorrhea, was considered a major cause of childhood blindness; in Europe at that time, the prevalence of ophthalmia neonatorum among live births in maternity hospitals was greater than 10%, resulting in corneal damage in 20% and blindness in approximately 3% of these infected infants [39, 40]. An observational study from Nairobi, Kenya in the 1980s reported that 16% of a series of 64 infants with gonococcal ON had corneal involvement [37].

Treatment-related complications are rare but oral erythromycin is associated with an increased risk of developing pyloric stenosis [41]. The risk of chemical conjunctivitis with erythromycin is between 10 and 13% [3, 42] and chemical conjunctivitis is a well-known side effect of prophylactic topical agents used at birth such as silver nitrate.

4.10 Prognosis

Detection and timely treatment of infected mothers is essential to prevent permanent ocular damage; if left untreated or partially treated, corneal ulceration, perforation, and blindness can occur. Approximately 10,000 cases of blindness per year are secondary to ophthalmia neonatorum worldwide [43]. Fortunately, in most cases, neonatal ophthalmia neonatorum caused by non-gonococcal bacteria is a mild disease and has a good prognosis; however, up to 50% of babies born to mothers with chlamydia infection may develop neonatal conjunctivitis [30], and from those, up to 20% are at risk of having pneumonia [44]. Chemical conjunctivitis secondary to silver nitrate or other topical prophylactic agents is self-limiting.

References

1. Rapoza PA, Quinn TC, Kiessling LA, Green WR, Taylor HR. Assessment of neonatal conjunctivitis with a direct immunofluorescent monoclonal antibody stain for Chlamydia. JAMA. 1986;255(24):3369–73.
2. Teoh DL, Reynolds S. Diagnosis and management of pediatric conjunctivitis. Pediatr Emerg Care. 2003;19(1):48–55.
3. Zuppa AA, D'Andrea V, Catenazzi P, Scorrano A, Romagnoli C. Ophthalmia neonatorum: what kind of prophylaxis? J Matern Fetal Neonatal Med. 2011;24(6):769–73.
4. Zloto O, Gharaibeh A, Mezer E, Stankovic B, Isenberg S, Wygnanski-Jaffe T. Ophthalmia neonatorum treatment and prophylaxis: IPOSC global study. Graefes Arch Clin Exp Ophthalmol. 2016;254(3):577–82.
5. International Statistical Classification of Diseases and Related Health Problems (ICD-10). https://icd.who.int/browse10/2010/en.
6. Pilling R, Long V, Hobson R, Schweiger M. Ophthalmia neonatorum: a vanishing disease or underreported notification? Eye. 2009;23(9):1879–80.

7. Kreisel K, Weston E, Braxton J, Llata E, Torrone E. Keeping an eye on chlamydia and gonorrhea conjunctivitis in infants in the United States, 2010-2015. Sex Transm Dis. 2017;44(6):356–8.
8. Pak KY, Kim SI, Lee JS. Neonatal bacterial conjunctivitis in Korea in the 21st century. Cornea. 2017;36(4):415–8.
9. Di Bartolomeo S, Mirta DH, Janer M, Rodríguez Fermepin MR, Sauka D, Magariños F, de Torres RA. Incidence of Chlamydia trachomatis and other potential pathogens in neonatal conjunctivitis. Int J Infect Dis. 2001;5(3):139–43.
10. Smolkin T, Roth-Ahronson E, Kranzler M, Geffen Y, Mashiach T, Kugelman A, Makhoul IR. Optimizing accessibility of a hand-wash gel to infant's cradle: effect on neonatal conjunctivitis. Pediatr Infect Dis J. 2019;38(1):e7–11.
11. Jin J. Prevention of gonococcal eye infection in newborns. JAMA. 2019;321(4):414.
12. Castro Ochoa KJ, Mendez MD. Ophthalmia neonatorum. In: StatPearls. Treasure Island, FL: StatPearls Publishing; 2020.
13. Centers for Disease Control and Prevention. STDs in Women and Infants. https://www.cdc. gov/std/stats17/womenandinf.htm.
14. Newlands S, Dickson J, Pearson J, Mansell C, Wilson G. Neonatal conjunctivitis in the New Zealand Midland region. N Z Med J. 2018;131(1486):9–17.
15. Gul SS, Jamal M, Khan N. Ophthalmia neonatorum. J Coll Physicians Surg Pak. 2010;20(9):595–8.
16. Zikic A, Schünemann H, Wi T, Lincetto O, Broutet N, Santesso N. Treatment of neonatal chlamydial conjunctivitis: a systematic review and meta-analysis. J Pediatric Infect Dis Soc. 2018;7(3):e107–15.
17. Singh G, Galvis A, Das S. Case 1: eye discharge in a 10-day-old neonate born by cesarean delivery. Pediatr Rev. 2018;39(4):210.
18. Moore DL, MacDonald NE, Canadian Paediatric Society, Infectious Diseases and Immunization Committee. Preventing ophthalmia neonatorum. Can J Infect Dis Med Microbiol. 2015;26(3):122–5.
19. Matejcek A, Goldman RD. Treatment and prevention of ophthalmia neonatorum. Can Fam Physician. 2013;59(11):1187–90.
20. Prevention of neonatal ophthalmia. In: Pickering LK, Baker CJ, Kimberlin DW, Long SS (eds). Red Book: 2012 Report of the Committee on Infectious Diseases. 29th ed. American Academy of Pediatrics Elk Grove Village (IL): American Academy of Pediatrics; 2012. pp. 880–882.
21. Yeo KT, Octavia S, Lim K, Lin C, Lin R, Thoon KC, Tee NWS, Yung CF. Serratia marcescens in the neonatal intensive care unit: a cluster investigation using molecular methods. J Infect Public Health. 2019; S1876-0341(19)30384-3.
22. Darville T. Chlamydia trachomatis infections in neonates and young children. Semin Pediatr Infect Dis. 2005;16(4):235–44.
23. Rafiei Tabatabaei S, Afjeiee SA, Fallah F, Tahami Zanjani N, Shiva F, Tavakkoly Fard A, Shamshiri AR, Karimi A. The use of polymerase chain reaction assay versus cell culture in detecting neonatal chlamydial conjunctivitis. Arch Iran Med. 2012;15(3):171–5.
24. Balla E, Petrovay F, Erdősi T, Balázs A, Henczkó J, Urbán E, Donders GGG. Distribution of Chlamydia trachomatis genotypes in neonatal conjunctivitis in Hungary. J Med Microbiol. 2017;66(7):915–8.
25. Gallo Vaulet L, Entrocassi C, Corominas AI, Rodríguez Fermepin M. Distribution study of Chlamydia trachomatis genotypes in symptomatic patients in Buenos Aires, Argentina: association between genotype E and neonatal conjunctivitis. BMC Res Notes. 2010;3:34.
26. Workowski KA, Bolan GA, Centers for Disease Control and Prevention. Sexually transmitted diseases treatment guidelines, 2015. MMWR Recomm Rep. 2015;64:RR–03): 1-137.
27. Recommendations for prevention of neonatal ophthalmia. Infectious diseases and immunization committee, Canadian Paediatric Society. Can Med Assoc J. 1983;129(6):554–5.
28. MacDonald N, Mailman T, Desai S. Gonococcal infections in newborns and in adolescents. Adv Exp Med Biol. 2008;609:108–30.

29. Fransen L, Nsanze H, Klauss V, Stuyft PV, D'Costa L, Brunham RC, Piot P. Ophthalmia neonatorum in Nairobi, Kenya: the roles of Neisseria gonorrhoeae and Chlamydia trachomatis. J Infect Dis. 1986;153(5):862–9.
30. Hammerschlag MR. Chlamydial and gonococcal infections in infants and children. Clin Infect Dis. 2011;53(Suppl-3):S99–S102.
31. Kapoor VS, Whyte R, Vedula SS. Interventions for preventing ophthalmia neonatorum. Cochrane Database Syst Rev. 2016;2016(9):CD001862.
32. World Health Organisation. Guidelines for the management of sexually transmitted infections 2004. https://apps.who.int/medicinedocs/en/d/Jh2942e/.
33. Tarabishy AB, Jeng BH. Bacterial conjunctivitis: a review for internists. Cleve Clin J Med. 2008;75(7):507–12.
34. U.S. Preventive Services Task Force. Ocular prophylaxis for gonococcal ophthalmia neonatorum: reaffirmation recommendation statement. Am Fam Physician. 2012;85(2):195–8.
35. Snowe RJ, Wilfert CM. Epidemic reappearance of gonococcal ophthalmia neonatorum. Pediatrics. 1973;51(1):110–4.
36. Woods CR. Gonococcal infections in neonates and young children. Semin Pediatr Infect Dis. 2005;16(4):258–70.
37. Fransen L, Klauss V. Neonatal ophthalmia in the developing world. Epidemiology, etiology, management and control. Int Ophthalmol. 1988;11(3):189–96.
38. Aruljyothi L, Radhakrishnan N, Prajna VN, Lalitha P. Clinical and microbiological study of paediatric infectious keratitis in South India: a 3-year study (2011-2013). Br J Ophthalmol. 2016;100(12):1719–23.
39. Schaller UC, Klauss V. Is Credé's prophylaxis for ophthalmia neonatorum still valid? Bull World Health Organ. 2001;79(3):262–3.
40. Stephenson S. Ophthalmia neonatorum with especial reference to its causation and prevention. London: George Pulman and Sons Ltd, The Ophthalmoscope Press; 1907.
41. Eberly MD, Eide MB, Thompson JL, Nylund CM. Azithromycin in early infancy and pyloric stenosis. Pediatrics. 2015;135(3):483–8.
42. Isenberg SJ, Apt L, Wood M. A controlled trial of povidone-iodine as prophylaxis against ophthalmia neonatorum. N Engl J Med. 1995;332(9):562–6.
43. Isenberg SJ, Apt L, Wood M. The influence of perinatal infective factors on ophthalmia neonatorum. J Pediatr Ophthalmol Strabismus. 1996;33(3):185–8.
44. Hammerschlag MR, Chandler JW, Alexander ER, English M, Koutsky L. Longitudinal studies on chlamydial infections in the first year of life. Pediatr Infect Dis. 1982;1(6):395–401.

Clinical Work-Up of Corneal Ulcers

5

Prashant Garg and Aravind Roy

5.1 Introduction

Microbial keratitis is a potentially blinding disorder in the developing world. It is defined as a breach in continuity of the corneal epithelium with underlying stromal infiltration and associated tissue necrosis. In a study from south India, the reported incidence of corneal ulceration was 113 per 10,000 population [1]. When these estimates are extrapolated to all of India, 840,000 new cases of corneal ulceration are expected to develop annually and the projections approach 1.5–2 million for Africa and Asia [2]. In comparison, the incidence of corneal ulcerations in the developed world range from 11–27.6/100000 in the United States, 3.6–40.3/100000 in the United Kingdom, and 6.3/100000 in the developed city of Hong Kong [3].

This high number of cases of corneal ulceration in developing world is reflected in corneal blindness as well. Corneal ulceration is the most important cause of corneal blindness and ocular morbidity in Africa and Asia. It is very well recognized that early institution of appropriate treatment plays a crucial role in preventing or limiting vision loss from this condition. Towards that, the identification of causative microorganism becomes crucial.

However, the management of corneal ulcer in developing nations poses several challenges. These are: (a) poor health education in community and nonavailability of health care system forcing rural population to resort to using homemade and often harmful remedies; (b) easy access to over-the-counter drugs, including corticosteroids, without prescriptions; and (c) irrational empirical management even by

P. Garg (✉)
Cornea & Anterior Segment Service, L V Prasad Eye Institute, Hyderabad, Telangana, India
e-mail: prashant@lvpei.org

A. Roy
Cornea & Anterior Segment Service, L V Prasad Eye Institute,
Vijayawada, Andhra Pradesh, India
e-mail: aravindroy@lvpei.org

© Springer Nature Singapore Pte Ltd. 2021
S. Das, V. Jhanji (eds.), *Infections of the Cornea and Conjunctiva*,
https://doi.org/10.1007/978-981-15-8811-2_5

ophthalmologists. All of these limitations result in an inordinate delay in the institution of appropriate treatment, which in turn results in loss of vision and at times loss of eye.

5.2 Aims of Clinical Evaluation

Whenever we approach a case of microbial keratitis the clinical evaluation must help us in: (1) assessing severity of the disease; (2) suggesting probable etiological agent; and (3) finding associated complications and predisposing or aggravating factors. A detailed history and thorough ocular examination helps achieving these goals.

5.3 History

A careful and detailed history must include: (1) symptoms with severity and duration; (2) mode of onset; (3) pace of evolution of symptoms, i.e., rapidly progressive versus slowly progressive; (4) prior and current medical treatment with frequency and duration; and (5) response to treatment.

If the patient is a contact lens user ascertain the type of lens, age of the lens, pattern of lens worn including the history of overnight wear, and contact lens care regimen. Ascertain past history of any ocular disease and ocular surgery, and details of systemic illness and treatment. While eliciting history, carefully observe the patient. Some of the important observations include lesions around the eye, any proptosis or exophthalmos, blink rate and its completeness, and ocular deviation. Many of these conditions predispose for corneal infection and result in delayed healing or nonhealing.

5.4 Clinical Examination

Every patient of corneal ulcer must be subjected to a thorough and complete ocular examination including lid, lacrimal sac, tear film, conjunctiva, sclera, anterior chamber, and posterior segment. While evaluating corneal ulcer, make note of the following points:

Θ	Location of ulcer:	• Central
		• Peripheral (within 3 mm of limbus)
		• Total
Θ	Epithelial infiltrate:	• Defect size
		• Single/multiple
		• Size
		• Nature
		• Edge
		• Depth
		• Thinning
		• Perforation—size and site

Θ	Vascularization:	• Type and qudrant
Θ	Endothelium:	• Keratic precipitates
		• Exudates
		• Endothelial ring
Θ	Surrounding cornea:	• Satellite lesions
		• Immune ring
Θ	Limbal or scleral involvement	
Θ	Make note of anterior chamber depth and reaction including the presence/absence of hypopyon	

5.5 Documentation and Diagrammatic Representation

It is important to document all these findings as a schematic diagram or using slit-lamp photograph. Making a diagrammatic representation of corneal lesions with appropriate color coding helps to follow the course of the disease systematically, improves observation skills, and is inexpensive compared to photographs while providing important clinical data. Ulcer severity is described in terms of the dimensions of the lesion. This involves recording the maximum length and width in two axes and denoting their orientation. The degree of corneal thinning is expressed as a percentage of the corneal thickness with indication of the location of the maximum thinning. Hypopyon is expressed as the maximum vertical height with any accompanying endothelial exudates or fibrin in the anterior chamber. Corneal edema is denoted by blue, scar and degeneration by black, infiltrates and keratic precipitates by orange, vessels by red lines and ghost vessels by dashed red lines, lens and vitreous by green, contact lenses by dashed black line, and sutures by solid black line [4]. It is a standard notation to represent a frontal view and a slit view of the cornea.

5.6 Interpretation of Clinical Evaluation Findings

Once clinical evaluation is complete, the following must be assessed:

(a) Severity of the microbial keratitis and associated complication
(b) Probable etiological agent
(c) Possible predisposing or risk factor

5.6.1 Assessment of Severity of Infectious Keratitis

The assessment of severity is important because a nonsevere case can be managed empirically on an outpatient basis with a close follow-up while severe cases must be managed as inpatient preferably by a cornea specialist with experience in infectious diseases and having access to microbiology setup (Table 5.1).

5.6.2 Identification of Probable Etiological Agent (Generating a Differential Diagnosis)

The second aim of clinical evaluation is to identify probable etiological agent. Table 5.2 will help in identifying probable etiological agent.

Table 5.1 Grades of severity of microbial keratitis

Features		Severity grade	
		Non-severe	Severe
Rate of progression		Slow	Rapid
Infiltrate			
Θ	Area	<6 mm in diameter	>6 mm diameter
Θ	Depth	Superficial 2/3	Inner 1/3
Θ	Perforation	Unlikely	Imminent or present
Θ	Scleral involvement	Absent	Present

Table 5.2 Possible etiologic agents for slowly progressive versus rapidly progressive microbial keratitis

Differential diagnosis of microbial keratitis	
Slowly progressive localized infiltrate	Rapidly progressive diffuse suppurative infiltrate
(A) Bacteria	
(a) Gram-positive	(a) Gram-positive
(i) *Staphylococcus epidermidis*	(i) *Staphylococcus aureus*
(ii) α-hemolytic streptococci other than *S. pneumoniae*	(ii) *Streptococcus pneumoniae*
(iii) Actinomycetales	(iii) ß-hemolytic streptococci
– *Actinomyces*	
– *Nocardia*	
– *Mycobacterium*	
(b) Gram-negative	(b) Gram-negative
(i) *Moraxella*	(i) *Pseudomonas*
(ii) *Serratia*	(ii) *Enterobacteriaceae*
	(c) Mixed infection
	(d) Drug toxicity
(B) Fungi	
(a) Filamentous fungi	
(i) *Fusarium*	
(ii) *Aspergillus*	
(iii) Dematiaceous Fungi	
(b) Yeast-like	
(i) *Candida*	
(C) Protozoa	
(a) *Acanthamoeba*	
(b) *Microsporidia*	

5.6.2.1 Distinctive Features of Specific Bacteria

Gram-positive cocci and bacilli produce a localized round or oval ulceration with grayish white stromal infiltrate having distinct borders and minimal surrounding corneal edema.

Θ	*S. epidermidis*:	• Indolent course
Θ	*S. aureus*:	• Marked suppuration
		• Deep stromal abscess
		• Endothelial plaque
		• Large hypopyon
Θ	*S. pneumoniae* and other ß-hemolytic streptococci:	• Focal suppurative stromal infiltrate
		• Serpiginous leading edge
		• Cellular infiltration into the deep stroma
		• Radiating folds in Descemet's membrane
		• Retrocorneal fibrin deposition
Θ	α-hemolytic streptococci other than *S. pneumoniae*:	• Indolent localized ulceration
Θ	*Nocardia* and *Actinomyces*:	• Indolent ulcer
		• Superficial localized infiltrate
		• Ill-defined edges
		• Calcareous bodies at the edge (wreath pattern)
Θ	Atypical *Mycobacteria*:	• History of metallic foreign body or surgery
		• Slow progression
		• Waxing and waning course
		• Lack of response to conventional antibiotics
		• Localized infiltrate with a paucity of suppuration

Gram-negative infections typically follow a rapid inflammatory destructive course.

Θ	*Pseudomonas aeroginosa* and other enteric bacilli:	• Rapidly progressive ulcer
		• Severe conjunctival reaction
		• Dense stromal suppuration
		• Copious mucopurulent firmly adherent exudate
		• Ground glass appearance of surrounding cornea
Θ	*Moraxella*:	• Indolent ulcer in a debilitated patient or compromised cornea
		• Superficial focal infiltrate with irregular margins
		• Mild to moderate anterior chamber reaction
Θ	*Neisseria gonorrhoeae*:	• Rapidly paced keratitis in neonate or sexually active adult
		• Marked conjunctival hyperemia and chemosis
		• Thick copious purulent discharge
		• Dense suppurative stromal infiltrate
		• Preauricular lymphadenopathy

5.6.2.2 Distinctive Features of Fungi, Acanthamoeba, Microsporidia

Θ	Fungi:	• Slowly progressive keratitis
		• History of trauma with vegetable matter
		• Dry raised slough
		• Hyphate edges
		• Satellite lesions
		• Pigmented infiltrate
Θ	Acanthamoeba:	• Pain out of proportion to clinical signs
		• Slowly progressive course
		• History of exposure to contaminated water/contact lens
		• Epitheliopathy
		• Patchy stromal infiltrate which may be arranged in a ring shape
		• Radial keratoneuritis
Θ	Microsporidia:	• Pain, redness, Lacrimation, photophobia, foreign body sensation
		• Keratoconjunctivitis with multifocal, small, punctate, raised epithelial or subepithelial corneal lesions
		• History of exposure to contaminated water may be present
		• Stromal keratitis: Indolent, waxing and waning course, patchy deep stromal infiltrate, persists for months to years

5.6.3   Identify Predisposing or the Risk Factors

(a) Contact lens wear
(b) Traumatic corneal injury
(c) Protracted epithelial ulceration
(d) Corneal surgery
(e) Herpes simplex keratitis

5.7   How Clinical Features Are Pointers for Specific Microbiology Workup?

A good clinical examination and logical interpretation of its findings help a clinician in ordering specific microbiology tests. This is especially true for the diagnosis of rare forms of microbial keratitis (MK), viz., Acanthamoeba, atypical mycobacteria, and microsporidia.

For example, a patient with history of contact lens presenting without of proportion pain, exposure to tap or contaminated water associated with epitheliopathy or stromal keratitis should direct a clinician for suspecting Acanthamoeba. In developing nations where contact lens usage is less prevalent, clinical picture is different. In such nations trauma during agricultural activity and exposure to dirty contaminated water, soil, or mud are found to be common risk factors [5, 6]. The clinical picture is characterized by lack of disproportionate pain. However, a large majority of these cases are treated as herpes simplex keratitis but without much response before the diagnosis of Acanthamoeba keratitis. One third or more of cases present with a typical ring infiltrate, radial keratopathy is associated in 2.7% of cases, and when present is pathognomic of Acanthamoeba keratitis (AK). In typical clinical setting presentation with pseudo dendritiform epitheliopathy or stromal keratitis that resembles HSV keratitis but does not resolve with antivirals or a dry, superficial, necrotic nonresolving keratitis with ring infiltrates and prior history of several weeks to months of treatment with antibiotics and antifungals that resembles fungal keratitis are clinical cues for possible underlying AK [6].

Atypical mycobacterium may present as late indolent corneal ulceration usually 3 weeks to 2 months post trauma, typically with a metallic foreign body. The corneal may have mid-stromal infiltrates with fluffy satellite infiltrates around the main lesion. When present a cracked windshield appearance of the corneal stroma is pathognomic [7].

Microsporidia may present as keratoconjunctivitis or as stromal keratitis. Keratoconjunctivitis may be a self-limiting condition presenting as diffuse superficial keratopathy with a typical stuck on appearance of coarse punctate epithelial lesions. They can be easily scraped off the cornea and appear as scattered rice grains under the 10% KOH-calcofluor white wet mount [8]. On the contrary microsporidial stromal keratitis has a very unusual chronic and indolent clinical course with episodes of waxing and waning. The lesions typically present as multifocal deep stromal infiltrates with or without endothelial plaques and may involve the full thickness of the corneal stroma with or without an overlying epithelial defect. Typically patients have a history of months to years and corneal scraping/biopsy provides a definitive diagnosis of underlying microsporidia keratitis. Treatment is surgical with penetrating keratoplasty which has good outcomes in such cases [9].

5.8   Why Clinical Examination Alone Is Not Reliable?

There are several clinical features that are characteristic of each particular variety of MK. For example, fungal keratitis is typically associated with a dry necrotic slough with feathery irregular margins. In a study based on clinical scoring patterns [10], trained ophthalmologists noted feathery irregular margins in 79% of fungal keratitis and 48% of bacterial keratitis. The probability of a particular type of MK is more when a set of typical clinical characteristics are present. Often this may not be the case due to variable time points of presentation, prior treatment with medications, or late presentation with complications such as perforation. Often ophthalmologists do not have access to microbiology or rely only on clinical features while managing MK. It is important to consider that there may be a significant overlap of clinical features among MK due to different etiologic agents and there are no reliable clinical features that assist in identifying causative organisms. Hence, it is recommended to send specimens for microbiology evaluation [10, 11].

5.9 Why Microbiological Evaluation of Microbial Keratitis Is Important?

Clinical diagnosis alone may not be sufficient to arrive at a probable etiologic cause of the infectious microorganisms. This could be due to overlapping clinical features of different types of corneal ulcerations and varied therapeutic interventions prior to presentation. A study reported lack of training and outlook as an important determinant rather than nonavailability of resources to investigate causes of microbial keratitis [11]. Clinical scoring to guide the treatment of microbial keratitis conducted simultaneously from two study locations recommended treating ophthalmologists to scrape corneal ulcers and subject to microbiological evaluation where available [10].

Microbiology laboratory techniques include corneal scraping and smear examination and inoculation into various media to allow growth of colonies for subsequent identification. We recommend instillation of preservative-free proparacaine 0.5% in the eye followed by using a sterile No.15 Bard-Parker blade on a handle to scrape the edges and base of an ulcer. Scraped material is subjected to 10% KOH-calcofluor white wet mount, Gram, and Giemsa staining on a sterile glass slide. The material is also inoculated into solid and liquid media in ensuring that the media is not cut or disturbed. Serial "C" streaks are made on the media plates to allow distribution of the sample adequately and enable distinct growth of colonies. Inoculum is gently touched to the center of non-nutrient agar without disturbing the media. Smear examinations provide a rapid diagnosis of causative organisms. Culture methods involve inoculation into appropriate media to allow the growth of relevant organisms for a period of 7 days before a negative report is generated [12].

Microbiological cultures are significant if: (a) growth of same organisms from two or more solid media, (b) microscopy consistent with confluent growth of same organism from one media, and (c) growth of same organism on repeated scraping [10]. Several media are used in the routine identification of causative organisms of ocular suppuration, these include: sheep blood agar, chocolate agar, Sabouraud's dextrose agar, potato dextrose agar, non-nutrient agar with *E. coli* overlay, thiolglycolate broth, brain heart infusion broth (Fig. 5.1). A study recommended that the detection rate of fungi and Acanthamoeba was higher in smears compared to bacteria [13]. They reported the sensitivity of gram stain to be 89.8% for fungi and 73.3% for Acanthamoeba compared to 56.6% to bacteria. The low sensitivity to bacteria was attributed to prior antibiotic usage and other patient-related factors [13]. Polymerase chain reaction (PCR) was a useful diagnostic technique to help detect organisms. PCR samples are collected during scraping and collected in sterile tubes containing 0.1 ml of balanced salt solution [14].

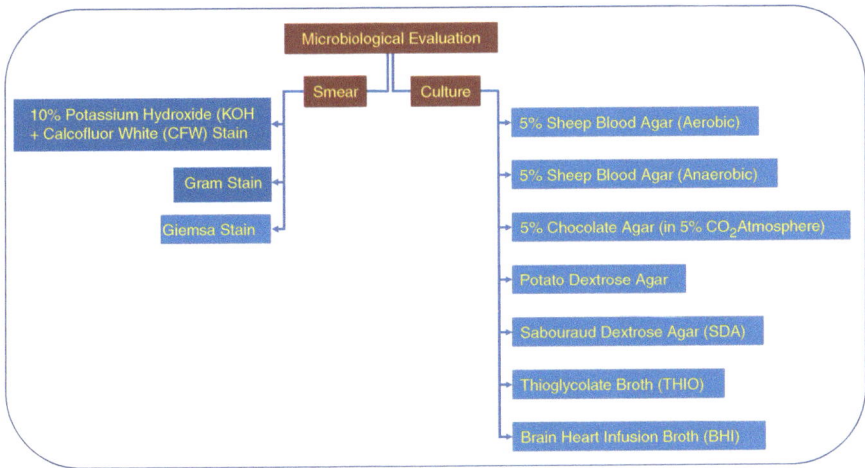

Fig. 5.1 Microbiological evaluation of microbial keratitis

5.10   Role of Confocal Microscopy for Evaluation of Microbial Keratitis

Confocal microscopy is a noninvasive diagnostic test for detection of fungal and acanthamoeba infection in the deeper corneal stroma [15]. The confocal has x- and y-axis resolution of 1.5 and 6.0 μm, and hence bacteria cannot be detected. However, fungi (3–8 μm) and Acanthamoeba cysts (12–15 μm) owing to their larger size can be detected by confocal microscopy. Both of these organisms have a chronic and indolent clinical course and require long-term treatment. Vaddavalli [16] et al. reported the sensitivity and specificity of confocal for detecting Acanthamoeba to be 88.3% and 91.1% and for fungus 89.2% and 92.7%. They recommend confocal microscopy under the following clinical scenarios:

(a) Deep corneal infiltrates that are not accessible to scraping and may require invasive procedures such as a corneal biopsy.
(b) Patients pretreated with anti-fungal or anti-Acanthamoeba medications are usually microbiologically negative; therefore, confocal may assist in arriving at an etiologic diagnosis.
(c) Post-LASIK interface keratitis and keratitis after radial or astigmatic keratectomy may have organisms embedded into the deeper corneal stroma and may be imaged with confocal microscopy.

Confocal microscopy has several limitations; besides the cost of the equipment, it is difficult to acquire images in a painful inflamed eye and is dependent on the operator skill and experience [17].

5.11 Conclusions

In conclusion, microbial keratitis presents as an ophthalmic emergency and unless managed appropriately may lead to loss of vison and eye. Typical history and characteristic clinical features assist the ophthalmologist in arriving at a probable etiologic diagnosis. It is equally important to confirm clinical findings with microbiology or confocal imaging where possible so as to target definitive treatment as per causative organisms.

References

1. Gonzales CA, Srinivasan M, Whitcher JP, Smolin G. Incidence of corneal ulceration in Madurai District, South India. Ophthalmic Epidemiol. 1996;3(3):159–66.
2. Whitcher JP, Srinivasan M, Upadhyay MP. Corneal blindness: a global perspective. Bull World Health Organ. 2001;79(3):214–21.
3. Ung L, Bispo PJM, Shanbhag SS, Gilmore MS, Chodosh J. The persistent dilemma of microbial keratitis: Global burden, diagnosis, and antimicrobial resistance. Surv Ophthalmol. 2019;64(3):255–71.
4. Waring GO, Laibson PR. A systematic method of drawing corneal pathologic conditions. Arch Ophthalmol. 1977;95(9):1540–2.
5. Sharma S, Garg P, Rao GN. Patient characteristics, diagnosis, and treatment of non-contact lens related Acanthamoeba keratitis. Br J Ophthalmol. 2000;84(10):1103–8.
6. Garg P, Kalra P, Joseph J. Non-contact lens related Acanthamoeba keratitis. Indian J Ophthalmol. 2017;65(11):1079–186.
7. Huang SC, Soong HK, Chang JS, Liang YS. Non-tuberculous mycobacterial keratitis: a study of 22 cases. Br J Ophthalmol. 1996;80(11):962–8.
8. Sharma S, Das S, Joseph J, Vemuganti GK, Murthy S. Microsporidial keratitis: need for increased awareness. Surv Ophthalmol. 2011;56(1):1–22.
9. Sabhapandit S, Murthy SI, Garg P, Korwar V, Vemuganti GK, Sharma S. Microsporidial stromal keratitis: clinical features, unique diagnostic criteria, and treatment outcomes in a large case series. Cornea. 2016;35(12):1569–74.
10. Thomas PA, Leck AK, Myatt M. Characteristic clinical features as an aid to the diagnosis of suppurative keratitis caused by filamentous fungi. Br J Ophthalmol. 2005;89(12):1554–8.
11. Agrawal V, Biswas J, Madhavan HN, Mangat G, Reddy MK, Saini JS, Sharma S, Srinivasan M. Current perspectives in infectious keratitis. Indian J Ophthalmol. 1994;42(4):171–92.
12. Garg P, Rao GN. Corneal ulcer: diagnosis and management. Community Eye Health. 1999;12(30):21–3.
13. Gopinathan U, Sharma S, Garg P, Rao GN. Review of epidemiological features, microbiological diagnosis and treatment outcome of microbial keratitis: experience of over a decade. Indian J Ophthalmol. 2009;57(4):273–9.
14. Alkatan HM, Al-Essa RS. Challenges in the diagnosis of microbial keratitis: a detailed review with update and general guidelines. Saudi J Ophthalmol. 2019;33(3):268–76.
15. Kaufman SC, Musch DC, Belin MW, Cohen EJ, Meisler DM, Reinhart WJ, Udell IJ, Van Meter WS. Confocal microscopy: a report by the American Academy of Ophthalmology. Ophthalmology. 2004;111(2):396–406.
16. Vaddavalli PK, Garg P, Sharma S, Sangwan VS, Rao GN, Thomas R. Role of confocal microscopy in the diagnosis of fungal and acanthamoeba keratitis. Ophthalmology. 2011;118(1):29–35.
17. Garg P. Fungal, mycobacterial, and nocardia infections and the eye: an update. Eye. 2012;26(2):245–51.

Bacterial Keratitis

6

Darlene Miller, Kara M. Cavuoto, and Eduardo C. Alfonso

6.1 Introduction

Bacterial keratitis is an infection of the cornea initiated by the invasion and multiplication of bacteria [1]. It is a leading cause of corneal ulceration, opacification, visual morbidity, and blindness and remains a major healthcare burden world wide [2]. The true burden is not known. Estimates in the United States range from 25,000 to 71,000 cases annually, while global rates may exceed 2.0–3.5 million cases each year [2, 3]. These rates may not reflect the true prevalence. These estimates are based on data collected and analyzed for unique populations more than 15 years ago.

The main function of the cornea is to bend, refract, and focus light. It must remain clear and free of scars to accomplish this task [1, 4]. Although constantly exposed to environmental insults, including microbes, the cornea is well protected by anatomical and local ocular surface epithelial, tear film, and immune defenses [5]. These work together to prevent microbial adherence and invasion. Once there is a breach in the ocular surface immune defense via trauma, contact lens wear, and topical antibiotics/steroids, any organism may gain access, multiply, and establish sight-threatening disease [1, 4, 5]. Active invasion of the corneal epithelium and stroma is considered an ocular emergency. The etiological agent and appropriate antimicrobial therapy must be rapidly identified and implemented to preserve vision [1].

D. Miller · K. M. Cavuoto · E. C. Alfonso (✉)
Bascom Palmer Eye Institute, Miller School of Medicine, University of Miami, Miami, FL, USA
e-mail: dmiller@med.miami.edu; KCavuoto@med.miami.edu; ealfonso@med.miami.edu

© Springer Nature Singapore Pte Ltd. 2021
S. Das, V. Jhanji (eds.), *Infections of the Cornea and Conjunctiva*,
https://doi.org/10.1007/978-981-15-8811-2_6

6.2 Etiology

Bacteria are the most common cause of infectious keratitis [1, 4, 6]. Gram-positive organisms, *Staphylococci*, *Streptococci*, and *Corynebacterium*, constitute greater than 70% of reported corneal ulcers worldwide. *Pseudomonas* species and other gram-negative rods are more often associated with contact lens, surgery, and/or trauma [2, 6, 7].

Etiology may differ by geography, patient populations, culture frequency, and laboratory expertise and practice. In a recent meta-analysis by Teweldemedhin et al., coagulase-negative staphylococci (4.4–66.6%), *Pseudomonas aeruginosa* (6.8–55%), and *Staphylococcus aureus* (2–22.4%) were identified as the most commonly reported culture-derived corneal pathogens [8]. *Streptococcus pneumoniae* (1.3–24.7%) and *Streptococcus viridans* (0.4–14.3%) were also among the top five reported pathogens [8].

6.3 Risk Factors

Contact lens wear is the most common risk factor for bacterial keratitis in urbanized populations (Table 6.1) [3]. In the United States, 41 million patients are at risk [3]. Contact lens wear risks include trauma in the form of mini-abrasions, ocular surface integrity interruption (hypoxia, tear film disruption), and changes to the ocular surface microbiota [1, 9]. Forty percent of the culture-proven cases have been associated with sleeping and/or swimming in contact lens [3, 8].

Other risk factors associated with this population include trauma with contaminated water, soil, and vegetative matter [1, 4]. Exposure to contaminated soil, plant matter, and water can deliver heavy microbial loads, foreign bodies, and a diverse

Table 6.1 Risk factors for bacterial keratitis

Risk factor	Breach of ocular surface integrity	Compromise/alter ocular immune defenses	Microbiome (microbiota) dysbiosis
Contact lens wear	+++[a]	++	++
Keratoprosthetics	++++	+++	+++
Ocular surgery	++++	++	+
Trauma (blunt, chemical, vegetative matter, contaminated water, soil)	++++	+++	++
Topical medications (antibiotics, steroids, preservatives, anesthetics, glaucoma medications)	++	++	++++
Ocular surface disorders	+++	+++	+++
Crosslinking	++++	+++	++++
Photodynamic therapy	++++	+++	++++
Gut dysbiosis	+	++	++

+ = [a]light impact; ++ = moderate impact; +++, ++++ = heavy impact microbiota to the ocular surface including *Pseudomonas aeruginosa*, *Stenotrophomonas maltophilia*, and *Achromobacter xylosoxidans*. This group of organisms has a large arsenal of virulence factors (biofilm formation, toxins, proteases, resistance genes) that aid in virulence, invasion, and drug resistance [10–12].

Disruption of the ocular surface integrity via surgery, keratoprosthesis placement, and/or trauma provides easy access of microorganisms to corneal tissue and disruption of the tear film [1, 4]. Both mechanisms predispose to bacterial invasion and disease. Chronic ocular surface disorders increase the risk of tear film deficiency, altered immune defenses (immunosuppression, steroids), and ocular microbiota (microbiome) dysbiosis (antibiotics, anesthetics, steroids) which lead to increased risk of bacterial infection [1, 4].

In nonurbanized populations, environmental/agrarian trauma, chronic ocular surface disease, malnutrition, and poor and/or delayed access to appropriate ophthalmic care are the major predisposing factors for bacterial keratitis and corneal opacification/blindness [2, 4].

6.4   Role of Ocular and Gut Dysbiosis in Bacterial Keratitis

The ocular surface microbiota plays an important role in the protection of the ocular surface from invasion by opportunistic and/or true bacterial pathogens [13, 14]. Core members include Firmicutes (predominantly, *Staphylococci*, *Streptococci*), Actinobacteria (*Corynebacteria*), and Proteobacteria (*Pseudomonas*, *Haemophilus*, *Neisseria*). They engage in crosstalk with the corneal and conjunctival epithelial cells to provide and coordinate immune, spatial, and chemical protection of the ocular surface [13, 15]. The major outcomes from this partnership include: (a) barrier preservation, (b) inhibition of inflammation, (c) accelerated tissue repair, and (d) exclusion of pathogens.

Increasing metagenomic studies support this role [5]. Dysbiosis of the ocular microbiome by contact lens wear, instillation of topical antibiotics, surgery, and corticosteroid use can lead to increase susceptibility to bacterial virulence and invasion [15, 16].

As the ocular surface is part of the systemic mucosal system, it is in communications with and impacted by the health and dysbiosis of this organ [14, 17]. Kugadas et al. demonstrated in mice that there was an interconnection between gut and ocular surface dysbiosis and increased susceptibility to bacteria (*Pseudomonas*) induced keratitis [18]. In health, the ocular surface microbiota strengthens the ocular innate immune barriers by significantly increasing the concentration of immune effectors in the tear film. When depleted by administration of gentamicin, the normally resistant Swiss Webster mice became susceptible to the infection. Both the ocular and the gut microbiota contributed to the maintenance of the barrier protection with the ocular surface having a moderate but significant effect [18].

Jayasudha and colleagues also documented a connection between gut dysbiosis and susceptibility to bacterial keratitis [19]. In a recent study, they compared the fecal samples from normal controls and patients with bacterial keratitis and found a distinct difference in the relative abundance of protective anti-inflammatory genera in the gut versus microbial recovered from patients with bacterial keratitis [19].

Taken together, ocular microbiome dysbiosis may be an important unrecognized and underappreciated risk factor in bacterial keratitis.

6.5   Bacterial Keratitis in Children

Bacterial keratitis is a rare condition in children, with children contributing <15% of all cases [20–22]. The condition is difficult to treat in this population, as children may not be able to convey symptoms accurately and cooperation for evaluation and treatment may be limited. Additionally, there is a high risk of poor visual outcomes in keratitis, not only due to the disease itself but also due to the sequelae of corneal scarring leading to deprivational and/or anisometropic amblyopia.

The mean age for children presenting with bacterial keratitis typically ranges between 10 and 13 years old with a relatively even distribution between males and females [20–25]. Although these patient demographics have remained stable over time, the risk factors for bacterial keratitis in children have changed and vary with geographic location. Studies published in the 1980s and 1990s found that the main risk factor for bacterial keratitis was trauma [25, 26], whereas more recent publications indicate that contact lens wear is the most common factor contributing 40.7–77.6% of cases [20, 21, 23]. Geographic location also appears to affect risk, as in contrast to these recent studies from the United States and Taiwan, studies from Brazil and Mexico found that ocular trauma remains the most common risk factor [25, 27]. It is possible that the age of the patient population plays a role in the difference, as one study of 81 eyes reported trauma and ocular disease were significantly more common in children <12 years old whereas contact lens wear was more common in older children [20].

The causative organism in bacterial keratitis in children differs based upon the most common risk factor in a given patient population. In the studies that reported contact lens wear as the most common risk factor, *Pseudomonas aeruginosa* was the most common organism representing 30.6–46.2% of isolates [20, 21, 23]. In studies where trauma was the most common risk factor, gram-positive organisms such as coagulase-negative *Staphylococcus* [24] or *Staphylococcus epidermidis* [25, 27] represented the majority (23.4–28.6%) of organisms isolated.

Regardless of the pathologic organism, studies published in the 1990s reported that surgical intervention for eye salvage or visual rehabilitation would be indicated in 14–28% of pediatric keratitis cases [22, 26]. For instance, Cruz et al. found that 7 of 51 eyes (14%) required surgery [26]. However, more recent studies showed this percentage to be much lower, ranging from 0 to 6% [23, 27, 28]. In a series of 107 cases, Rossetto et al. found that zero penetrating keratoplasties were performed to treat perforation [23].

Overall, bacterial keratitis in children remains a potentially serious cause of ocular morbidity. The trend towards increasing incidence in older children who wear contact lenses is likely a reflection of global management of refractive error. As the prevalence of myopia is increasing, contact lens use is more prevalent and techniques such as orthokeratology are being employed more frequently. Future studies investing this trend will be useful.

6.6 Pathology

The ocular surface is well protected against microbial insult and invasion [4, 5]. Local immune defenses of the tight epithelial barrier coupled with the wide array of antimicrobial substances in the tear film and a stable microbiome help to maintain ocular surface integrity and health [5, 13, 17]. Disturbance or disruption of any of these can lead to imbalance and ocular surface disease including bacterial keratitis. Any organism gaining access to corneal tissue can establish disease.

In general, bacterial keratitis progress in stages [1]. These include infiltration, ulceration, regression, and healing. Patient outcome for all four stages is dependent on the bacterial species, ocular surface health, host defense response, diagnostic (microbiological, clinical) accuracy, and rapid, appropriate therapy [1, 4].

6.7 Clinical Assessment

6.7.1 Signs and Symptoms

There is no consensus of characteristics that identify infectious keratitis as bacterial in origin [1, 4, 27]. Signs and symptoms are dependent on a combination of the ocular surface health, invading pathogen and host defenses and response. Some common and suggestive signs and symptoms may include conjunctival injection and chemosis, decreased vision, pain, photophobia, tearing, and purulent discharge [1, 4]. A detailed history coupled with a complete ophthalmic examination is the foundation for an accurate and informative clinical assessment in the differential diagnosis of bacterial keratitis [1, 4, 21].

6.7.2 History

The history checklist should include onset of symptoms, recent and past ocular trauma, contact lens wear, and associated activities such as swimming, sleeping, lens changing schedule, and cleaning regimen [1]. In addition, information on previous eye disorders, ocular surgeries, and medications should be recorded. An updated medical history including allergies, systemic medications, family history, and organ system review should also be obtained [1].

6.7.3 Physical Examination

A thorough physical examination checklist should include slit-lamp photos and assessments for vision, intraocular pressure, and pupil evaluation [1, 4]. The location, size, and depth of the corneal infiltrate plus the anterior chamber reaction (cells, flare, fibrin, or hypopyon) must be recorded. Additional predisposing factors for infections such as foreign bodies, blepharitis, entropion, trichiasis, or lagophthalmos should be documented [1, 4].

6.7.4 Laboratory Assessment

Ideally, all corneal ulcers should be cultured for definitive identification of the causative agent(s) before the administration of topical, broad-spectrum antibiotics [6]. However, the most recent American Academy of Ophthalmology Bacterial Keratitis Practice Patterns guidelines indicate microbiological workup only for sight-threatening ulcers (large, central) and/or severe keratitis involving atypical appearance and/or those unresponsive to empirical therapy [1]. Smears should be collected and examined for rapid diagnosis and early implementation of therapy [1].

Current treatment recommendations for small infiltrates with no stromal involvement are to treat first with a broad spectrum commercially available (fluoroquinolone, aminoglycoside) topical antibiotic and culture later if at all. Most corneal ulcers are managed this way both in the community and by corneal specialists [1, 4, 29, 30].

6.7.5 Laboratory Workup

Rapid laboratory identification and in vitro susceptibility profiles are essential for providing appropriate and effective antibacterial therapy. Cultures and smears may offer the best support for (1) central, large ulcers with significant stromal involvement, (2) ulcers following surgery, (3) chronic ulcers, nonresponsive to empirical treatment, (4) ulcers with multiple infiltrates, and (5) ulcers with atypical clinical features [1].

Routine media and smears for microbiological assessment are outlined in Tables 6.2 and 6.3. Corneal scrapings may be obtained using a spatula, blade, and/or flocked swab.

Table 6.2 Routine microbiology stains for bacterial keratitis

Stain	Organisms	Notes
Gram	Aerobic and anaerobic bacteria, fungi, amoeba, and microsporidia. **Note**: Nocardia species stain weakly gram-positive	Documents morphology (rods, cocci) and distinguishes between gram-positive and gram-negative organisms. Both morphology and staining are impacted by topical antibiotic use **Turnaround time**: 5 min
Giemsa	Inflammatory cells, bacteria, amoeba, fungi, and microsporidia	Determines types of inflammatory/immune cells, presence of bacteria, fungi, amoeba, and microsporidia **Turnaround time**: 2 min
Acid fast	Mycobacteria, Nocardia, Streptomyces, and Microsporidia	Kinyoun, Ziehl-Neelsen, and/or acid fast (AFB) fluorescent stains. Requires a fluorescent microscope **Turnaround time**: 15 min
Acridine orange	Bacteria and fungi	Requires a fluorescent microscope **Turnaround time**: 3–5 min

The reported culture-dependent frequency, diversity, and relative abundance of the major bacterial corneal pathogens have remained essentially the same over the last 30 years in South Florida and worldwide. Frequency, diversity, and relative abundance differ however by geographic locations, patient populations, time periods, culture positive criteria, and practice locations [2, 6]. Data collected are highlighted in Tables 6.4, 6.5, 6.6, and 6.7 (Figs. 6.1 and 6.2).

Table 6.3 Common media for recovery of frequent bacterial keratitis isolates

Media for bacterial keratitis	Recovery spectrum
Routine	
– Chocolate agar	Fastidious organisms including *Neisseria gonorrheae*, *Haemophilus influenzae*, Moraxella species, and Bartonella species Aerobic and anaerobic bacteria including *Staphylococcus aureus*, coagulase-negative Staphylococci, *Streptococcus pneumoniae*, and *Pseudomonas aeruginosa* Less common organisms including Mycobacteria, Streptomyces, and Nocardia species
– 5% sheep blood agar	Aerobic and anaerobic bacteria including *Staphylococcus aureus*, coagulase-negative Staphylococci, *Streptococcus pneumoniae*, and *Pseudomonas aeruginosa* Less common organisms including Mycobacteria, Streptomyces, and Nocardia species
– Thioglycolate broth	Aerobic and anaerobic bacteria including *Cutibacterium acnes*, Bacteroides, and Clostridium species Important to include with cultures collected from pretreated patients serves to dilute out the antibiotic and/or other medications
Supplemental	
– Anaerobic media (CDC Anaerobic blood agar, Kanamycin-Vancomycin agar, Phenyl ethyl alcohol agar-anaerobic)	Anaerobic bacteria including *Cutibacterium acnes*, Peptotostreptococcus, Bacteroides, and Clostridium species
– MacConkey agar	Aerobic and facultative gram-negative rods including *Pseudomonas aeruginosa*, *Serratia marcescens*, *Stenotrophomonas maltophilia*, *Achromobacter xylosoxidans*, and Enterobacteriaceae Most useful with cultures from patients with contact lens-associated ulcers
– ESwab Mini-Flocked liquid-based Ames medium	Molecular testing—including PCR and next generation metagenomic studies. Place at 20 C with 15 min of collection and at 80 C for long-term storage
– Lowenstein-Jensen medium	Mycobacteria, Streptomyces, and Nocardia species
Transport	
– ESwab Mini-Flocked liquid-based Ames medium	Multipurpose collection and transport medium for the recovery of fastidious, aerobic and anaerobic bacteria up to 48 h Also used as a medium for metagenomic studies

Table 6.4 Culture-dependent corneal pathogen, BPEI 2015-June 30, 2019

Firmicutes (gram-positive)	# of isolates	%
Abiotrophia defective	1	0.2%
Aerococcus urinae	1	0.2%
Enterococcus faecalis	14	2.9%
Gemella haemolysans	1	0.2%
Gemella morbillorum	3	0.6%
Globicatella sanguinis	1	0.2%
Granulicatella adiacens	4	0.8%
Lactococcus lactis spp lactis	1	0.2%
Lactococcus raffinolactis	1	0.2%
Micrococcus luteus	1	0.2%
Staphylococcus aureus	226	47.6%
Staphylococcus auricularis	1	0.2%
Staphylococcus capitus	1	0.2%
Staphylococcus epidermidis	81	17.1%
Staphylococcus haemolyticus	4	0.8%
Staphylococcus hominis ssp. hominis	6	1.3%
Staphylococcus lentus	1	0.2%
Staphylococcus lugdunensis	1	0.2%
Staphylococcus pseudintermedius	1	0.2%
Staphylococcus sciuri	1	0.2%
Staphylococcus warneri	3	0.6%
Streptococcus agalactiae	4	0.8%
Streptococcus dysgalactiae ssp. equisimilis	4	0.8%
Streptococcus gordonii	1	0.2%
Streptococcus intermedius	3	0.6%
Streptococcus mitis	2	0.4%
Streptococcus mitis/streptococcus oralis	48	10.1%
Streptococcus oralis	1	0.2%
Streptococcus parasanguinis	1	0.2%
Streptococcus plunimalium	2	0.4%
Streptococcus pneumoniae	35	7.4%
Streptococcus pseudoporcinus	2	0.4%
Streptococcus pyogenes	3	0.6%
Streptococcus sanguinis	7	1.5%
Streptococcus sanguis	1	0.2%
Streptococcus viridans group except S. pneumoniae	7	1.5%
Total isolates	**475**	**100.0%**

Table 6.5 Culture-dependent corneal pathogen, BPEI 2015-June 30, 2019

Actinobacteria (gram-positive, weakly gram-positive)	# of isolates	%
Corynbacterium propinquum	2	5.4%
Dermacoccus nishinomiyaensis	1	2.7%
Gardnerella vaginalis	2	5.4%
Kocuria kristinae	4	10.8%
Kocuria rosea	4	10.8%
Kocuria varians	1	2.7%
Mycobacterium abscessus	4	10.8%
Mycobacterium chelonae	1	2.7%
Mycobacterium fortuitum species group	1	2.7%
Nocardia asteroides complex	5	13.5%
Nocardia farcinica	1	2.7%
Nocardia species	8	21.6%
Streptomyces species	3	8.1%
Total isolates	**37**	**100.0%**

Table 6.6 Culture-dependent corneal pathogen, BPEI 2015-June 30, 2019

Proteobacteria (gram-negative)	# of isolates	%
Ochromobacter anthropic	1	0.2%
Achromobacter denitrificans	2	0.3%
Achromobacter xylosoxidans	7	1.2%
Burkholderia cepacia	1	0.2%
Burkholderia cepacia group	4	0.7%
Acinetobacter baumannii complex	3	0.5%
Acinetobacter iwoffii	1	0.2%
Acinetobacter radioresistens	1	0.2%
Aeromonas hydrophila/caviae	1	0.2%
Citrobacter koseri	12	2.0%
Enterobacter aerogenes	2	0.3%
Enterobacter cloacae complex	7	1.2%
Escherichia coli	2	0.3%
Klebsiella oxytoca	6	1.0%
Klebsiella pneumonia ssp pneumoniae	9	1.5%
Moraxella (Branhamella) catarrhalis	2	0.3%
Moraxella group	23	3.8%
Moraxella lacunata	1	0.2%
Moraxella lincolnii	1	0.2%
Moraxella osloensis	3	0.5%
Moraxella species	4	0.7%
Morganella morganii ssp morganiii	1	0.2%
Pantoea ssp	4	0.7%
Proteus hauseri	1	0.2%
Proteus mirabilis	17	2.8%
Pseudomonas aeruginosa	396	65.8%

Table 6.6 (continued)

Proteobacteria (gram-negative)	# of isolates	%
Pseudomonas alcaligenes	1	0.2%
Pseudomonas fluorescens	4	0.7%
Pseudomonas luteola	1	0.2%
Pseudomonas mendocina	1	0.2%
Pseudomonas oryzihabitans	1	0.2%
Pseudomonas putida	1	0.2%
Pseudomonas stutzeri	1	0.2%
Rhizobium radiobacter	1	0.2%
Serratia fonticola	1	0.2%
Serratia liquefaciens	1	0.2%
Serratia liquefaciens group	4	0.7%
Serratia marcescens	65	10.8%
Stenotrophomonas maltophilia	7	1.2%
Vibrio alginolyticus	1	0.2%
Total isolates	**602**	**100.0%**

Table 6.7 Culture-dependent corneal pathogen, BPEI 2015-June 30, 2019

Bacteroidetes (gram-negative)	# of isolates	%
Chryseobacterium indologenes	2	33.3%
Elizabethkingia meningoseptica	1	16.7%
Sphingomonas paucimobilis	3	50.0%
Total isolates	**6**	**100.0%**

Fig. 6.1 Trends in the culture-dependent recovery of top corneal pathogens, 1990-June 30, 2019

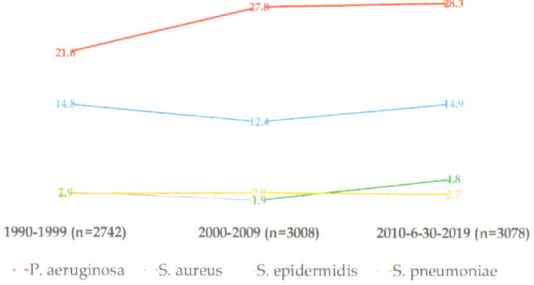

The most commonly reported bacteria corneal pathogens include gram-positive species belonging to two major phyla (Firmicutes and Actinobacteria) [2, 6, 10, 17]. The frequency and abundance vary with patient populations, time period, culture frequency, and empirical treatment.

Fig. 6.2 Culture-dependent diversity and relative abundance of corneal pathogens-BPEI, 2015-6-30-2019

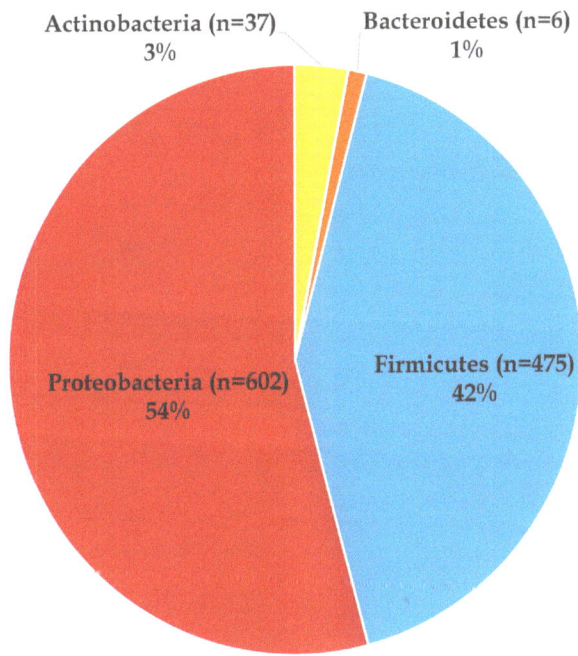

Actinobacteria (n=37)
3%

Bacteroidetes (n=6)
1%

Proteobacteria (n=602)
54%

Firmicutes (n=475)
42%

6.7.5.1 Firmicutes (Gram-Positive Cocci and Rods)

The Firmicutes are a phylum or group of bacteria with characteristics associated with gram-positive cell wall structure (Table 6.4). They usually stain purple with the gram stain due to a thick peptidoglycan layer [10]. They are found in a variety of habitats including the skin and mucus membranes of humans. These are the most reported bacterial species recovered from culture dependent and culture independent bacterial keratitis surveys. *Staphylococci, Streptococci, Micrococcus, Lactobacillus, Bacilli, and Clostridia* are among the most common genera among this group [6, 10]. This was the second most common phylum (42.4%) reported at our Institute and included 36 different species across 10 genera.

Staphylococci are among the leading causes of bacterial keratitis in the United States and worldwide. Reported prevalence ranges from 1 to 45% [2, 6]. Infections are diverse and include contact lens-associated keratitis (Fig. 6.3) and marginal keratitis. Coagulase-negative *Staphylococci* constitutes the major corneal pathogen recovered from patients with ocular surface disease including bullous keratopathy, chronic herpetic keratitis, and atopic keratoconjunctivitis [1]. Currently, there are more than 30 species of coagulase-negative Staphylococci [31]. However, *S. epidermidis* is the most commonly identified and reported species, especially in older patients, bandage contact lens wears, and those with a compromised ocular surface, altered immune response, and microbiome dysbiosis. This group of Firmicutes is among the most frequent bacteria identified by both culture-dependent and culture-independent studies as core members of the ocular surface microbiome [6, 7, 10, 17].

Fig. 6.3 14-year old who
presented with contact
lens-associated bacterial
keratitis

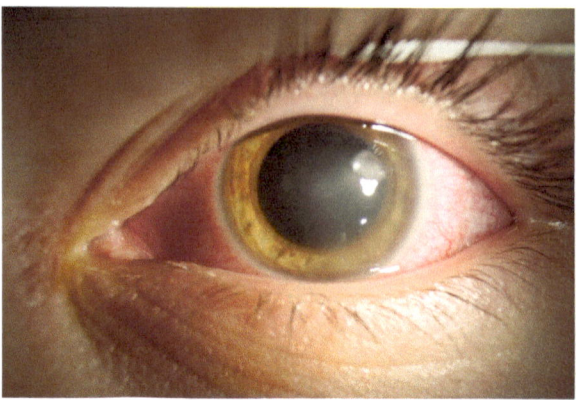

Fig. 6.4 *Staphylococcus
aureus* keratitis

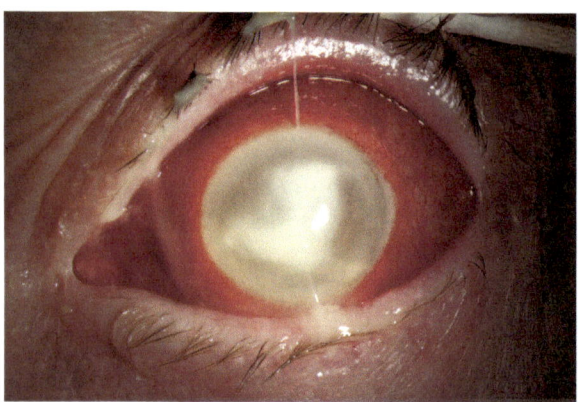

Coagulase-positive species, mainly *S. aureus*, are the second most frequently reported cause of bacterial keratitis in several reports from the United States and Europe, with rates ranging from 3 to 49% (Fig. 6.4) [6]. Both methicillin-sensitive (MSSA) and methicillin resistant (MRSA) *Staphylococcus aureus isolates are frequently* recovered from healthcare exposure. In a recent report from South Florida, 81.3% of the 75 evaluated isolates were healthcare–associated following corneal transplantation, contact lens wear, and/or cataract surgery. There was no significant difference between MRSA ($n = 47$, 74.5%) and MSSA ($n = 28$, 92.8%), p-0.0507 [32]. Similar results were reported from Taiwan [33].

Streptococci including *S. pneumoniae* are among the most common gram-positive cocci reported from Asia and are frequently associated with patients with chronic ocular surface disorders (Fig. 6.5). The group includes the beta-hemolytic Streptococci, *S. pyogenes* (Group A), *S. agalactiae* (Group B), the alpha-hemolytic species including *S. pneumoniae* and the viridans group (i.e., *Streptococcus mitis, Streptococcus oralis*). Nonhemolytic (gamma) Streptococci and nutritionally deficient Streptococci (i.e., *Abiotrophia defective*) are also in this group. This group appears in chains and/or pairs in gram stain and/or Giemsa smears [6].

Fig. 6.5 *Streptococcus pneumoniae* keratitis

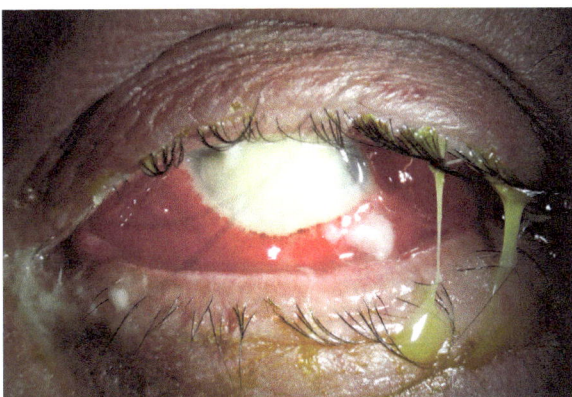

Fig. 6.6 *Pseudomonas aeruginosa* keratitis

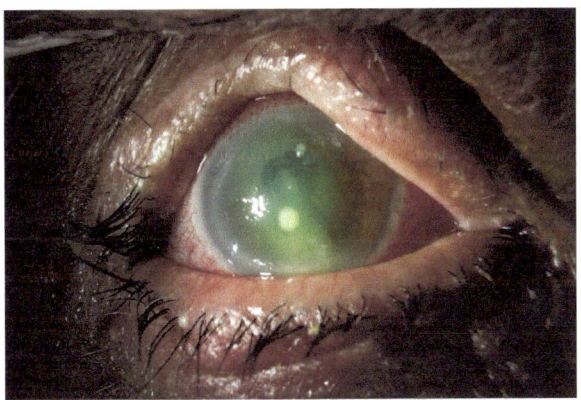

Streptococcus pneumoniae was the top corneal pathogen recovered in the Steroids for Corneal Ulcer Trial (SCUT) study and may be the most common gram-positive isolate in some parts of India [34]. *S. pneumoniae* isolates were recovered in less than 10% of the corneal isolates in South Florida.

The *Streptococcus viridans* group is frequently involved in infectious crystalline keratopathy, described as gray-white opacities (Fig. 6.6). It most commonly develops in patients on long-term steroid use, especially following penetrating keratopathy. These bacteria are difficult to culture because they are encased in a thick biofilm which protects them from removal and antibiotic therapy [10, 35].

6.7.5.2 Actinobacteria (Gram-Positive Rods)

Actinobacteria are gram-positive rods found in the environment including soil and water and on human skin (Table 6.5). Genera include the Corynebacterium and Cutibacterium (Propionibacterium, Mycobacteria, and the aerobic Actinomycetes). *Corynebacterium and Cutibacterium* are considered part of the ocular "core" microbiota but are also recovered in bacterial keratitis among contact lens wears, the elderly, and patients with compromised ocular surface disease and/or immunosuppression [36, 37]. Mycobacteria and Nocardia corneal ulcers are discussed in Chaps. 7 and 8 respectively. We have observed a decline in the number of culture dependent Corynebacterium associated corneal ulcers in the last 5 years, but an increase in Nocardia and Mycobacteria species.

6.7.5.3 Proteobacteria (Gram-Negative Cocci, Rods)

Reported prevalence of infectious keratitis due to gram-negative bacteria ranges from 1 to 50% [1, 2, 6]. The majority of these are members of the Proteobacteria (Table 6.6). Common members among these included *Pseudomonas aeruginosa*, *Serratia marcescens*, and *Moraxella* species [4, 6–8, 15]. This was the largest and most diverse group of microorganisms recovered in our cultures. *Pseudomonas aeruginosa* was the most frequent isolate and constituted 65% of the Proteobacteria and 54.3% of the total gram-negative isolates in general. Bacteroidetes were recovered in less than 1% of bacterial corneal ulcers.

Pseudomonas species, predominantly, *Pseudomonas aeruginosa*, are leading causes of gram-negative bacterial keratitis. It is the leading cause associated with cosmetic contact lenses wear in the United States, the United Kingdom, and France [1, 4, 6]. It is also recovered from patients exposed to trauma with contaminated water, soil, and/or vegetation. In both conventional and metagenomic surveys, it has been recovered from healthy and diseased corneas as well as contact lenses from asymptomatic and symptomatic patients [15]. It presents as an acute, virulent, and progressive infection that can lead to corneal melting and perforation within 48 h (Fig. 6.7). It has an array of virulent factors including toxins, proteases, and antibiotic-resistant genes that aids it in establishing and maintaining corneal infection [1, 4].

Bacteroidetes

Members of this group are recovered from patients with chronic ocular surface disease and/or chronic local/systemic ocular disease (Table 6.7). These are found in a wide variety of environmental niches (soil, water) and in the gut and on the skin of humans and animals [10]. These ulcers can be indolent and difficult to treat.

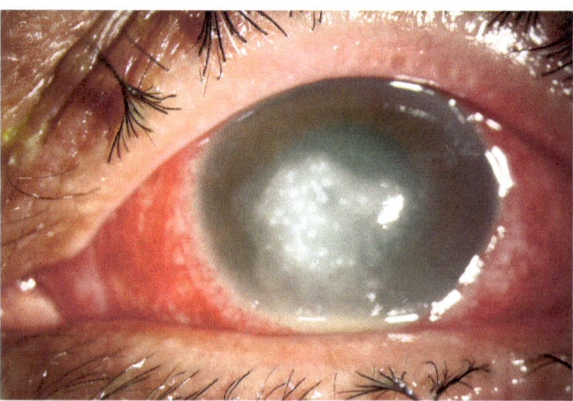

Fig. 6.7 *Streptococcus mitis* crystalline keratitis

6.8 Use of Metagenomics to Detect Bacterial Keratitis

Although several investigators have attempted to use shotgun metagenomics to reduce turnaround time and improved identification of the etiological agent in bacterial keratitis, challenges exist [38]. Currently, there are no standard protocols for specimen collection, storage, or genomic platform. Availability is also an issue.

The main challenge, however, is coordinating and selecting the true ocular pathogen from the diversity of microorganisms recovered and associated with this sensitive method and/or documenting the roles of the other community members to the disease process. In a recent report by Seitzman et al., they confirmed that shotgun metagenomics could amplify the etiological agent identified by culture in a proof-of-concept exercise [39]. This was done by eliminating "contaminating and background taxa." However, 15 of the 20 (75%) most common taxa have been recovered from bacteria. The most challenging task in establishing an etiological agent interpreting metagenomic results. No culture-negative cases were included in the study. As with culture results, metagenomic analysis must be coordinated with the clinical picture.

6.8.1 Antimicrobial Therapy

Empirical therapy, with broad spectrum, commercially available topical antibiotics Empirical therapy is the current standard of care for treating bacterial keratitis [1]. Both the AAO's current Bacterial Keratitis Practice guidelines and the Royal College of Ophthalmologists Focus, United Kingdom guidelines recommend monotherapy with a fluoroquinolone as the initial therapy for bacterial keratitis. Alternatives include combination/fortified therapy with a cephalosporin and aminoglycosides. Vancomycin should be reserved for documented multidrug-resistant gram-positive isolates. Efficacy and susceptibility profiles may be significantly different according to location, patient populations, and dispensing frequency [1, 40].

Evidence and support for these recommendations were provided by a 2014 Cochrane-like review that found no difference in the effectiveness between monotherapy with a fluoroquinolone and combination therapy with commonly used fortified antibiotics (cephalosporins and aminoglycosides) [41, 42].

However, increasing drug resistance to the fluoroquinolones and emerging resistance to commonly used fortified drops in the United States have been documented by two national surveys since 2005. The Ocular Tracking Resistance in US Today (TRUST) was the first national surveillance study tracking emerging antibiotic resistance among *Staphylococcus aureus*, *Streptococcus pneumoniae*, and *Haemophilus influenzae* ocular isolates collected over a 3-year period 2005–2008. Susceptibility rates among the fluoroquinolones for MSSA and MRSA were less than 90% and 20% respectively. Susceptibility for *S. pneumoniae* and *Haemophilus influenzae* remained at >90% [43].

The Antibiotic Resistance Monitoring in Ocular Microorganisms (ARMOR) replaced and expanded the TRUST study in 2009. Data from the cumulative ARMOR (2009–2018) report confirms the continuation of increasing fluoroquinolone resistance among ocular Staphylococcal isolates and increasing resistance among both *Pseudomonas aeruginosa* and *Streptococcus pneumoniae*. Nonsusceptibility rates to the aminoglycosides ranged from 2.9% *P. aeruginosa* to 17.5% coagulase-negative Staphylococci. The rate for S. aureus was 15.6%. For MSSA and CoNMSSA nonsusceptible rates were less than 7%, which methicillin resistance was associated with rates higher than 25% [44]. Multidrug-resistant isolates to ciprofloxacin and ofloxacin have been reported from several developing countries [45]. Wilcox reported resistance rates ranging from 10 to 24% of isolates from Africa, Asia, and South America [46].

In general, bacterial ocular isolates recovered from keratitis in the United States remain susceptible to combination therapy with fortified antimicrobials, cephalosporins and aminoglycosides and/or aminoglycosides and vancomycin [6, 47].

Increasing or sustained fluoroquinolone resistance (ciprofloxacin, ofloxacin, levofloxacin, and moxifloxacin) among methicillin susceptible and resistant Staphylococci and emerging resistance among *Pseudomonas aeruginosa*, *Serratia marcescens*, and *Streptococcus pneumoniae* remain worrisome [6]. The current recommendation of initial fluoroquinolone treatment for bacterial keratitis may need to be revisited for this location and regions with rates greater than 20% resistance. Antibiotic drug selection should be based on clinical impression, probable pathogens, antibiotic exposure history, and current local susceptibility profiles.

In vitro susceptibility testing may improve antimicrobial therapy. Although there is no current and/or standard ocular breakpoints, Oldenburg et al. documented a correlation with general MIC breakpoints and outcomes for keratitis for moxifloxacin [48]. The conclusion from the SCUT study was that moxifloxacin mediates the relationship between causative organisms and clinical outcomes in bacterial keratitis and is likely on the causal pathway between the organism and outcome [34, 48].

6.9   Steroids and Bacterial Keratitis

The use of corticosteroids as adjunctive therapy in the management of bacterial keratitis is still somewhat controversial. Some clarity about their benefit was provided by the Steroids for Corneal Ulcers Trial (SCUT), a large, randomized, double-blinded, placebo study developed to evaluate the role of corticosteroids treatment of bacterial corneal ulcers [49].

In general, topical corticosteroids appeared safe but provided no significant improvement in the treatment of bacterial keratitis. They did appear to be beneficial for ulcers that were central, deep or large, non-Nocardia or classically invasive *Pseudomonas aeruginosa*, patients with low baseline vision, and when started early after the initiation of antibiotics [49, 50].

6.10   Conclusions

Bacterial keratitis remains a common, major global and public health concern. Despite improvements in surgical techniques, topical antibiotic spectrum, and patient and provider education, minimal progress has been achieved in reducing the incidence and/or prevalence of bacterial keratitis in urban and nonurban populations.

Local, regional, and international rates and pathogen spectrum have remained relatively stable over the last 30 years with little improvement in clinical assessment/diagnosis or rapid laboratory detection. Increasing exposure to healthcare (contact lens—cosmetic, therapeutic; ocular surgeries) coupled with the aggressive use of broad-spectrum antibiotics, corticosteroids, and other immunosuppressive agents increase the risk of bacterial keratitis. This strategy does not seem to be effective in reducing the antimicrobial resistance. Rates or complications associated with this current "standard of care."

A new paradigm is needed. It needs to include the integration of improved clinical and laboratory techniques/technology for rapid and accurate diagnosis with the understanding of the dynamic interactions at the ocular surface health, between the ocular and gut microbiome diversity and immune defenses in cornea health and disease. Two new opportunities to reach this goal include the use of artificial intelligence and selection of next generation sequencing.

6.10.1 Artificial Intelligence and Neural Networks

The use of artificial intelligence and neural networks could serve as an adjunct to supplement both the clinical and laboratory diagnosis of bacterial keratitis. A combination of imaging (confocal, slit lamp), microbiology slides as well as integration of clinical and microbiology laboratory data from electronic medical records and/or microbiology laboratory database could be integrated into a neural network to generate a computer-assisted diagnosis of bacterial keratitis.

6.10.2 Next Generation Sequencing

Use of molecular techniques such as shotgun metagenomics and standard bioinformatics interpretations could provide information on the interaction of the ocular microbiome, ocular surface epithelium and local immune (tears) defenses and their contribution to patient diverse outcomes in bacterial keratitis.

Acknowledgments With contributions from Nayef K. Alshammari, Feras Mohder, Anne-Marie E. Okoduwa, and Mike Zein.

References

1. Lin A, Rhee MK, Akpek EK, Amescua G, Farid M, Garcia-Ferrer FJ, Varu DM, Musch DC, Dunn SP, Mah FS, American Academy of Ophthalmology Preferred Practice Pattern Cornea and External Disease Panel. Bacterial keratitis preferred practice pattern. Ophthalmology. 2019;126(1):P1–P55.
2. Ung L, Bispo PJM, Shanbhag SS, Gilmore MS, Chodosh J. The persistent dilemma of microbial keratitis: global burden, diagnosis, and antimicrobial resistance. Surv Ophthalmol. 2019;64(3):255–71.
3. Collier SA, Gronostaj MP, MacGurn AK, Cope JR, Awsumb KL, Yoder JS, Beach MJ. Estimated burden of keratitis—United States, 2010. MMWR Morb Mortal Wkly Rep. 2014;63(45):1027–30.

 4. Hong A, Shute T, Huang A. Bacterial keratitis. In: Mannis M, Holland E, editors. Cornea, fundamentals, diagnosis and management. 4th ed. New York: Elsevier; 2017. p. 875–901.
 5. Boost M, Cho P, Wang Z. Disturbing the balance: effect of contact lens use on the ocular proteome and microbiome. Clin Exp Optom. 2017;100(5):459–72.
 6. Miller D. Update on the epidemiology and antibiotic resistance of ocular infections. Middle East Afr J Ophthalmol. 2017;24(1):30–42.
 7. Karsten E, Watson SL, Foster LJR. Diversity of microbial species implicated in keratitis: a review. Open Ophthalmol J. 2012;6:110–24.
 8. Teweldemedhin M, Gebreyesus H, Atsbaha AH, Asgedom SW, Saravanan M. Bacterial profile of ocular infections: a systematic review. BMC Ophthalmol. 2017;17(1):212.
 9. Fleiszig SM, Evans DJ. Pathogenesis of contact lens-associated microbial keratitis. Optom Vis Sci. 2010;87(4):225–32.
10. Ryan KJ. Sherris medical microbiology. 7th ed. New York: McGraw-Hill Education; 2018.
11. Spierer O, Miller D, O'Brien TP. Comparative activity of antimicrobials against Pseudomonas aeruginosa, Achromobacter xylosoxidans and Stenotrophomonas maltophilia keratitis isolates. Br J Ophthalmol. 2018;102(5):708–12.
12. Wiley L, Bridge DR, Wiley LA, Odom JV, Elliott T, Olson JC. Bacterial biofilm diversity in contact lens-related disease: emerging role of Achromobacter, Stenotrophomonas, and Delftia. Invest Ophthalmol Vis Sci. 2012;53(7):3896–905.
13. Miller D, Iovieno A. The role of microbial flora on the ocular surface. Curr Opin Allergy Clin Immunol. 2009;9(5):466–70.
14. Cavuoto KM, Banerjee S, Galor A. Relationship between the microbiome and ocular health. Ocul Surf. 2019;17(3):384–92.
15. Ozkan J, Willcox MD. The ocular microbiome: molecular characterisation of a unique and low microbial environment. J Current Eye Res. 2019;44(7):685–94.
16. Thomason CA, Mullen N, Belden LK, May M, Hawley DM. Resident microbiome disruption with antibiotics enhances virulence of a colonizing pathogen. Sci Rep. 2017;7(1):16177.
17. Lu LJ, Liu J. Human microbiota and ophthalmic disease. Yale J Biol Med. 2016;89(3):325–30.
18. Kugadas A, Christiansen SH, Sankaranarayanan S, Surana NK, Gauguet S, Kunz R, Fichorova R, Vorup-Jensen T, Gadjeva M. Impact of microbiota on resistance to ocular pseudomonas aeruginosa-induced keratitis. PLoS Pathog. 2016;12(9):e1005855.
19. Jayasudha R, Chakravarthy SK, Prashanthi GS, Sharma S, Garg P, Murthy SI, Shivaji S. Alterations in gut bacterial and fungal microbiomes are associated with bacterial keratitis, an inflammatory disease of the human eye. J Biosci. 2018;43(5):835–56.
20. Hsiao CH, Yeung L, Ma DH, Chen YF, Lin HC, Tan HY, Huang SC, Lin KK. Pediatric microbial keratitis in Taiwanese children: a review of hospital cases. Arch Ophthalmol. 2007;125(5):603–9.
21. Lee YS, Tan HY, Yeh LK, Lin HC, Ma DH, Chen HC, Chen SY, Chen PY, Hsiao CH. Pediatric microbial keratitis in Taiwan: clinical and microbiological profiles, 1998-2002 versus 2008-2012. Am J Ophthalmol. 2014;157(5):1090–6.
22. Ormerod D, Murphree AL, Gomez DS, Schanzlin DJ, Smith RE. Microbial keratitis in children. Ophthalmology. 1986;93(4):449–55.
23. Rossetto JD, Cavuoto KM, Osigian CJ, Chang TCP, Miller D, Capo H, Spierer O. Paediatric infectious keratitis: a case series of 107 children presenting to a tertiary referral centre. Br J Ophthalmol. 2017;101(11):1488–92.
24. Yu MC, Höfling-Lima AL, Furtado GH. Microbiological and epidemiological study of infectious keratitis in children and adolescents. Arq Bras Oftalmol. 2016;79(5):289–93.
25. Kunimoto DY, Sharma S, Reddy MK, Gopinathan U, Jyothi J, Miller D, Rao GN. Microbial keratitis in children. Ophthalmology. 1998;105(2):252–7.
26. Cruz OA, Sabir SM, Capo H, Alfonso EC. Microbial keratitis in childhood. Ophthalmology. 1993;100(2):192–6.
27. Chirinos-Saldaña P, Bautista de Lucio VM, Hernandez-Camarena JC, Navas A, Ramirez-Miranda A, Vizuet-Garcia L, Ortiz-Casas M, Lopez-Espinosa N, Gaona-Juarez C, Bautista-

Hernandez LA, Graue-Hernandez EO. Clinical and microbiological profile of infectious keratitis in children. BMC Ophthalmol. 2013;13:54.
28. Al-Otaibi AG. Non-viral microbial keratitis in children. Saudi J Ophthalmol. 2012;26(2):191–7.
29. Park J, Lee KM, Zhou H, Rabin M, Jwo K, Burton WB, Gritz DC. Community practice patterns for bacterial corneal ulcer evaluation and treatment. Eye Contact Lens. 2015;41(1):12–8.
30. Austin A, Schallhorn J, Geske M, Mannis M, Lietman T, Rose-Nussbaumer J. Empirical treatment of bacterial keratitis: an international survey of corneal specialists. BMJ Open Ophthalmol. 2016;2:e000047.
31. Becker K, Heilmann C, Peters G. Coagulase-negative staphylococci. Clin Microbiol Rev. 2014;27(4):870–926.
32. Peterson JC, Durkee H, Miller D, Maestre-Mesa J, Arboleda A, Aguilar MC, Relhan N, Flynn HW Jr, Amescua G, Parel JM, Alfonso E. Molecular epidemiology and resistance profiles among healthcare- and community-associated Staphylococcus aureus keratitis isolates. Infect Drug Resist. 2019;12:831–43.
33. Hsiao CH, Ong SJ, Chuang CC, Ma DHK, Huang YC. A comparison of clinical features between community-associated and healthcare-associated methicillin-resistant Staphylococcus aureus keratitis. J Ophthalmol. 2015;2015:923941.
34. Lalitha P, Srinivasan M, Manikandan P, Bharathi MJ, Rajaraman R, Ravindran M, Cevallos V, Oldenburg CE, Ray KJ, Toutain-Kidd CM, Glidden DV, Zegans ME, McLeod SD, Acharya NR, Lietman TM. Relationship of in vitro susceptibility to moxifloxacin and in vivo clinical outcome in bacterial keratitis. Clin Infect Dis. 2012;54(10):1381–7.
35. Porter AJ, Lee GA, Jun AS. Infectious crystalline keratopathy. Surv Ophthalmol. 2018;63(4):480–99.
36. Das S, Rao AS, Sahu SK, Sharma S. Corynebacterium spp as causative agents of microbial keratitis. Br J Ophthalmol. 2016;100(7):939–43.
37. Ovodenko B, Seedor JA, Ritterband DC, Shah M, Yang R, Koplin RS. The prevalence and pathogenicity of Propionibacterium acnes keratitis. Cornea. 2009;28(1):36–9.
38. Borroni D, Romano V, Kaye SB, Somerville T, Napoli L, Fasolo A, Gallon P, Ponzin D, Esposito A, Ferrari S. Metagenomics in ophthalmology: current findings and future prospectives. BMJ Open Ophthalmol. 2019;4:e000248.
39. Seitzman GD, Hinterwirth A, Zhong L, Cummings S, Chen C, Driver TH, Lee MD, Doan T. Metagenomic deep sequencing for the diagnosis of corneal and external disease infections. Ophthalmology. 2019;126(12):1724–6.
40. Tuft S, Burton M. Microbial keratitis. Royal College Ophthalmologists, Autumn; 2013.
41. McDonald EM, Ram FS, Patel DV, McGhee CN. Topical antibiotics for the management of bacterial keratitis: an evidence-based review of high quality randomised controlled trials. Br J Ophthalmol. 2014;98(11):1470–7.
42. Austin A, Lietman T, Rose-Nussbaumer J. Update on the management of infectious keratitis. Ophthalmology. 2017;124(11):1678–89.
43. Asbell PA, Colby KA, Deng S, McDonnell P, Meisler DM, Raizman MB, Sheppard JD Jr, Sahm DF. Ocular TRUST: nationwide antimicrobial susceptibility patterns in ocular isolates. Am J Ophthalmol. 2008;145(6):951–8.
44. Asbell PA, Sanfilippo CM, Sahm DF, DeCory HH. Trends in antibiotic resistance among ocular microorganisms in the United States from 2009 to 2018. JAMA Ophthalmol. 2020;138(5):439–50.
45. Fernandes M, Vira D, Medikonda R, Kumar N. Extensively and pan-drug resistant Pseudomonas aeruginosa keratitis: clinical features, risk factors, and outcome. Graefes Arch Clin Exp Ophthalmol. 2016;254(2):315–22.
46. Willcox MD. Management and treatment of contact lens-related Pseudomonas keratitis. Clin Ophthalmol. 2012;6:919–24.
47. Thomas RK, Melton R, Asbell PA. Antibiotic resistance among ocular pathogens: current trends from the ARMOR surveillance study (2009-2016). Clin Optom. 2019;11:15–26.

48. Oldenburg CE, Lalitha P, Srinivasan M, Manikandan P, Bharathi MJ, Rajaraman R, Ravindran M, Mascarenhas J, Nardone N, Ray KJ, Glidden DV. Moxifloxacin susceptibility mediates the relationship between causative organism and clinical outcome in bacterial keratitis. Invest Ophthalmol Vis Sci. 2013;54(2):1522–6.
49. Srinivasan M, Mascarenhas J, Rajaraman R, Ravindran M, Prajna L, Glidden DV, Ray KJ, Hong KC, Oldenburg CE, Lee SM, Zegans ME, McLeod SD, Lietman TM, Nisha R, Acharya NR, Steroids for Corneal Ulcers Trial Group. Corticosteroids for bacterial keratitis: the Steroids for Corneal Ulcers Trial (SCUT). Arch Ophthalmol. 2012;130(2):143–50.
50. Ni N, Srinivasan M, McLeod SD, Acharya NR, Lietman TM, Rose-Nussbaumer J. Use of adjunctive topical corticosteroids in bacterial keratitis. Curr Opin Ophthalmol. 2016;27(4):353–7.

7

Isa S. K. Mohammed and Bennie H. Jeng

7.1 Introduction

Atypical Mycobacteria (AM), also known as nontuberculous Mycobacteria, are aerobic, nonmotile, nonspore-forming bacilli that can be responsible for multiple ocular infections, most commonly keratitis [1, 2]. Although there are many known species of AM, the majority responsible for keratitis are rapidly growing and non-chromogenic Runyon group IV organisms: *Mycobacterium chelonae* (42.7%), *Mycobacterium fortuitum* (14.7%), and *Mycobacterium abscessus* (11.1%) [3]. In addition to causing keratitis, AM infections have also been known to involve the orbit, periocular skin, and lacrimal system, and they can cause scleritis, conjunctivitis, endophthalmitis, choroiditis, iridocyclitis, and panuveitis [3]. Human infections are acquired from environmental exposure, often from soil, dust, or water [4].

The majority of AM ocular infections are keratitis [4]. Historically, AM have been known to cause corneal ulcers via nonsurgical trauma directly inoculating AM into the corneal stroma [5]. Post-corneal transplant AM keratitis was first reported in the 1980s, followed by multiple cases of post-laser in situ keratomilieusis (LASIK) AM keratitis in the 1990s, both sporadic and epidemic [6–8]. Presently, the plurality (47.6%) of AM cases occur post-LASIK, and the most common cause of post-LASIK keratitis is AM. Other common causes of AM include foreign bodies (17.6%), implants (17.3%), trauma (14.8%), and contact lens wear (6.4%) [3].

The common causes of AM keratitis often involve some degree of penetrating trauma to the corneal epithelium [4]. Soft contact lens wearers who develop abrasions are at risk [9], as well as patients who undergo suture removal [10]. Additionally, post-clear corneal cataract surgery wound ulcers secondary to AM have been reported [11, 12]. However, nearly one-third of AM keratitis cases

I. S. K. Mohammed · B. H. Jeng (✉)
Department of Ophthalmology and Visual Sciences, University of Maryland School of Medicine, Baltimore, MD, USA
e-mail: Isa.Mohammed@som.umaryland.edu; bjeng@som.umaryland.edu

© Springer Nature Singapore Pte Ltd. 2021
S. Das, V. Jhanji (eds.), *Infections of the Cornea and Conjunctiva*,
https://doi.org/10.1007/978-981-15-8811-2_7

present with no associated epithelial defect and with corneal scrapings showing normal epithelium and no growth of organisms [13] making diagnosis challenging.

Topical corticosteroids may increase the risk of AM keratitis. In a rabbit model, *M. fortuitum* was cultured from corneal lesions from rabbit corneas treated with subconjunctival methylprednisolone at the time of inoculation with *M. fortuitum*, whereas controls who did not receive the steroids showed no active disease at 3–4 weeks, and no organisms could be identified from culture [14]. It has been noted that steroids were used in more than half of the cases of reported AM keratitis (57.4%) [3]. Postoperative subconjunctival and topical corticosteroids not only increase the risk of AM keratitis but can also exacerbate AM keratitis and are associated with cases that are recalcitrant to antibiotic therapy [13, 15, 16]. Additionally, corneal grafts require postoperative topical corticosteroids and are therefore also at risk for AM keratitis, and these cases may warrant regraft, or penetrating keratoplasty if the keratitis occurs following endothelial keratoplasty [17–20]. *M. chelonae* has even been implicated in AM keratitis after routine phacoemulsification cataract surgery [21].

7.2   Clinical Features

AM keratitis can be difficult to diagnose, and this often results in delayed treatment [22]. In one series, delayed diagnosis was reported in 55.5% of cases, with these being attributed to misdiagnosis, misidentification of the causative organism on culture, delay in taking cultures, or slow or no growth of the organism [3]. Cases have been misidentified as Nocardia and Corynebacterium species or misdiagnosed as herpes keratitis and fungal keratitis. The duration of delay ranged from 1 week to 30 weeks, with an average of 8 weeks.

Cases of AM keratitis typically follow an indolent course and are prolonged by the use of topical steroids [14]. Often, cases of AM keratitis are preceded by a history of trauma, both surgical and nonsurgical, including foreign body removal [5, 23]. Pain is variable, and vision is often decreased. A white central ulcer with white satellite infiltrates is characteristic of *M. fortuitum* and *M. chelonae* [5, 17, 24]. (Fig. 7.1) These satellite lesions can mimic those seen in fungal keratitis. A hypopyon may develop if untreated (Fig. 7.2), but it is less common with an intact epithelium [25]. A "cracked windshield" appearance of lines radiating from the central area of ulceration is also typical of AM keratitis. Unlike infectious crystalline keratopathy, this sign is seen transiently early in the disease course [4]. Despite the predilection to develop in cases of epithelial breakdown, the infection can be deep in the stroma without an epithelial defect due to direct inoculation, often from prior surgical trauma [13, 26]. These cases are associated with irregular margins and satellite lesions, and usually involve Runyon group I or II AM [27]. AM keratitis can extend to the corneoscleral junction [25, 26] and can appear like any other bacterial, herpetic stromal, or fungal keratitis. Some cases, especially those involving *M. marinum*, *M. chelonae*, and *M. gordonae*, can present with dendritic or geographic epithelial defects with minimal stromal infiltration that simulate a nonsuppurative herpetic keratitis, leading to an incorrect diagnosis [5, 27, 28].

Fig. 7.1 (**a**) Atypical mycobacterial keratitis at presentation; (**b**) during topical treatment; and (**c**) after resolution of active infection. (Courtesy: Sujata Das)

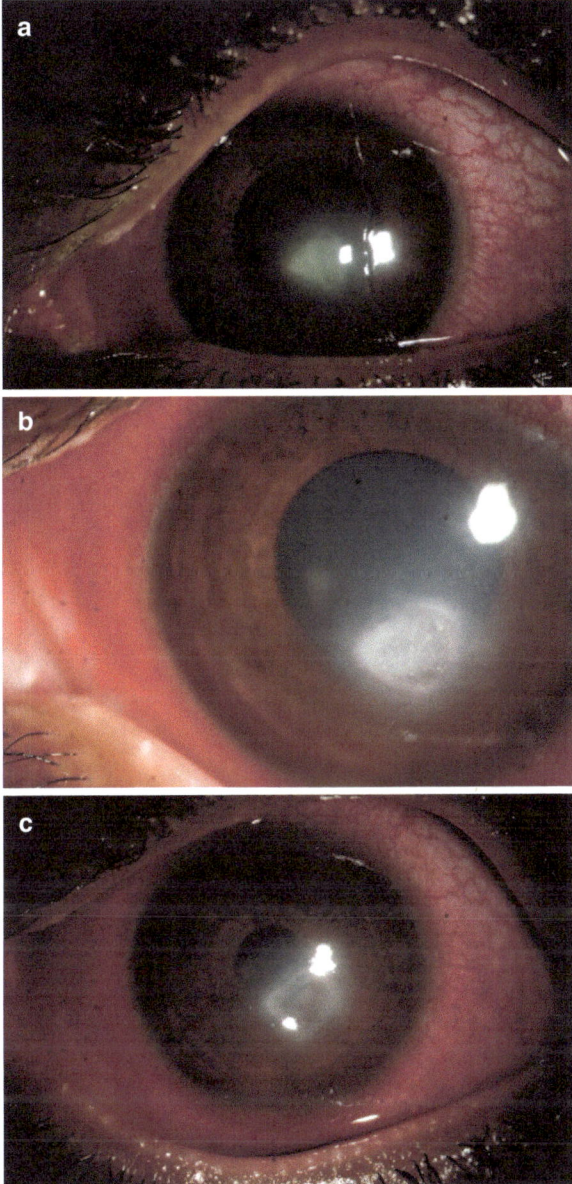

7.3   Diagnosis

A combination of standard and special stains and media are often needed to make a microbiological diagnosis of AM keratitis. Gram and Giemsa stains typically reveal nonspecific polymorphonuclear leukocytes or partially stained bacilli that may be easily misdiagnosed [29]. Specific stains such as Ziehl–Neelsen show

Fig. 7.2 Slit lamp photograph of left eye with *Mycobacterium abscessus* keratitis. Note two satellite lesions in addition to the dense white infiltrate in the central cornea. Also, note the hypopyon

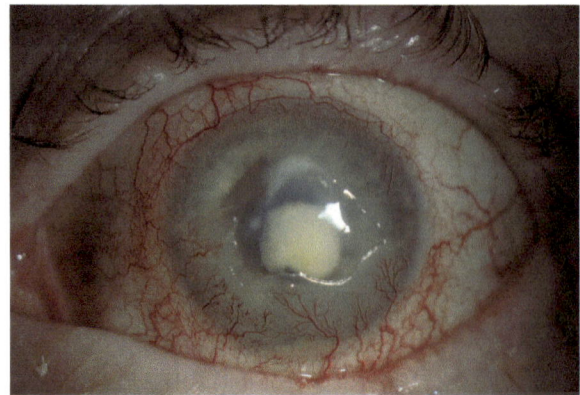

Fig. 7.3 Corneal button excised for recalcitrant *Mycobacterium abscessus* keratitis. Note staining of bacilli with Ziehl–Neelsen stain

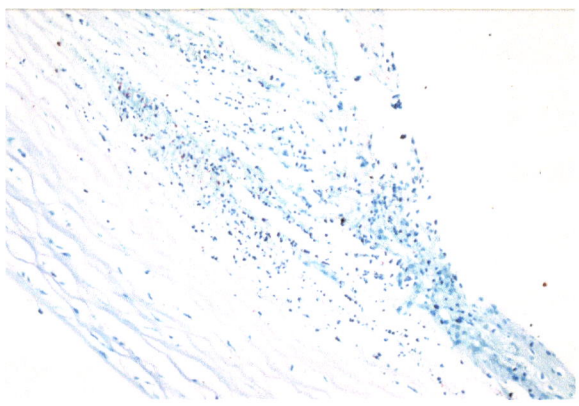

gram-variable bacilli which do not decolorize with 20% sulfuric acid (Fig. 7.3). Fluorescein-conjugated stains such as auramine-rhodamine fluorescent acid-fast stain and fluorescent conjugated lectins are also useful [4]. With regards to cultures, blood agar, chocolate agar, MacConkey agar, Lowenstein–Jensen medium, and liquid broth such as Middlebrook 7H9 broth in conjunction with a mycobacterial growth indicator tube are recommended [30]. Multiple culture media increases yield, particularly of slower-growing varieties (Runyon groups I and II). Given variation in growth rates between different species, culture times vary from 2 to 4 days, but they should be maintained for up to 8 weeks [31]. Recently, AM has been further characterized by PCR pulsed-field gel electrophoresis, which can aid in the diagnosis of AM keratitis [32, 33]. Of samples from one series of AM keratitis cases that isolated a causative organism, 64.1% were from superficial corneal scrapings, 9.5% were from corneal biopsy, 13.6% were from flap lift post-LASIK, and 5.5% were from corneal buttons post-transplant [3]. The sample source depends on clinical context.

7.4   Management and Outcomes

Recurrence of AM keratitis is common, despite an initial response to treatment [34], and the prognosis is guarded, as up to 50% of patients may have severe vision loss in cases of post-LASIK AM keratitis [8]. Thus, a high suspicion is needed in post-LASIK keratitis in order to recognize and start treatment promptly [7, 35–38].

As in all cases of microbial keratitis, antibiotics play a crucial role in AM keratitis, and the choice of antibiotics is based off of sensitivity data and outcomes from the treatment of non-ocular (systemic) AM infections [4]. Slower growing AM are sensitive to agents used to treat *M. tuberculosis,* such as rifabutin, rifampin, and streptomycin, whereas rapidly growing AM are sensitive to macrolides, fluoroquinolones, and aminoglycosides. Cases often require a combination of two or more antibiotics. Triple therapy with topical clarithromycin or amikacin, azithromycin, and often a fourth generation fluoroquinolone, in conjunction with appropriate corneal debridement has been suggested in the literature [7, 33, 39]. Two antibiotics have been used in 55.2% of eyes, with a plurality of combinations including amikacin (50 mg/mL) (39.4%) [3]. Only in the minority of cases (27.6%) has amikacin been used as monotherapy [3]. Clarithromycin (10 mg/mL) is ideally reconstituted from lyophilized parenteral drug, but it is no longer available in the US [40]. Currently, it is formulated from an oral suspension, which has been shown to have decreased bioavailability in rabbit corneas with intact corneal epithelium [40]. Azithromycin (2 mg/mL) can be reconstituted from lyophilized drug used parenterally or from a mucoadhesive commercial preparation. Azithromycin 1% is a commercially available topical formulation, but its efficacy is not known for AM keratitis. Finally, moxifloxacin or gatifloxacin has been used in AM keratitis with varying success. In vitro susceptibility testing has shown that based on the MIC cut off, fluoroquinolones are less likely to be useful in AM keratitis. In a series of 15 cases of AM keratitis, all isolates were sensitive to amikacin, azithromycin, and clarithromycin, but only 9/15 (60%) were sensitive to gatifloxacin and 6/15 (40%) were sensitive to ciprofloxacin [41].

Systemic antibiotics may be used in recalcitrant cases [39], with oral clarithromycin or oral doxycycline being commonly used. In one series of 203 cases of AM keratitis, topical antibiotic therapy alone was used in 53.2% of cases, whereas systemic and topical antibiotics were combined in 41.9% of cases [3]. There are no set guidelines regarding duration of treatment, but cases of AM keratitis often require 6 weeks to 6 months of topical and systemic antibiotic therapy [4]. Discontinuation of topical corticosteroids is also recommended as reduced local host immune mechanisms prolong the duration of AM keratitis [13].

Surgical management is a mainstay of treatment, and it is required in 55.1% of eyes in one series [3]. Of the 73.1% of eyes that had an initial lack of response to medical therapy, 79.3% required surgical intervention [3]. Surgical debridement is often necessary given the potential for biofilm formation, which may allow for evasion of immune defense mechanisms and an ability to withstand antimicrobial therapy [6, 42]. Surgical intervention varies depending on the location of the infection with corneal scraping, unroofing of abscesses [7], and excimer photo-therapeutic keratectomy described [43]. Flap lift and irrigation are commonly performed in post-LASIK cases [44, 45], with removal of corneal flap noted in 17.3% of AM cases [3]. When looking specifically at cases of post-LASIK AM keratitis, removal of the flap for resolution of the infections was needed in 80.3% of cases. Removal of the flap allowed for improved penetration of the topical antibiotics into the cornea and a shortened disease course [36, 46]. Flap removal results in a hyperopic shift, but vision has been shown to return to 20/50 with correction after healing [7, 37, 47].

Lamellar keratectomy or penetrating keratoplasty may be indicated in recalcitrant cases (Fig. 7.3). Penetrating keratoplasty was required in 14.1% of cases [3], in situations where there was no response to medical therapy or there were recurrent, severe exacerbations with attempted weaning of topical antibiotics [13]. Surgically, it is imperative to maintain clean margins as recurrence in the graft can occur if adequate margins are not obtained [10, 48]. In such cases, AM keratitis can recur in the corneal graft, and may ultimately require a regraft [20].

Untreated infections may extend from the deep stroma to the epithelium and cause a secondary breakdown of the corneal epithelium or may spread to internal ocular structures, highlighting the need for timely diagnosis and treatment [13]. Resolution of AM keratitis occurred in 80.9% of cases in one series, with visual acuity of 20/40 or better in 54.9% of cases, and visual acuity of 20/200 or worse in 19.6% [3]. In 1.3% of cases, there is loss of eye, and patients who undergo surgical interventions are more likely to end up with visual impairment [3]. Among cases that resolved without severe vision loss, 25.8% had a prolonged course that required either multiple medical therapies or more than one surgical intervention.

7.5   Conclusion

The majority of AM keratitis is caused by Runyon group IV mycobacteria and poses diagnostic and therapeutic challenges. A high degree of suspicion is needed to diagnose AM keratitis, with close attention in cases of keratitis in the setting of previous trauma or surgery or recalcitrance to traditional antibiotics. Specific cultures in addition to standard media may be needed, including acid-fast stains, Ziehl–Neelsen, auramine-rhodamine fluorescence, and fluorescent conjugated lectins. Special media such as Lowenstein–Jensen medium and Middlebrook 7H9 broth are useful, as well as PCR. Cultures should be kept for at least 2 weeks to detect slow-growing AM, but may need to be kept for up to 8 weeks. While AM keratitis is sensitive to topical antibiotics, it often requires combination therapy including amikacin, clarithromycin, and azithromycin. In addition, systemic antibiotics may need to be used adjunctively in many cases. Due to the development of biofilms, surgical debridement is sometimes needed for definitive management.

References

1. Garg P. Fungal, Mycobacterial, and Nocardia infections and the eye: an update. Eye. 2012;26(2):245–51.
2. Girgis DO, Karp CL, Miller D. Ocular infections caused by non-tuberculous mycobacteria: update on epidemiology and management. Clin Exp Ophthalmol. 2012;40(5):467–75.
3. Kheir WJ, Sheheitli H, Abdul Fattah M, Hamam RN. Nontuberculous mycobacterial ocular infections: a systematic review of the literature. Biomed Res Int. 2015;2015:164989.
4. Moorthy RS, Valluri S, Rao NA. Nontuberculous mycobacterial ocular and adnexal infections. Surv Ophthalmol. 2012;57(3):202–35.
5. Dugel PU, Holland GN, Brown HH, Pettit TH, Hofbauer JD, Simons KB, Ullman H, Bath PE, Foos RY. Mycobacterium fortuitum keratitis. Am J Ophthalmol. 1988;105(6):661–9.
6. Alvarenga L, Freitas D, Hofling-Lima AL, Belfort R Jr, Sampaio J, Sousa L, Yu M, Mannis M. Infectious post-LASIK crystalline keratopathy caused by nontuberculous mycobacteria. Cornea. 2002;21(4):426–9.
7. Chandra NS, Torres MF, Winthrop KL, Bruckner DA, Heidemann DG, Calvet HM, Yakrus M, Mondino BJ, Holland GN. Cluster of Mycobacterium chelonae keratitis cases following laser in-situ keratomileusis. Am J Ophthalmol. 2001;132(6):819–30.
8. Chang MA, Jain S, Azar DT. Infections following laser in situ keratomileusis: an integration of the published literature. Surv Ophthalmol. 2004;49(3):269–80.
9. Khooshabeh R, Grange JM, Yates MD, McCartney AC, Casey TA. A case report of Mycobacterium chelonae keratitis and a review of mycobacterial infections of the eye and orbit. Tuber Lung Dis. 1994;75(5):377–82.
10. Newman PE, Goodman RA, Waring GO 3rd, Finton RJ, Wilson LA, Wright J, Cavanagh HD. A cluster of cases of Mycobacterium chelonei keratitis associated with outpatient office procedures. Am J Ophthalmol. 1984;97(3):344–8.
11. Servat JJ, Ramos-Esteban JC, Tauber S, Bia FJ. Mycobacterium chelonae-Mycobacterium abscessus complex clear corneal wound infection with recurrent hypopyon and perforation after phacoemulsification and intraocular lens implantation. J Cataract Refract Surg. 2005;31(7):1448–51.
12. Mah-Sadorra JH, Cohen EJ, Rapuano CJ. Mycobacterium chelonae wound ulcer after clear-cornea cataract surgery. Arch Ophthalmol. 2004;122(12):1888–9.
13. Ford JG, Huang AJ, Pflugfelder SC, Alfonso EC, Forster RK, Miller D. Nontuberculous mycobacterial keratitis in south Florida. Ophthalmology. 1998;105(9):1652–8.
14. Paschal JF, Holland GN, Sison RF, Berlin OG, Bruckner DA, Dugel PU, Foos RY. Mycobacterium fortuitum keratitis. Clinicopathologic correlates and corticosteroid effects in an animal model. Cornea. 1992;11(6):493–9.
15. Palani D, Kulandai LT, Naraharirao MH, Guruswami S, Ramendra B. Application of polymerase chain reaction-based restriction fragment length polymorphism in typing ocular rapid-growing nontuberculous mycobacterial isolates from three patients with postoperative endophthalmitis. Cornea. 2007;26(6):729–35.
16. Valenton M. Wound infection after cataract surgery. Jpn J Ophthalmol. 1996;40(3):447–55.
17. Zimmerman LE, Turner L, McTigue JW. Mycobacterium fortuitum infection of the cornea. A report of two cases. Arch Ophthalmol. 1969;82(5):596–601.
18. Laflamme MY, Poisson M, Chéhadé N. Mycobacterium chelonei keratitis following penetrating keratoplasty. Can J Ophthalmol. 1987;22(3):178–80.
19. Busin M, Ponzin D, Arffa RC. Mycobacterium chelonae interface infection after endokeratoplasty. Am J Ophthalmol. 2003;135(3):393–5.
20. Aylward GW, Stacey AR, Marsh RJ. Mycobacterium chelonei infection of a corneal graft. Br J Ophthalmol. 1987;71(9):690–3.
21. Martinez JD, Amescua G, Lozano-Cárdenas J, Suh LH. Bilateral Mycobacterium chelonae keratitis after phacoemulsification cataract surgery. Case Rep Ophthalmol Med. 2017;2017:6413160.

22. Broadway DC, Kerr-Muir MG, Eykyn SJ, Pambakian H. Mycobacterium chelonei keratitis: a case report and review of previously reported cases. Eye. 1994;8(1):134–42.
23. Turner L, Stinson I. Mycobacterium fortuitum: as a cause of corneal ulcer. Am J Ophthalmol. 1965;60(2):329–31.
24. Levenson DS, Harrison CH. Mycobacterium fortuitum corneal ulcer. Arch Ophthalmol. 1966;75(2):189–91.
25. Bullington RH Jr, Lanier JD, Font RL. Nontuberculous mycobacterial keratitis. Report of two cases and review of the literature. Arch Ophthalmol. 1992;110(4):519–24.
26. Schönherr U, Naumann GO, Lang GK, Bialasiewicz AA. Sclerokeratitis caused by Mycobacterium marinum. Am J Ophthalmol. 1989;108(5):607–8.
27. Gangadharam PR, Lanier JD, Jones DE. Keratitis due to Mycobacterium chelonei. Tubercle. 1978;59(1):55–60.
28. Moore MB, Newton C, Kaufman HE. Chronic keratitis caused by Mycobacterium gordonae. Am J Ophthalmol. 1986;102(4):516–21.
29. Garg P, Athmanathan S, Rao GN. Mycobacterium chelonei masquerading as Corynebacterium in a case of infectious keratitis: a diagnostic dilemma. Cornea. 1998;17(2):230–2.
30. Katoch VM. Infections due to non-tuberculous mycobacteria (NTM). Indian J Med Res. 2004;120(4):290–304.
31. Brown-Elliott BA, Wallace RJ Jr. Clinical and taxonomic status of pathogenic nonpigmented or late-pigmenting rapidly growing mycobacteria. Clin Microbiol Rev. 2002;15(4):716–46.
32. Shrestha NK, Tuohy MJ, Hall GS, Reischl U, Gordon SM, Procop GW. Detection and differentiation of Mycobacterium tuberculosis and nontuberculous mycobacterial isolates by real-time PCR. J Clin Microbiol. 2003;41(11):5121–6.
33. Chen KH, Sheu MM, Lin SR. Rapid identification of mycobacteria to the species level by polymerase chain reaction and restriction enzyme analysis—a case report of corneal ulcer. Kaohsiung J Med Sci. 1997;13(9):583–8.
34. Willis WE, Laibson PR. Intractable Mycobacterium fortuitum corneal ulcer in man. Am J Ophthalmol. 1971;71(2):500–4.
35. Daines BS, Vroman DT, Sandoval HP, Steed LL, Solomon KD. Rapid diagnosis and treatment of mycobacterial keratitis after laser in situ keratomileusis. J Cataract Refract Surg. 2003;29(5):1014–8.
36. Freitas D, Alvarenga L, Sampaio J, Mannis M, Sato E, Sousa L, Vieira L, Yu MC, Martins MC, Hoffling-Lima A, Belfort R Jr. An outbreak of Mycobacterium chelonae infection after LASIK. Ophthalmology. 2003;110(2):276–85.
37. Fulcher SF, Fader RC, Rosa RH Jr, Holmes GP. Delayed-onset mycobacterial keratitis after LASIK. Cornea. 2002;21(6):546–54.
38. Winthrop KL, Steinberg EB, Holmes G, Kainer MA, Werner SB, Winquist A, Vugia DJ. Epidemic and sporadic cases of nontuberculous mycobacterial keratitis associated with laser in situ keratomileusis. Am J Ophthalmol. 2003;135(2):223–4.
39. John T, Velotta E. Nontuberculous (atypical) mycobacterial keratitis after LASIK: current status and clinical implications. Cornea. 2005;24(3):245–55.
40. Kuehne JJ, Yu AL, Holland GN, Ramaswamy A, Taban R, Mondino BJ, Yu F, Rayner SA, Giese MJ. Corneal pharmacokinetics of topically applied azithromycin and clarithromycin. Am J Ophthalmol. 2004;138(4):547–53.
41. Reddy AK, Garg P, Babu KH, Gopinathan U, Sharma S. In vitro antibiotic susceptibility of rapidly growing nontuberculous mycobacteria isolated from patients with microbial keratitis. Curr Eye Res. 2010;35(3):225–9.
42. Holland SP, Pulido JS, Miller D, Ellis B, Alfonso E, Scott M, Costerton JW. Biofilm and scleral buckle-associated infections. A mechanism for persistence. Ophthalmology. 1991;98(6):933–8.
43. Fogla R, Rao SK, Padmanabhan P. Interface keratitis due to Mycobacterium fortuitum following laser in situ keratomileusis. Indian J Ophthalmol. 2003;51(3):263–5.
44. Garg P, Bansal AK, Sharma S, Vemuganti GK. Bilateral infectious keratitis after laser in situ keratomileusis: a case report and review of the literature. Ophthalmology. 2001;108(1):121–5.

45. Solomon A, Karp CL, Miller D, Dubovy SR, Huang AJ, Culbertson WW. Mycobacterium interface keratitis after laser in situ keratomileusis. Ophthalmology. 2001;108(12):2201–8.

46. Seo KY, Lee JB, Lee K, Kim MJ, Choi KR, Kim EK. Non-tuberculous mycobacterial keratitis at the interface after laser in situ keratomileusis. J Refract Surg. 2002;18(1):81–5.

47. Chung MS, Goldstein MH, Driebe WT Jr, Schwartz BH. Mycobacterium chelonae keratitis after laser in situ keratomileusis successfully treated with medical therapy and flap removal. Am J Ophthalmol. 2000;129(3):382–4.

48. Mirate DJ, Hull DS, Steel JH Jr, Carter MJ. Mycobacterium chelonei keratitis: a case report. Br J Ophthalmol. 1983;67(5):324–6.

Nocardia Keratitis

Pranita Sahay, Prafulla K. Maharana, and Namrata Sharma

8.1 Introduction

Corneal infection caused by rare organisms is often difficult to manage [1]. A large part of the difficulty in dealing with such an organism is a lack of a standardized method for their diagnosis, atypical presentation leading to a delay in suspicion, and a lack of standard treatment protocol. In some cases, the infection itself runs an indolent course despite being sensitive to the antibiotics used. *Nocardia* keratitis belongs to one such category of microbial keratitis, which, although the term rare may not be justified, runs an atypical course, and often associated with poor outcomes.

Nocardia, initially classified as a fungus, is now identified as a gram-positive bacteria [1, 2]. Ocular infections with *Nocardia* are rare and include keratitis, scleritis, and endophthalmitis [3]. In 1944, the first case of *Nocardia* keratitis was reported by Benedict et al., following which several case reports and few case series from various parts of the world have been reported [2–4]. The diagnosis of this entity is often missed, as the clinical picture is not well known to all considering its rare occurrence. Also, the presentation may sometimes be nonspecific or mimic other common clinical entities like fungal or atypical mycobacterial infection, further adding to the problem [2]. This results in a delayed diagnosis and improper management in most of the cases. Hence, in this chapter, we attempt to familiarize our readers with the microbiology, clinical features, investigations, and management of cases presenting with *Nocardia* Keratitis.

P. Sahay
Department of Ophthalmology, Lady Hardinge Medical College & Smt Sucheta Kriplani Hospital, New Delhi, India

P. K. Maharana · N. Sharma (✉)
Cornea, Cataract and Refractive Surgery Services, Dr. Rajendra Prasad Centre for Ophthalmic Sciences, All India Institute of Medical Sciences, New Delhi, India

8.2   Epidemiology

Nocardia is ubiquitous. It is extensively found worldwide and is saprophytic. It is an essential component of the normal soil microflora as well as water. It may also be found in air, dust, and decaying vegetation [2]. Ocular infection often occurs as a result of contamination from these sources, mostly associated with ocular trauma, as *Nocardia* is not a part of the normal ocular flora. Most of the cases of *Nocardia* keratitis have been reported from Asian Countries. The prevalence of *Nocardia* keratitis varies from 1.7 to 8.3% of all cases of bacterial keratitis, as reported in studies from South India [5, 6]. Also, a rising trend has been observed in this region. However, such cases have been less commonly reported from other parts of the world. Therefore, eliciting a travel history to Asia is important in case of clinical suspicion of Nocardial infection [7]. Of the important clinical isolates, *N. asteroides* is commonly found in the temperate region and *N. brasiliensis* in the tropical and subtropical areas.

8.3   Microbiology

The taxonomy of *Nocardia* has undergone numerous revisions over the past leading to a lot of confusion and controversy [8]. Initially, all cases were referred to as *Nocardia asteroides* only; however, it was found that it is a group of bacteria with a heterozygous pattern of antimicrobial drug susceptibilities and was referred as *N. asteroides* complex. Later, *N. asteroides* complex was separated and reorganized into different species on the basis of drug susceptibility patterns. To date, more than 50 species belonging to this group have been identified. Common species identified to be of clinical significance for human infections include *Nocardia abscessus, Nocardia brevicatena-paucivorans* complex, *Nocardia nova* complex (which includes *Nocardia nova, Nocardia veterana, Nocardia africana, Nocardia kruczakiae*), *Nocardia transvalensis* complex, *Nocardia farcinica*, and *Nocardia asteroides* [8, 9]. *N. asteroides* and *N. brasiliensis* are the most common species involved in ocular infection [2, 10–12]. Other species of clinical importance are *N. farcinica*, *N. abscessus*, *N. cyriageorgica*, *N. gypsoides*, *N. levis*, and *N. caviae* [11, 13, 14].

Nocardia is a gram-positive, immobile, aerobically growing bacteria. However, it appears as a filamentous bacterium with a hyphae-like branching on direct microscopy, unlike other gram-positive bacteria. It has numerous branching with thin beaded filaments (<2.5 µm) [2, 14]. The branching is observed at the right angle. It shows variable acid fastness, largely due to variability in the cell wall mycolic acid. Both acid-fast and non-acid-fast variants of *Nocardia* have been observed with Ziehl–Neelson staining. The sensitivity for detecting *Nocardia* is 87% with gram stain and 100% with 10% KOH wet mount [15]. This microorganism does not have fastidious requirements for growth and can be cultured in conventional bacteriologic media like blood agar or chocolate agar.

8.4   Risk Factors

The risk factors for *Nocardia* keratitis are similar to other forms of infective keratitis. Ocular trauma is the most common predisposing factor as *Nocardia* is found in soil, dust, and vegetative matter [3, 11]. Sridhar et al. reported a definite history of trauma in 25% of their cases in a series, including 16 culture-proven cases of *Nocardia* keratitis [16]. Lalitha et al. reported a previous history of trauma in as high as 84% of cases in a series of 32 eyes of *Nocardia* keratitis [11]. Similarly, DeCroos et al. in the most extensive series published on *Nocardia* keratitis involving 111 cases of culture-proven *Nocardia* keratitis reported ocular exposure to soil or plant matter in 48% of their cases [3]. Next to trauma, ocular surgery accounts for most cases of *Nocardia* keratitis reported in the literature. *Nocardia* keratitis has been reported following keratorefractive surgery (LASIK/PRK), penetrating keratoplasty, implantation of intracorneal ring segments, extracapsular cataract extraction, phacoemulsification, and Descemet membrane endothelial keratoplasty (DMEK) [3, 17–20]. Other reported risk factors include contact lens wear and topical steroid use [2].

8.5   Clinical Presentation

The growth rate of *Nocardia* is relatively slow; hence, fulminant infection with this microorganism is rare. The onset is usually indolent. The progression is slow. The infection usually runs a prolonged and benign clinical course. Most cases are unilateral except the cases following refractive surgery where it can present bilaterally. Similar to other forms of keratitis, males are affected more than females [3, 16].

The most common presenting symptoms are ocular pain, redness, watering blepharospasm, and lid swelling. The pain can be out of proportion to the clinical findings. Conjunctival congestion with a papillary reaction is often noted.

Corneal involvement may occur in several forms. Most commonly, it presents as patchy infiltrates, predominantly involving the anterior corneal stroma. These infiltrates are often arranged in a characteristic "wreath-like pattern" with satellite lesions (Fig. 8.1) [3]. The adjacent epithelium and subepithelial area are also involved. An overlying epithelial defect is seen in most of the cases. The infiltrates are usually situated in the mid-periphery of the cornea. The surrounding cornea remains clear in most of the cases. It can be associated with keratic precipitates, endothelial ring deposits, anterior chamber reaction, and hypopyon. With time vessels extend from the periphery towards the lesion. Over time, the granular infiltrates may coalesce to form a grayish plaque and subsequently, a corneal ulcer. A reduced corneal sensation can be seen in some cases. However, it must be remembered that this classical picture is seen in only around 30% of the cases [3]. In few cases, the ulcer margin is surrounded by raised and multiple yellow-white "pinhead-shaped superficial corneal infiltrate." [2, 16]

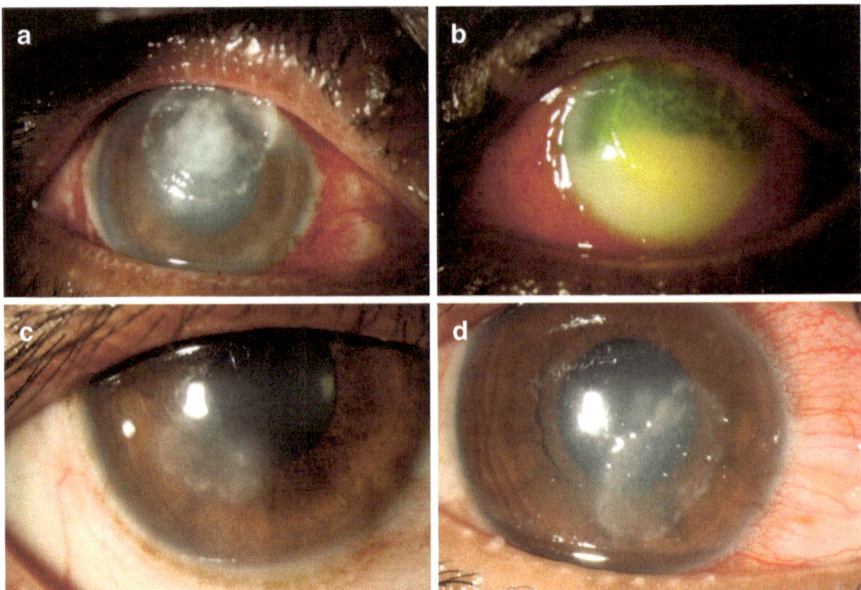

Fig. 8.1 Slit-lamp photograph showing: (**a**) superficial infiltrate with pinhead-like lesions in the periphery arranged in wreath-like pattern; (**b**) superficial infiltrate with hypopyon; (**c**) a case of *Nocardia* keratitis with superficial paracentral stromal infiltrate; and (**d**) superficial patchy stromal infiltrate. (Courtesy: Sujata Das)

Almost half of the cases of *Nocardia* keratitis present with atypical features. These include pseudo-dendritic corneal ulcer, satellite lesions, large corneal ulcer with overhanging edges, persistent epithelial defect, cotton wool appearance, full-thickness corneal infiltrate, and deep stromal infiltrate with endothelial plaque [21, 22]. Post-LASIK infections present as a well-defined whitish nodule surrounded by corneal infiltrate at the interface [18]. Lalitha et al. observed that cases presenting within 2 weeks of onset usually have a characteristic clinical presentation while those presenting later have atypical features, although a similar finding was not observed in other studies. It may be due to the fact that the atypical presentations are usually less symptomatic in contrast to the classical presentation and hence a delayed presentation.

8.6   Differential Diagnosis

Fungal and Mycobacterial keratitis is the common differentials for *Nocardia* keratitis, as all of them share an indolent clinical course [2, 11]. However, classical features of fungal keratitis, such as feathery margins, endothelial plaque, and dry look, often help in differentiating the two forms of keratitis. Likewise, infiltrates with indistinct fluffy or feather-like appearance with radiating projections in cases of atypical mycobacteria helps in differentiating it from *Nocardia* keratitis. Viral keratitis is another differential as pseudo-dendrites are sometimes seen with *Nocardia* keratitis. Nevertheless, lack of infiltrates and rapid response to topical acyclovir often rule out *Nocardia*.

8.7 Investigations

8.7.1 Microscopy

Corneal scraping specimen is collected for microbiological investigation. Proper communication with the microbiologist regarding suspicion for *Nocardia* is essential. Microscopic examination of the prepared smears is done with gram stain, Giemsa stain, KOH stain, calcofluor white stain, and modified Kinyoun stain (1% sulfuric acid) [3]. *Nocardia* appears as a gram-positive bacteria with branching filaments having a beaded appearance [2]. *Nocardia* is partially acid-fast on modified Kinyoun stain (1% sulfuric acid); however, it completely decolorizes on treatment with 20% sulfuric acid, which helps to differentiate it from Mycobacteria [14]. KOH wet mount also reveals branching thin filaments. It is essential to emphasize here that; although *Nocardia* can be seen by various smear examinations, Gram staining is the most sensitive method for its diagnosis, and the modified acid-fast stain is not reliable. The modified acid-fast stain should be used only to confirm the acid fastness of organisms suspected to be *Nocardia* by Gram staining.

8.7.2 Culture

It is not a fastidious microorganism and hence can be cultured in conventional media like blood agar, chocolate agar, and BACTEC blood culture broth media. Selective media for *Nocardia* includes colistin-nalidixic acid agar, modified Thayer-Martin agar, and buffered charcoal-yeast extract (BCYE) and selective BCYE agars. Selective media can be used to optimize the identification of *Nocardia* when suspicion for the same is high or smear has already revealed *Nocardia*. Colonies appear by 48–72 hrs but sometimes may take as long as 2 weeks. Hence, one should wait for at least 2 weeks before declaring a negative culture to avoid a false negative report. A zone of ß-hemolysis may be observed around the colonies by third day in sheep or bovine blood agar; however, *N. asteroides* are mostly nonhemolytic in sheep blood agar [2]. Since *Nocardia* is not a part of the natural human ocular flora or laboratory environment, its growth, even on a single solid media, is considered positive, unlike other microorganisms [1]. It grows in the form of pellicle on the surface of liquid media, which breaks into small particles on shaking [2].

8.7.3 Confocal Microscopy

The use of confocal microscopy has recently been described as a noninvasive tool for the identification of Nocardial infection. It is especially useful in cases where the lesion is difficult to access for corneal scraping, such as deep corneal infiltrate with an absence of an overlying epithelial defect, keratitis after LASIK, implantation of intracorneal ring segments, following keratoplasty, and in self-sealing wounds after cataract surgery. *Nocardia* appears as hyperreflective, short, thin, and right-angled branching filaments in the background of bright round-to-oval inflammatory cells [19, 23]. They are best visualized at the edge of the infiltrate since the scattered light from the inflammatory cells is least here [23]. These filamentous structures of *Nocardia* can be confused with other linear structures seen on confocal microscopy such as fungal filaments and corneal nerves. Fungal filaments are highly reflective, double-walled, elongated, septate with varying size between 3 to 8 μm (Nocardia, <1.5 μm), runs the entire length of the scanned image and have a uniform width with an irregular branching pattern. While, corneal nerves appear as bright, elongated, uniform (stromal nerves) or beaded (subbasal plexus) structures with acute-angled branching pattern and size between 5 and 20 μm in thickness [23].

8.7.4 Molecular Diagnostic-Based Methods

Identification of this organism at the species level requires advanced molecular tests. These tests include polymerase chain reaction (PCR) and gene sequencing with restriction endonuclease analysis of 16S rRNA gene and restriction fragment length polymorphism analysis of heat shock protein (HSP) gene, DNA sequencing, and pyrosequencing. However, the lack of availability of these testing facilities is often a limiting factor [24].

8.8 Management

Medical management with topical amikacin 2.5% is considered the first-line therapy in Nocardia keratitis [11]. Most of the species are sensitive to topical amikacin with low minimum inhibitory concentration (MIC) values compared to other drugs; however, strains resistant to amikacin have also been reported [25]. Aminoglycosides such as gentamicin and tobramycin are the second-line treatment of this infection. Cotrimoxazole, ciprofloxacin, gatifloxacin, vancomycin, and linezolid are the other treatment options for this microorganism [14, 25, 26]. Systemic treatment with cotrimoxazole has been described for cases not responding to topical therapy [25]. Complete healing with topical poly Hexa-methyl biguanide (PHMB) 0.02% has been reported in a case of *Nocardia* sclerokeratitis [27]. The mean healing time for *Nocardia* keratitis is approximately 38 days [3]. Topical corticosteroids should be avoided in these cases as they increase the risk of corneal perforation and endophthalmitis.

Medical management usually results in clinical resolution in most of the cases. However, surgical intervention is warranted in cases not responding to medical therapy or showing signs of progression despite maximum medical therapy. Lamellar keratectomy can be performed to reduce the infection load and increase the drug penetration cases showing poor response to medical treatment. Therapeutic penetrating keratoplasty is performed for cases with full-thickness corneal ulcers, impending perforation, and perforated corneal ulcers [2, 11].

8.9 Complications

Delay in diagnosis can sometimes result in the extension of the corneal infection to cause *Nocardia* scleritis. Management of such cases often requires surgical intervention in addition to topical amikacin therapy [3]. The surgical intervention in these cases includes scleral debridement to reduce the infective load, tissue adhesive application for impending perforation, and conjunctival excision. The mean healing time is 2 months, which is much longer than that for cases with only corneal involvement [3]. Use of topical PHMB 0.02% and intravenous amikacin has also been reported for this condition [3, 27]. Nocardial infection can also result in endophthalmitis [3]. However, there are no reports of direct extension of corneal infection resulting in endophthalmitis. Management of these cases include pars plana vitrectomy with intravitreal antibiotic injection in addition to topical amikacin therapy [3]. The outcome for both Nocardia keratitis and endophthalmitis is poor. Corneal perforation as a result of a progression of keratitis is another dreaded complication of this condition that may affect the long-term visual outcome and result in blindness if left untreated.

8.10 Outcome

The variability in clinical presentation and lack of familiarity among clinicians and microbiologists with this rare condition often results in a delayed diagnosis. This delay in diagnosis, in conjunction with the lack of response of this microorganism to the routinely used antimicrobial drugs often results in variable outcomes despite the indolent course of the disease [3, 11, 16]. However, complete healing with medical treatment is observed in most of the cases.

The use of steroids is known to worsen the course of *Nocardia* keratitis and, in extreme cases, may result in corneal perforation or endophthalmitis [12, 28]. The 12-month follow-up results of steroids in corneal ulcer treatment trial (SCUT) highlighted that the use of topical steroids in *Nocardia* keratitis resulted in a relatively larger scar size when compared to the nonsteroid group while cases of non-*Nocardia* keratitis treated with steroids showed a nonsignificant reduction in the scar size [28].

Lalitha et al., in a retrospective case series of 32 patients of *Nocardia* keratitis, reported complete healing with medical therapy in 30 cases with the requirement for surgical intervention in only two cases [11]. In this study, 25% of cases were treated with sulfacetamide with or without gentamicin/ciprofloxacin, 31% of cases with gentamicin/ciprofloxacin, and 44% cases with amikacin. Visual acuity improved in 44% cases while it remained the same in 50% cases. The authors observed a faster healing rate in cases treated with topical amikacin. DeCross et al., in the largest case series of *Nocardia* keratitis (111 cases), reported complete healing with medical therapy in 82% cases [3]. Topical amikacin 2.5% was the first line of treatment in all the cases. Systemic cotrimoxazole was added in cases of poor response to topical amikacin therapy. Surgery was performed in cases with poor response to medical treatment and cases having a large corneal ulcer, scleral involvement, corneal thinning, or corneal perforation at the time of presentation. The authors observed that younger age and better visual acuity at presentation resulted in a better final visual acuity [3].

8.11   Conclusion

Nocardia keratitis is a rare cause of infectious keratitis in the world and is more commonly found in Asian countries. It has an indolent course and is often misdiagnosed due to its atypical clinical presentation and lack of familiarity of clinicians with this condition. Pinhead-shaped superficial corneal infiltrate and wreath-like pattern of patchy anterior stromal infiltrate is typical of *Nocardia* keratitis. Grampositive branching filamentous bacteria with 1% acid-fast staining are the key findings for its microbiological diagnosis. Topical amikacin remains the mainstay of treatment, and most of the cases respond well to medical therapy. Early diagnosis and appropriate therapy can salvage vision in most of the cases.

References

1. Sahay P, Goel S, Nagpal R, Maharana PK, Sinha R, Agarwal T, Sharma N, Titiyal JS. Infectious keratitis caused by rare and emerging micro-organisms. Curr Eye Res. 2020;45(7):761–73.
2. Sridhar MS, Gopinathan U, Garg P, Sharma S, Rao GN. Ocular nocardia infections with special emphasis on the cornea. Surv Ophthalmol. 2001;45(5):361–78.
3. DeCroos FC, Garg P, Reddy AK, Sharma A, Krishnaiah S, Mungale M, Mruthyunjaya P, Hyderabad Endophthalmitis Research Group. Optimizing diagnosis and management of nocardia keratitis, scleritis, and endophthalmitis: 11-year microbial and clinical overview. Ophthalmology. 2011;118(6):1193–200.
4. Benedict WL, Iverson HA. Chronic keratoconjunctivitis associated with Nocardia. Arch Ophthalmol. 1944;32(2):89–92.
5. Srinivasan M, Gonzales CA, George C, Cevallos V, Mascarenhas JM, Asokan B, Wilkins J, Smolin G, Whitcher JP. Epidemiology and aetiological diagnosis of corneal ulceration in Madurai, South India. Br J Ophthalmol. 1997;81(11):965–71.
6. Garg P, Rao GN. Corneal ulcer: diagnosis and management. Community Eye Health. 1999;12(30):21–3.
7. Trichet E, Cohen-Bacrie S, Conrath J, Drancourt M, Hoffart L. Nocardia transvalensis keratitis: an emerging pathology among travelers returning from Asia. BMC Infect Dis. 2011;11:296.
8. Wilson JW. Nocardiosis: updates and clinical overview. Mayo Clin Proc. 2012;87(4):403–7.
9. Brown-Elliott BA, Brown JM, Conville PS, Wallace RJ Jr. Clinical and laboratory features of the Nocardia spp. based on current molecular taxonomy. Clin Microbiol Rev. 2006;19(2):259–82.
10. Srinivasan M, Sharma S. Nocardia asteroides as a cause of corneal ulcer. Case report. Arch Ophthalmol. 1987;105(4):464.
11. Lalitha P, Tiwari M, Prajna NV, Gilpin C, Prakash K, Srinivasan M. Nocardia keratitis: species, drug sensitivities, and clinical correlation. Cornea. 2007;26(3):255–9.
12. Lalitha P, Srinivasan M, Rajaraman R, Ravindran M, Mascarenhas J, Priya JL, Sy A, Oldenburg CE, Ray KJ, Zegans ME, McLeod SD, Lietman TM, Acharya NR. Nocardia keratitis: clinical course and effect of corticosteroids. Am J Ophthalmol. 2012;154(6):934–9.

13. Sharma N, O'Hagan S. The role of oral co-trimoxazole in treating Nocardia farcinica keratitis: a case report. J Ophthalmic Inflamm Infect. 2016;6(1):21.
14. Lalitha P. Nocardia keratitis. Curr Opin Ophthalmol. 2009;20(4):318–23.
15. Bharathi MJ, Ramakrishnan R, Meenakshi R, Padmavathy S, Shivakumar C, Srinivasan M. Microbial keratitis in South India: influence of risk factors, climate, and geographical variation. Ophthalmic Epidemiol. 2007;14(2):61–9.
16. Sridhar MS, Sharma S, Reddy MK, Mruthyunjay P, Rao GN. Clinicomicrobiological review of Nocardia keratitis. Cornea. 1998;17(1):17–22.
17. Srirampur A, Mansoori T, Reddy AK, Katta KR, Chandrika TN. Management of Nocardia interface keratitis after descemet membrane endothelial keratoplasty. Cornea. 2019;38(12):1599–601.
18. Garg P, Sharma S, Vemuganti GK, Ramamurthy B. A cluster of Nocardia keratitis after LASIK. J Refract Surg. 2007;23(3):309–12.
19. Javadi MA, Kanavi MR, Zarei-Ghanavati S, Mirbabaei F, Jamali H, Shoja M, Mahdavi M, Naghshgar N, Yazdani S, Faramarzi A. Outbreak of Nocardia keratitis after photorefractive keratectomy: clinical, microbiological, histopathological, and confocal scan study. J Cataract Refract Surg. 2009;35(2):393–8.
20. Garg P. Fungal, Mycobacterial, and Nocardia infections and the eye: an update. Eye. 2012;26(2):245–51.
21. Perry HD, Nauheim JS, Donnenfeld ED. Nocardia asteroides keratitis presenting as a persistent epithelial defect. Cornea. 1989;8(1):41–4.
22. Denk PO, Thanos S, Thiel HJ. Amikacin may be drug of choice in Nocardia keratitis. Br J Ophthalmol. 1996;80(10):928–9.
23. Vaddavalli PK, Garg P, Sharma S, Thomas R, Rao GN. Confocal microscopy for Nocardia keratitis. Ophthalmology. 2006;113(9):1645–50.
24. Saubolle MA, Sussland D. Nocardiosis: review of clinical and laboratory experience. J Clin Microbiol. 2003;41(10):4497–501.
25. Johansson B, Fagerholm P, Petranyi G, Claesson Armitage M, Lagali N. Diagnostic and therapeutic challenges in a case of amikacin-resistant Nocardia keratitis. Acta Ophthalmol. 2017;95(1):103–5.
26. Callegan MC, Ramirez R, Kane ST, Cochran DC, Jensen H. Antibacterial activity of the fourth-generation fluoroquinolones gatifloxacin and moxifloxacin against ocular pathogens. Adv Ther. 2003;20(5):246–52.
27. Prajna NV, Anitha M, Divya R, George C, Srinivasan M. Effect of topical 0.02% polyhexamethylene biguanide on nocardial keratitis associated with scleritis. Indian J Ophthalmol. 1998;46(4):251–2.
28. Srinivasan M, Mascarenhas J, Rajaraman R, Ravindran M, Lalitha P, O'Brien KS, Glidden DV, Ray KJ, Oldenburg CE, Zegans ME, Whitcher JP, McLeod SD, Porco TC, Lietman TM, Acharya NR, Steroids for Corneal Ulcers Trial Group. The steroids for corneal ulcers trial (SCUT): secondary 12-month clinical outcomes of a randomized controlled trial. Am J Ophthalmol. 2014;157(2):327–33.

Acanthamoeba Keratitis

9

Nóra Szentmáry and Berthold Seitz

9.1 Introduction

In Europe, *Acanthamoeba* keratitis (AK) mostly occurs in contact lens wearers. However, in China and India, it may also occur due to direct trauma in rural areas. *Acanthamoeba* keratitis is often misdiagnosed and treated as herpetic, bacterial, or mycotic keratitis, as clinical signs and symptoms may be similar to other kinds of keratitis. In addition, AK is a rare clinical entity. Therefore, diagnosis is often delayed and ophthalmologists tend to observe a heterogeneous and protracted clinical course. Nevertheless, an early diagnosis is essential for the success of the treatment [1, 2].

9.2 Physiology and Life Cycle

Acanthamoeba are ubiquitous, free-living protozoa, present in air, soil, dust, drinking water, and also seawater. There is a dormant resilient cyst and an infective trophozoite form. The so-called vegetative form or trophozoite has a size of 25–40 μm and it is fed from bacteria, algae, and yeasts. Enterobacteria are especially preferred through *Acanthamoeba* but some *Acanthamoeba* species house bacteria as endosymbionts [3].

N. Szentmáry (✉)
Dr. Rolf M. Schwiete Center for Limbal Stem Cell and Aniridia Research, Saarland University, Homburg/Saar, Germany

Department of Ophthalmology, Semmelweis University, Budapest, Hungary
e-mail: nora.szentmary@uks.eu

B. Seitz
Department of Ophthalmology, Saarland University Medical Center, Homburg/Saar, Germany
e-mail: berthold.seitz@uks.eu

© Springer Nature Singapore Pte Ltd. 2021
S. Das, V. Jhanji (eds.), *Infections of the Cornea and Conjunctiva*,
https://doi.org/10.1007/978-981-15-8811-2_9

125

The double-walled cysts have a 13–20 μm size and survive antibiotics, low temperatures (for example, 15 months at −15 °C), high doses of UV-light, and γ-radiation. In case of adverse conditions, *Acanthamoeba* trophozoites form cysts which may survive over 24 years.

Acanthamoeba are classified through their rDNA-sequence-types (T1–T12) (Stothard). AK most often occurs through the T4 genotype. Nevertheless, AK due to genotypes T2, T3, T5, T6, T8, T9, T10, T11, and T15 has also been described [4–10].

9.3   Pathophysiology

In case of a corneal infection, *Acanthamoeba* are first attached to the corneal epithelial cells through the Mannose-binding Protein. This binding supports secretion of metalloproteinase, serin- and cysteinproteinase through *Acanthamoeba*, which results in cytotoxic effects on human corneal epithelial cells and keratocytes and supports deeper corneal penetration of *Acanthamoeba* [11–13]. *Acanthamoeba* may also migrate along corneal nerves and damage these [14–15].

9.4   Epidemiology, Risk Factors, and Prevention

The first reports on *Acanthamoeba* keratitis were published in the 70s [16–17]. With increasing use of contact lenses, AK incidence increased in the 80s [18–20] and it was 1/30,000 contact lens wearer in the 90s (Great Britain, Hong Kong) [21]. Nowadays about 5% of contact lens-associated keratitis is caused by *Acanthamoeba* [22–23].

Main risk factors are extended use of contact lenses (therefore, daily lenses have a lower risk) [24–26], use of contact lenses during bath, and cleaning them with tap water [27]. Additional risk factors are corneal surface damage, exposition to contaminated water, and low socioeconomic status [28–29]. A study has proven that only hydrogen-peroxide containing contact lens cleaners are effective against all *Acanthamoeba* strains [30].

9.4.1   Clinical Symptoms

In early stages of the disease, about 75–90% of all patients are misdiagnosed, as typical *Acanthamoeba* keratitis symptoms are difficult to associate [5, 9]. Analysis of the German *Acanthamoeba Keratitis Registry* has shown that in 47.6% herpetic, in 25.2% mycotic, and in 3.9% bacterial keratitis was erroneously diagnosed by ophthalmologist, in *Acanthamoeba* keratitis patients [31]. Patient had the correct AK diagnosis not before 2.8 ± 4.0 months (range 0–23 months) after appearence of the first clinical symptoms, in Germany from 2001 to 2011 [31]. In about 23% of the cases, a mixed infection with virus, bacteria, or fungi is present [2, 32, 33–35]. Clinical signs of *Acanthamoeba* keratitis are the following: [33–46].

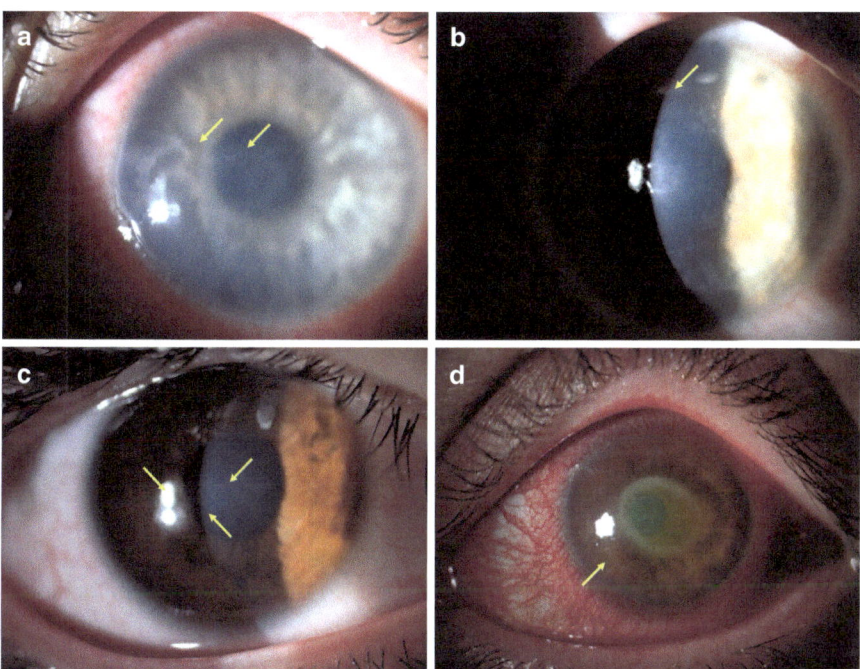

Fig. 9.1 Clinical signs in *Acanthamoeba* keratitis: (**a**) dirty epithelium, (**b**) multifocal stromal infiltrates, (**c**) *Acanthamoeba* dust, and (**d**) ring infiltrate with central epithelial defect

- Chameleon-like epithelial changes ("dirty epithelium," pseudodendritiformic epitheliopathy, epithelial microerosions, and microcysts) (Fig. 9.1a).
- Multifocal stromal infiltrates (Fig. 9.1b) or "dust-like" changes in the corneal stroma (Fig. 9.1c).
- Ring infiltrate ("Wessely immune ring") (Fig. 9.1d).
- Peripheral perineural infiltrate (Fig. 9.2).
- Common complications: broad-based anterior synechiae, secondary glaucoma, iris atrophy, mature cataract (Fig. 9.3), persistent epithelial defect.
- Rare complications: sterile anterior uveitis, scleritis (Fig. 9.3).
- Very rare complications: chorioretinitis and retinal vasculitis.

9.5 Diagnostics

- In case of clinical signs of *Acanthamoeba* keratitis, additional (laboratory) diagnostics always have to be performed. Confocal microscopy is used as in vivo diagnostics, in vitro diagnostics are polymerase chain reaction (PCR), histopathological examination, or microbiological culture [31, 32, 47–49]. The most important is to recognize clinical signs of *Acanthamoeba* keratitis, so that we use the appropriate diagnostic methods, as timely as possible.

Fig. 9.2 Perineuritis in *Acanthamoeba* keratitis (arrow), 4 weeks after first symptoms (contact lens wearer)

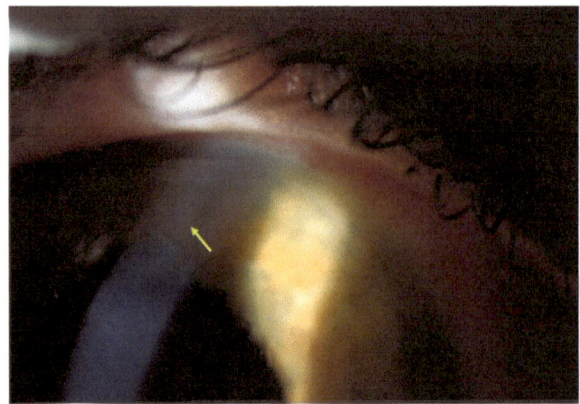

Fig. 9.3 Scleritis, persistent mydriasis, and mature cataract in severe *Acanthamoeba* keratitis

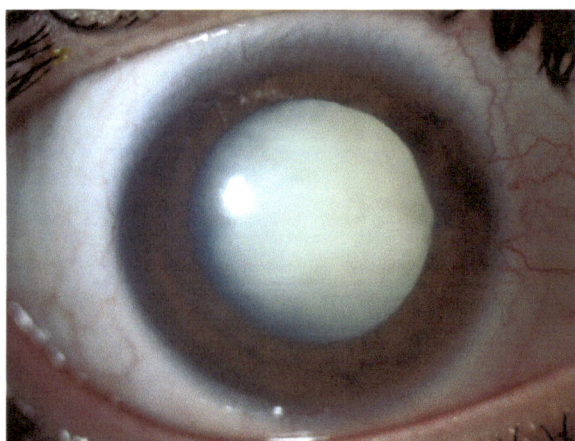

- Polymerase chain reaction (PCR) of corneal scrapings has with 84–100% the highest sensitivity and may give a result within 60 min [50–53].
- However, PCR may have the disadvantage that also not living *Acanthamoeba* genome may give a positive result [3].
- In vivo confocal microscopy has more than 90% sensitivity in experienced hands. However, only *Acanthamoeba* cysts are well recognized using this method [31, 48, 49].
- In vitro culture may have 0–70% sensitivity. This technique uses the fact that *Acanthamoeba* grows well on *Escherichia coli* (*E. coli*) and *Acanthamoeba* forms lines in an *E. coli* covered plate. This method has the disadvantage of giving results only within 3 weeks [54–56]. PCR or in vitro culture may also be used to analyze the contact lens case, which may add information to our diagnostics.
- Presence of *Acanthamoeba* may also be verified through *histopathological analysis*, with 31–65% sensitivity. Corneal scrapings or excision or explanted tissue from keratoplasty may be analyzed using periodic acid-Schiff, Masson, Gram, Giemsa, Grocott-methenamine-silver, or Calcofluor-white stainings. As sensitivity of this diagnostic method is lower than that of PCR, it is used rarely in clinical practice [33, 50, 57].

9.6   Differential Diagnosis

"Dirty epithelium" and pseudodendritiformic epitheliopathy have to be differentiated from an epithelial *herpetic* keratitis (dendritic or geographic). These do not have round spot-like widenings at the endings of the epithelial erosions, unlike herpetic epithelial keratitis.

In absence of bacterial or mycotic superinfection of an AK, the stromal infiltrates in AK are multifocal, dot-like (like unsharp-edged stromal stars), and in part transparent in an early stage of the disease. This may look like a "stromal dust," as it is mostly not accompanied by dense stromal infiltrates. In contrast, bacterial or mycotic stromal infiltrates are dense and typically monofocal and more whitish. Nevertheless, satellite infiltrates in fungal keratitis may imitate multifocal stromal infiltrates of AK.

The Wessely immune ring may be present in bacterial, myctotic, or *Acanthamoeba* keratitis.

9.7   Treatment

There are only case series on safety and effectivity of medical and surgical treatment of *Acanthamoeba* keratitis and there are up-to-date no completed randomized controlled clinical studies. Nevertheless, a first clinical trial is expected to be completed in 2021 (ClinicalTrials.gov Identifier: NCT03274895).

9.7.1   Conservative Treatment

9.7.1.1 Diamidine and Biguanlde

Diamidines, such as propamidine-isethionate (Brolene), hexamidine-diisethionate (Hexacyl), and dibromopropamidine (Golden Eye) are used in 0.1% concentration [58–60]. Biguanides, such as polyhexamethylene-biguanide (polyhexanide) (Lavasept) and chlorhexidine (Curasept) are applied in 0.02% concentration [2]. Nevertheless, an actual clinical trial is analyzing the potential effect of 0.08% polyhexanide in AK (NCT03274895).

The concentration-dependent effect of diamidines and biguanides on human epithelial cells, keratocytes, and endothelial cells has already been described and propamidine-isethionate as diamidine and chlorhexidine as biguanide seem to be the least cytotoxic. However, these may reduce proliferation and migration of human corneal cells more than other diamidines and biguanides [61].

9.7.1.2 Antibiotics

Neomycin kills trophozoites, prevents bacterial superinfection [62], and reduces bacterial load, as food source for *Acanthamoeba* [2].

9.7.1.3 Povidone-Iodine and Miltefosine

An in vitro experiment reported on a better anticystic effect of 1% povidone-iodine as propamidine-isethionate or polyhexamid. However, up to now, clinical studies did not verify these results [63]. Miltefosine was effective against *Acanthamoeba* in vitro [64].

9.7.1.4 Steroids

Topical use of steroids may masquerade clinical signs of *Acanthamoeba* keratitis, as long as these are used. In addition, they support excystment and an increase in number of throphozoites. On contrary, a patient with *Acanthamoeba* keratitis and severe inflammation may benefit from their use. Steroids should never be used without additional topical antiseptics and should never be applied at the early stage of *Acanthamoeba* keratitis treatment (never in the first week even after appropriate diagnosis) [65, 66]. In case of abrupt stopping topical steroids, a Wessely immune ring may develop within 2 days in patients with AK [67].

9.7.1.5 Antifungals

Miconazole and Clotrimazole have been previously used as topical treatment of AK [68, 69]. In addition, there are reports on local and systemic voriconazole used in these patients [68–70]. An in vitro study described better anticystic effect using natamycin in contrast to propamidine-isethionate or polyhexamethylene-biguanide [63]. However, data on clinical use of natamycin in AK patients is not available.

In Germany, we suggest topical application of polyhexamethylene-biguanide, propamidine-isethionate, and Neomycin as triple-therapy in case of AK [2]. During the first two days a "surprise attack" or "flash war" is initiated with polyhexamethylene-biguanide and propamidine-isethionate every quarter to half an hour day and night. Then, until the sixth day, polyhexamethylene-biguanide and propamidine-isethionate are applied every hour and only over the day (6^{00}–24^{00}). The following 4 weeks eyedrop use is reduced to every 2 h. Additionally, neomycin five times a day is also applied [62]. In therapy-resistant cases, we may change polyhexamethylene-biguanide to chlorhexidine or increase concentration (for polyhexamethylene-biguanide to 0.06%, for chlorhexidine to 0.2%).

To the best of our knowledge, combination therapy using diamidine, biguanide, and antibiotics should be continued in descending doses until 1 year. However, in case of nonhealing epithelial defects after penetrating keratoplasty, we may reduce the use of diamidine and biguanide with 1 drop every 2 months.

In our opinion, a specific treatment, following isolation of the pathognomic *Acanthamoeba* strain should be clinically applied in the future, following in vitro culture and testing.

9.8 Surgical Treatment

Through diagnostic and therapeutic epithelial abrasion we remove microorganisms and get a better penetration of topical medication [71]. If topical conservative treatment does not improve clinical signs and symptoms, corneal cryotherapy, amniotic membrane transplantation, or penetrating keratoplasty may be performed. In therapy-resistant cases, a cross linking treatment as photodynamic therapy may be used, in some cases repeatedly.

Corneal cryotherapy is an adjuvant treatment of topical therapy. The infected corneal areas or the recipient area before penetrating keratoplasty will be treated using a Cold Cryoprobe 2–3 times ("freeze-thaw-freeze") until ice crystals are formed in the corneal stroma [72]. As part of a penetrating keratoplasty, cryotherapy is circularly used (about 2–3 s at −80 °C to the recipient bed) before recipient trephination. The effect of this type of cryotherapy on limbal epithelial stem cells is up-to-date not clarified.

An Amniotic Membrane Transplantation (AMT) may be used, for persistent epithelial defects or ulcers as "Patch," "Graft," or "Sandwich" and may help to reach a quiet stage of the eye [73]. In many cases, AMT has to be repeated several times, to reach epithelial closure.

Photodynamic Therapy (PDT) may be an alternative treatment option in therapy-resistant infectious keratitis [74]. The successful use of Riboflavin-UVA cross-linking in Acanthamoeba keratitis has been summarized in a case series in 2011 [75]. Nevertheless, in case of stromal infiltrates, UVA-light penetration to the corneal stroma may be reduced. An accelerated cross linking in *Acanthamoeba* keratitis is not suggested as primary treatment [76].

In case of *Acanthamoeba* keratitis expansion in direction of the corneoscleral limbus, an early penetrating keratoplasty has to be considered, in order to perform the excision in uninfected corneal tissue. In case of progressive, therapy-resistant ulceration over weeks and months, with peripheral reparative neovascularization, we suggest an early (<5 months disease course) penetrating keratoplasty [77] (Figs. 9.4 and 9.5). The origin of frequent therapy-resistant epithelial defects at the transplanted tissue after PKP, is not clarified, yet. Potential treatment options of these epithelial defects are (1) autologous serum, (2) AMT, (3) Cacicol, or (4) Neurotrophic Growth Factor (NGF).

Following penetrating keratoplasty, we continue the use of the above described topical treatment for up to 1 year [2, 78]. However, there are also no controlled

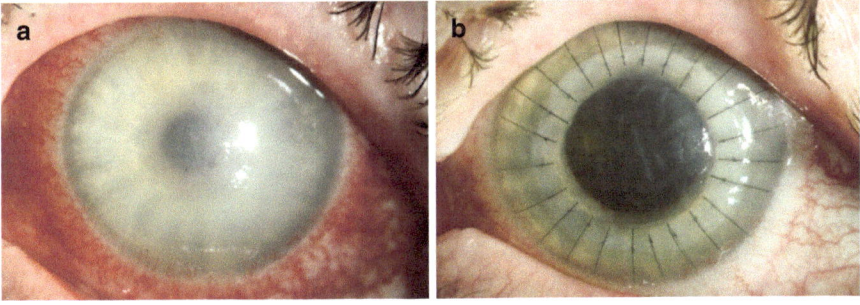

Fig. 9.4 (**a**) Multifocal stromal infiltrates (interstitial keratitis) in *Acanthamoeba* keratitis and (**b**) 2 days after central excimer laser penetrating keratoplasty with interrupted sutures

Fig. 9.5 Central, nonhealing epithelial defect, scleritis, iris atrophy, and mature cataract 14 months after penetrating keratoplasty in *Acanthamoeba* keratitis. There is no light perception. PKP has been performed 10 months after first symptoms of the contact lens-associated disease

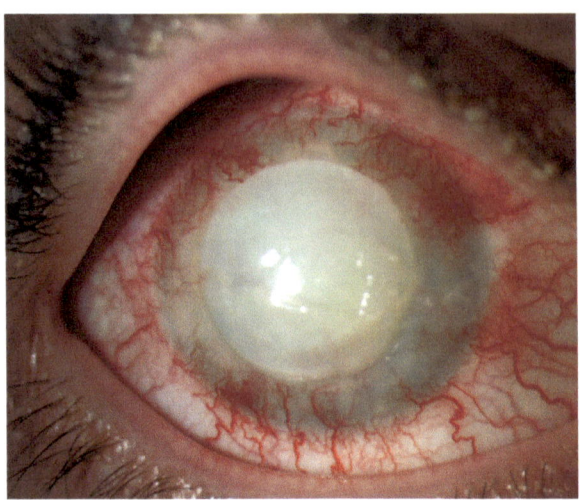

clinical trials related to this topic. Perhaps local therapy may be stopped earlier, in order to avoid persistent epithelial defects, peripheral anterior synechiae, and mature cataract. Confocal microscopy may be useful in diagnosis of AK recurrences [32].

In case of perforated corneal ulcers, a nonmechanical, excimer laser keratoplasty is best performed [78]. Using an elliptical excimer laser trephination with metal masks, we may remove the infected corneal area with a more homogeneous distance from the limbal vessels, especially in typically elliptical-shaped acanthamoeba keratitis [79].

Some authors suggest at least a 3-month-long observation period without inflammatory signs, following discontinuation of conservative therapy, before planning an elective penetrating keratoplasty, following AK. In such elective PKPs, transplant survival may be 100% following 5 years and 67% after 10 years [80–82].

9.9   Conclusion

In summary, *Acanthamoeba* keratitis presents in early stages with grey-dirty epithelium, pseudodendritiformic epitheliopathy, perineuritis, multifocal stromal infiltrates, ring infiltrates and in later stages with scleritis, iris atrophy, anterior synechiae, secondary glaucoma, mature cataract, and chorioretinitis. As conservative treatment, we use up to 1 year triple-topical therapy (polyhexamethylene-biguanide, propamidine-isethionate, neomycin). In therapy-resistant cases, surgical treatment options such as corneal cryotherapy, amniotic membrane transplantation, riboflavin-UVA cross linking, and penetrating keratoplasty may be applied.

Acknowledgments The work of Dr. Szentmáry at the Dr. Rolf M. Schwiete Center for Limbal Stem Cell and Aniridia Research was supported by the Dr. Rolf M. Schwiete Foundation.

References

1. Meltendorf C, Duncker G. [Acanthamoeba keratitis]. Klin Monbl Augenheilkd 2011;228(3):R29–43.
2. Szentmáry N, Goebels S, Matoula P, Schirra F, Seitz B. [Acanthamoeba keratitis—a rare and often late diagnosed disease]. Klin Monatsbl Augenheilkd 2012;229(5):521–8.
3. Weekers PH, Bodelier PL, Wijen JP, Vogels GD. Effects of grazing by the free-living soil amoebae Acanthamoeba castellanii, Acanthamoeba polyphaga, and Hartmannella vermiformis on various bacteria. Appl Environ Microbiol. 1993;59(7):2317–9.
4. Gupta S, Das SR. Stock cultures of free-living amebas: effect of temperature on viability and pathogenicity. J Parasitol. 1999;85(1):137–9.
5. De Jonckheere J, van de Voorde H. Differences in destruction of cysts of pathogenic and nonpathogenic Naegleria and Acanthamoeba by chlorine. Appl Environ Microbiol. 1976;31(2):294–7.
6. Khunkitti W, Lloyd D, Furr JR, Russell AD. Acanthamoeba castellanii: growth, encystment, excystment and biocide susceptibility. J Infect. 1998;36(1):43–8.
7. Brown TJ, Cursons RT. Pathogenic free-living amebae (PFLA) from frozen swimming areas in Oslo, Norway. Scand J Infect Dis. 1977;9(3):237–40.
8. Aksozek A, McClellan K, Howard K, Niederkorn JY, Alizadeh H. Resistance of Acanthamoeba castellanii cysts to physical, chemical, and radiological conditions. J Parasitol. 2002;88(3).621–3.
9. Mazur T, Hadaś E, Iwanicka I. The duration of the cyst stage and the viability and virulence of Acanthamoeba isolates. Trop Med Parasitol. 1995;46(2):106–8.
10. Stothard DR, Hay J, Schroeder-Diedrich JM, Seal DV, Byers TJ. Fluorescent oligonucleotide probes for clinical and environmental detection of Acanthamoeba and the T4 18S rRNA gene sequence type. J Clin Microbiol. 1999;37(8):2687–93.
11. Panjwani N. Pathogenesis of Acanthamoeba keratitis. Ocul Surf. 2010;8(2):70–9.
12. Clarke DW, Niederkorn JY. The pathophysiology of Acanthamoeba keratitis. Trends Parasitol. 2006;22(4):175–80.
13. Hadas E, Mazur T. Proteolytic enzymes of pathogenic and non-pathogenic strains of Acanthamoeba spp. Trop Med Parasitol. 1993;44(3):197–200.
14. Moore MB, McCulley JP, Kaufman HE, Robin JB. Radial keratoneuritis as a presenting sign in Acanthamoeba keratitis. Ophthalmology. 1986;93(10):1310–5.
15. Alfawaz A. Radial keratoneuritis as a presenting sign in acanthamoeba keratitis. Middle East Afr J Ophthalmol. 2011;18(3):252–5.
16. Naginton J, Watson PG, Playfair TJ, McGill J, Jones BR, Steele AD. Amoebic infection of the eye. Lancet. 1974;2(7896):1537–40.
17. Jones DB, Visvesvara GS, Robinson NM. Acanthamoeba polyphaga keratitis and Acanthamoeba uveitis associated with fatal meningoencephalitis. Trans Ophthalmol Soc U K. 1975;95(2):221–32.
18. Ku JY, Chan FM, Beckingsale P. Acanthamoeba keratitis cluster: an increase in Acanthamoeba keratitis in Australia. Clin Exp Ophthalmol. 2009;37(2):181–90.
19. Moore MB, McCulley JP, Newton C, Cobo LM, Foulks GN, O'Day DM, Johns KJ, Driebe WT, Wilson LA, Epstein RJ, et al. Acanthamoeba keratitis. A growing problem in soft and hard contact lens wearers. Ophthalmology. 1987;94(12):1654–61.
20. Schaumberg DA, Snow KK, Dana MR. The epidemic of Acanthamoeba keratitis: where do we stand? Cornea. 1998;17(1):3–10.
21. Seal DV. Acanthamoeba keratitis update-incidence, molecular epidemiology and new drugs for treatment. Eye. 2003;17(8):893–905.
22. Butler TK, Males JJ, Robinson LP, Wechsler AW, Sutton GL, Cheng J, Taylor P, McClellan K. Six-year review of Acanthamoeba keratitis in New South Wales, Australia: 1997-2002. Clin Exp Ophthalmol. 2005;33(1):41–6.

23. Acharya NR, Lietman TM, Margolis TP. Parasites on the rise: a new epidemic of Acanthamoeba keratitis. Am J Ophthalmol. 2007;144(2):292–3.
24. McAllum P, Bahar I, Kaiserman I, Srinivasan S, Slomovic A, Rootman D. Temporal and seasonal trends in Acanthamoeba keratitis. Cornea. 2009;28(1):7–10.
25. Radford CF, Lehmann OJ, Dart JK. Acanthamoeba keratitis: multicentre survey in England 1992-6. National Acanthamoeba Keratitis Study Group. Br J Ophthalmol. 1998;82(12):1387–92.
26. Chew HF, Yildiz EH, Hammersmith KM, Eagle RC Jr, Rapuano CJ, Laibson PR, Ayres BD, Jin YP, Cohen EJ. Clinical outcomes and prognostic factors associated with acanthamoeba keratitis. Cornea. 2011;30(4):435–41.
27. Hammersmith KM. Diagnosis and management of Acanthamoeba keratitis. Curr Opin Ophthalmol. 2006;17(4):327–31.
28. Stehr-Green JK, Bailey TM, Visvesvara GS. The epidemiology of Acanthamoeba keratitis in the United States. Am J Ophthalmol. 1989;107(4):331–6.
29. Sharma S, Garg P, Rao GN. Patient characteristics, diagnosis, and treatment of non-contact lens related Acanthamoeba keratitis. Br J Ophthalmol. 2000;84(10):1103–8.
30. Johnston SP, Sriram R, Qvarnstrom Y, Roy S, Verani J, Yoder J, Lorick S, Roberts J, Beach MJ, Visvesvara G. Resistance of Acanthamoeba cysts to disinfection in multiple contact lens solutions. J Clin Microbiol. 2009;47(7):2040–5.
31. Daas L, Szentmáry N, Eppig T, Langenbucher A, Hasenfus A, Roth M, Saeger M, Nölle B, Lippmann B, Böhringer D, Reinhard T, Kelbsch C, Messmer E, Pleyer U, Roters S, Zhivov A, Engelmann K, Schrecker J, Zumhagen L, Thieme H, Darawsha R, Meyer-Ter-Vehn T, Dick B, Görsch I, Hermel M, Kohlhaas M, Seitz B. [The German Acanthamoeba keratitis register: Initial results of a multicenter study]. Ophthalmologe 2015;112(9):752–63.
32. Dart JK, Saw VP, Kilvington S. Acanthamoeba keratitis: diagnosis and treatment update 2009. Am J Ophthalmol. 2009;148(4):487–99.
33. Claerhout I, Goegebuer A, Van Den Broecke C, Kestelyn P. Delay in diagnosis and outcome of Acanthamoeba keratitis. Graefes Arch Clin Exp Ophthalmol. 2004;242(8):648–53.
34. Awwad ST, Petroll WM, McCulley JP, Cavanagh HD. Updates in Acanthamoeba keratitis. Eye Contact Lens. 2007;33(1):1–8.
35. Perry HD, Donnenfeld ED, Foulks GN, Moadel K, Kanellopoulos AJ. Decreased corneal sensation as an initial feature of Acanthamoeba keratitis. Ophthalmology. 1995;102(10):1565–8.
36. Patel DV, McGhee CN. Acanthamoeba keratitis: a comprehensive photographic reference of common and uncommon signs. Clin Exp Ophthalmol. 2009;37(2):232–8.
37. Papathanassiou M, Gartry D. Sterile corneal ulcer with ring infiltrate and hypopyon after recurrent erosions. Eye. 2007;21(1):124–6.
38. Thomas KE, Purcell TL, Tanzer DJ, Schanzlin DJ. Delayed diagnosis of microsporidial stromal keratitis: unusual Wessely ring presentation and partial treatment with medications against Acanthamoeba. BMJ Case Rep. 2011; 2011.
39. Kremer I, Cohen EJ, Eagle RC Jr, Udell I, Laibson PR. Histopathologic evaluation of stromal inflammation in Acanthamoeba keratitis. CLAO J. 1994;20(1):45–8.
40. Clarke DW, Alizadeh H, Niederkorn JY. Failure of Acanthamoeba castellanii to produce intraocular infections. Invest Ophthalmol Vis Sci. 2005;46(7):2472–8.
41. Shigeyasu C, Shimazaki J. Ocular surface reconstruction after exposure to high concentrations of antiseptic solutions. Cornea. 2012;31(1):59–65.
42. Awwad ST, Heilman M, Hogan RN, Parmar DN, Petroll WM, McCulley JP, Cavanagh HD. Severe reactive ischemic posterior segment inflammation in acanthamoeba keratitis: a new potentially blinding syndrome. Ophthalmology. 2007;114(2):313–20.
43. Shi L, Hager T, Fries FN, Daas L, Holbach L, Hofmann-Rummelt C, Zemova E, Seitz B, Szentmáry N. Reactive uveitis, retinal vasculitis and scleritis as ocular end-stage of Acanthamoeba keratitis: a histological study. Int J Ophthalmol. 2019;12(12):1966–71.
44. Ehlers N, Hjortdal J. Are cataract and iris atrophy toxic complications of medical treatment of acanthamoeba keratitis? Acta Ophthalmol Scand. 2004;82(2):228–31.

45. Herz NL, Matoba AY, Wilhelmus KR. Rapidly progressive cataract and iris atrophy during treatment of Acanthamoeba keratitis. Ophthalmology. 2008;115(5):866–9.
46. Kelley PS, Dossey AP, Patel D, Whitson JT, Hogan RN, Cavanagh HD. Secondary glaucoma associated with advanced acanthamoeba keratitis. Eye Contact Lens. 2006;32(4):178–82.
47. Daas L, Viestenz A, Schnabel PA, Fries FN, Hager T, SzentmÁry N, Seitz B. Confocal microscopy as an early relapse marker for acanthamoeba keratitis. Clin Anat. 2018;31(1):60–3.
48. Pfister DR, Cameron JD, Krachmer JH, Holland EJ. Confocal microscopy findings of Acanthamoeba keratitis. Am J Ophthalmol. 1996;121(2):119–28.
49. Duguid IG, Dart JK, Morlet N, Allan BD, Matheson M, Ficker L, Tuft S. Outcome of acanthamoeba keratitis treated with polyhexamethyl biguanide and propamidine. Ophthalmology. 1997;104(10):1587–92.
50. Lehmann OJ, Green SM, Morlet N, Kilvington S, Keys MF, Matheson MM, Dart JK, McGill JI, Watt PJ. Polymerase chain reaction analysis of corneal epithelial and tear samples in the diagnosis of Acanthamoeba keratitis. Invest Ophthalmol Vis Sci. 1998;39(7):1261–5.
51. Qvarnstrom Y, Visvesvara GS, Sriram R, da Silva AJ. Multiplex real-time PCR assay for simultaneous detection of Acanthamoeba spp., Balamuthia mandrillaris, and Naegleria fowleri. J Clin Microbiol. 2006;44(10):3589–95.
52. Thompson PP, Kowalski RP, Shanks RM, Gordon YJ. Validation of real-time PCR for laboratory diagnosis of Acanthamoeba keratitis. J Clin Microbiol. 2008;46(10):3232–6.
53. Mathers WD, Sutphin JE, Folberg R, Meier PA, Wenzel RP, Elgin RG. Outbreak of keratitis presumed to be caused by Acanthamoeba. Am J Ophthalmol. 1996;121(2):129–42.
54. Reinhard T, Behrens-Baumann W. [Anti-infective drug therapy in ophthalmology—part 4: acanthamoeba keratitis]. Klin Monatsbl Augenheilkd 2006;223(6):485–92.
55. Aspöck H. Grundzüge der Diagnostik. In: Hiepe T, Lucius R, Gottstein B (Hrsg) Allgemeine Parasitologie mit den Grundzügen der Immunologie, Diagnostik und Bekämpfung. Stuttgart: Parey in MVS Medizinverlage; 2006. p. 339–457.
56. Bacon AS, Frazer DG, Dart JK, Matheson M, Ficker LA, Wright P. A review of 72 consecutive cases of Acanthamoeba keratitis, 1984-1992. Eye. 1993;7(Pt-6):719–25.
57. Sharma S, Athmanathan S, Ata-Ur-Rasheed M, Garg P, Rao GN. Evaluation of immunoperoxidase staining technique in the diagnosis of Acanthamoeba keratitis. Indian J Ophthalmol. 2001;49(3):181–6.
58. Larkin DF, Kilvington S, Dart JK. Treatment of Acanthamoeba keratitis with polyhexamethylene biguanide. Ophthalmology. 1992;99(2):185–91.
59. Ficker L, Seal D, Warhurst D, Wright P. Acanthamoeba keratitis—resistance to medical therapy. Eye. 1990;4(Pt-6):835–8.
60. Wright P, Warhurst D, Jones BR. Acanthamoeba keratitis successfully treated medically. Br J Ophthalmol. 1985;69(10):778–82.
61. Shi L, Stachon T, Seitz B, Wagenpfeil S, Langenbucher A, Szentmáry N. The effect of anti-amoebic agents on viability, proliferation and migration of human epithelial cells, keratocytes and endothelial cells, in vitro. Curr Eye Res. 2018;43(6):725–33.
62. Elder MJ, Kilvington S, Dart JK. A clinicopathologic study of in vitro sensitivity testing and Acanthamoeba keratitis. Invest Ophthalmol Vis Sci. 1994;35(3):1059–64.
63. Sunada A, Kimura K, Nishi I, Toyokawa M, Ueda A, Sakata T, Suzuki T, Inoue Y, Ohashi Y, Asari S, Iwatani Y. In vitro evaluations of topical agents to treat Acanthamoeba keratitis. Ophthalmology. 2014;121(10):2059–65.
64. Polat ZA, Walochnik J, Obwaller A, Vural A, Dursun A, Arici MK. Miltefosine and polyhexamethylene biguanide: a new drug combination for the treatment of Acanthamoeba keratitis. Clin Exp Ophthalmol. 2014;42(2):151–8.
65. McClellan K, Howard K, Niederkorn JY, Alizadeh H. Effect of steroids on Acanthamoeba cysts and trophozoites. Invest Ophthalmol Vis Sci. 2001;42(12):2885–93.
66. Carnt N, Robaei D, Watson SL, Minassian DC, Dart JK. The impact of topical corticosteroids used in conjunction with antiamoebic therapy on the outcome of Acanthamoeba keratitis. Ophthalmology. 2016;123(5):984–90.

67. Szentmáry N, Daas L, Shi L, Laurik KL, Lepper S, Milioti G, Seitz B. Acanthamoeba keratitis—clinical signs, differential diagnosis and treatment. J Curr Ophthalmol. 2018;31(1):16–23.
68. D'Aversa G, Stern GA, Driebe WT Jr. Diagnosis and successful medical treatment of Acanthamoeba keratitis. Arch Ophthalmol. 1995;113(9):1120–3.
69. Amoils SP, Heney C. Acanthamoeba keratitis with live isolates treated with cryosurgery and fluconazole. Am J Ophthalmol. 1999;127(6):718–20.
70. Oldenburg CE, Acharya NR, Tu EY, Zegans ME, Mannis MJ, Gaynor BD, Whitcher JP, Lietman TM, Keenan JD. Practice patterns and opinions in the treatment of acanthamoeba keratitis. Cornea. 2011;30(12):1363–8.
71. Brooks JG Jr, Coster DJ, Badenoch PR. Acanthamoeba keratitis. Resolution after epithelial debridement. Cornea. 1994;13(2):186–9.
72. Klüppel M, Reinhard T, Sundmacher R, Daicker B. [Therapy of advanced amoeba keratitis with keratoplasty à chaud and adjuvant cryotherapy]. Ophthalmologe 1997;94(2):99–103.
73. Seitz B, Resch MD, Schlötzer-Schrehardt U, Hofmann-Rummelt C, Sauer R, Kruse FE. Histopathology and ultrastructure of human corneas after amniotic membrane transplantation. Arch Ophthalmol. 2006;124(10):1487–90.
74. Szentmáry N, Goebels S, Bischoff M, Seitz B. [Photodynamic therapy for infectious keratitis]. Ophthalmologe 2012;109(2):165–70.
75. Khan YA, Kashiwabuchi RT, Martins SA, Castro-Combs JM, Kalyani S, Stanley P, Flikier D, Behrens A. Riboflavin and ultraviolet light a therapy as an adjuvant treatment for medically refractive Acanthamoeba keratitis: report of 3 cases. Ophthalmology. 2011;118(2):324–31.
76. Cristian C, Marco CDV, Arturo K, Claudio P, Miguel S, Rolf R, Remigio L, Leonidas T. Accelerated collagen cross-linking in the management of advanced Acanthamoeba keratitis. Arq Bras Oftalmol. 2019;82(2):103–6.
77. Laurik KL, Szentmáry N, Daas L, Langenbucher A, Seitz B. Early penetrating keratoplasty à chaud may improve outcome in therapy-resistant Acanthamoeba keratitis. Adv Ther. 2019;36(9):2528–40.
78. Hager T, Hasenfus A, Stachon T, Seitz B, Szentmáry N. Crosslinking and corneal cryotherapy in acanthamoeba keratitis—a histological study. Graefes Arch Clin Exp Ophthalmol. 2016;254(1):149–53.
79. Seitz B, Langenbucher A, Kus MM, Küchle M, Naumann GO. Nonmechanical corneal trephination with the excimer laser improves outcome after penetrating keratoplasty. Ophthalmology. 1999;106(6):1156–64; discussion 1165.
80. Szentmáry N, Langenbucher A, Kus MM, Naumann GO, Seitz B. Elliptical nonmechanical corneal trephination: intraoperative complications and long-term outcome of 42 consecutive excimer laser penetrating keratoplasties. Cornea. 2007;26(4):414–20.
81. Robaei D, Carnt N, Minassian DC, Dart JK. Therapeutic and optical keratoplasty in the management of Acanthamoeba keratitis: risk factors, outcomes, and summary of the literature. Ophthalmology. 2015;122(1):17–24.
82. Iovieno A, Gore DM, Carnt N, Dart JK. Acanthamoeba sclerokeratitis: epidemiology, clinical features, and treatment outcomes. Ophthalmology. 2014;121(12):2340–7.

Sujata Das, Smruti Rekha Priyadarshini, and Aravind Roy

10.1 Introduction

Microsporidia are eukaryotic unicellular organisms belonging to phylum Microspora and kingdom Protista [1 3]. Recently, it has been classified as fungi [4]. It infects both vertebrates and invertebrates. Microsporidiosis occurs worldwide. The prevalence varies depending on the region, method of diagnosis, and characteristic of population. This pathogen can affect eye, respiratory tract, intestine, muscles, kidneys, and central nervous system.

10.2 Organism

The number of microsporidian species are estimated to be between 1000 to 1500. The common genera involved in human disease are *Encephalitozoon (Septata)*, *Nosema*, *Vittaforma*, *Pleistophora*, *Trachipleistophora*, and *Anncaliia (Brachiola)* [4].

Microsporidia exists as a single highly organized spore [5]. The size of the spore varies from 1 to 40 μm. The intracellular spore is the infective form of the organism. A normal unit membrane and two rigid extracellular walls bind the spores. Within the spore membrane is the sporoplasm, which is infective material of microsporidia. The most obvious organelle associated with infection is the polar filament or the polar tube. The polar filament is attached to the apex of the spore via anchoring disk,

S. Das (✉) · S. R. Priyadarshini
Cornea and Anterior Segment Service, L V Prasad Eye Institute, Bhubaneswar, Odisha, India
e-mail: sujatadas@lvpei.org; drsmruti@lvpei.org

A. Roy
Cornea & Anterior Segment Service, L V Prasad Eye Institute,
Vijayawada, Andhra Pradesh, India
e-mail: aravindroy@lvpei.org

© Springer Nature Singapore Pte Ltd. 2021
S. Das, V. Jhanji (eds.), *Infections of the Cornea and Conjunctiva*,
https://doi.org/10.1007/978-981-15-8811-2_10

from which it extends to the posterior end of the spore. The number of coils and their arrangement is diagnostic of particular species [6]. Inside the host cell, there are two distinct phases in the development of microsporidia: a proliferative phase (merogony) and a sporogonic phase (sporogony).

10.3 Risk Factors

Although fecal-oral transmission is the likely route of intestinal microsporidiosis, the source of ocular infection is not clear. There are two distinct clinical microsporidial corneal infections: keratoconjunctivitis and stromal keratitis. Several cases of microsporidial keratoconjunctivitis have been reported in patients infected with human immunodeficiency virus (HIV) [7–10]. However, keratoconjunctivitis has been reported in healthy individuals in recent reports [11–14]. Systemic immunosuppression has been associated with keratoconjunctivitis [15]. The contact lens may act as a vector for an organism to reach the cornea, either by prolonging retention on the ocular surface or by the colonization of organism on contact lens reaching the eye [16, 17].

Topical corticosteroid may predispose to microsporidial infection by local immunosuppression. It has been reported in a corneal graft [18]. Association with trauma has been reported [12, 13]. Close contact with domestic animals may be a source of ocular infection [9, 19]. Exposure to muddy water has been described as a risk factor for keratoconjunctivitis [17].

10.4 Clinical Features

Microsporidia primarily affects the cornea and may present either in the form of superficial epithelial keratopathy or deep stromal keratitis. Rarely uvea and sclera have been reported to be involved [20]. In the past, the two clinical entities have been described, the superficial epithelial variant commonly seen in immunocompromised persons and the deep stromal keratitis seen in immunocompetent individuals [20]. Keratoconjunctivitis is mostly caused by the genus Encephalitozoon and stromal keratitis by Nosema and Microsporidium [13].

10.4.1 Keratoconjunctivitis

The first case of microsporidial infection was reported by Lowder et al. [21] in a young seropositive man who had a chronic history of conjunctivitis nonresponding to topical antibiotics. Patients present with history of "red eye" presumed to be of viral etiology and are often pretreated with steroids. They complain of unilateral or rarely bilateral pain, redness, photophobia, and watering along with blurring of vision. Past history of trauma or exposure to environmental agents such as dust, dirty water, soil, insects, or bathing in unclean river water may be present.

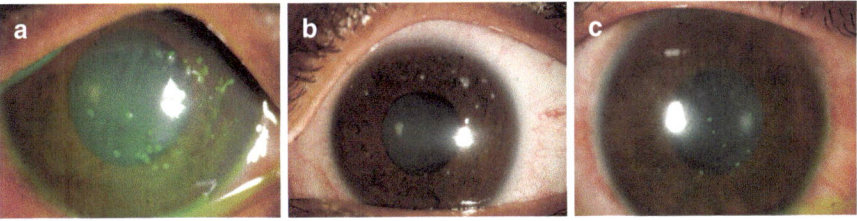

Fig. 10.1 Slit lamp photograph in diffuse illumination (**a–c**) showing diffuse, multifocal, coarse, minute, punctate raised epithelial lesions

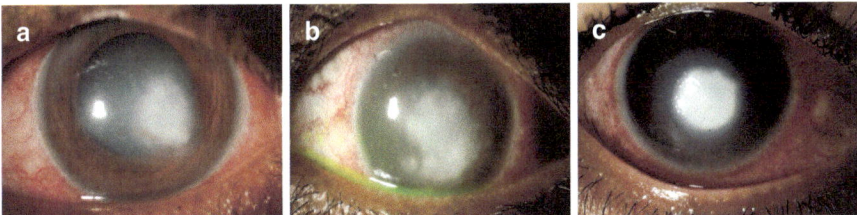

Fig. 10.2 Slit lamp photograph in diffuse illumination showing: (**a, b**) dense grayish infiltrate with surrounding edema and (**c**) well-defined central stromal infiltrate

Slit lamp biomicroscopy reveals diffuse, multifocal, elevated, coarse, and round-oval lesions with characteristic "stuck on" appearance (Fig. 10.1). These lesions may be epithelial, subepithelial, or involve anterior stroma. They may or may not stain positively with fluorescein. Surrounding conjunctiva appears mild-moderately congested, nonpurulent with papillary and/or follicular response [13]. Lewis et al. have reported a case of microsporidial keratoconjunctivitis in a 33-year-old immunocompetent patient who had follicular conjunctivitis and diffuse punctate lesions with anterior stromal involvement [22]. Fresh, pigmented keratic precipitates were reported in 20.1% of patients presenting with superficial keratoconjunctivitis and appeared 6.9 ± 2.7 days after presentation [12]. Multiple "target like" epithelial lesions along with classic punctate lesions were described by Raymond and coworkers [17]. Recent reports have shown that microsporidial keratoconjunctivitis can occur in healthy immunocompetent individuals contrary to previously published reports. It occurs more commonly than believed and the punctate lesions can be mistaken easily for adenoviral infection even to trained eyes.

10.4.2 Stromal Keratitis

Stromal keratitis has an indolent course and can affect individuals of any age. This entity is less common than the superficial variant. First reported in 1991, it clinically resembles HSV keratitis and often treated with antivirals and steroids with no response. Clinically, it presents with diffuse congestion, grayish white stromal infiltration, and edema without suppuration (Fig. 10.2). It may have a chronic course with corneal opacity with vascularization [23]. Anterior chamber involvement manifesting as cellular reaction is common.

Case report of microsporidial keratoconjunctivitis causing sclerouveitis and retinal detachment has been reported [24]. Spores of microsporidia were detected in vitrectomy samples. Endophthalmitis has been reported in patients suffering from Acute myelogenous leukemia [25]. Limbitis can also develop in requiring addition of topical corticosteroids.

10.5 Differential Diagnosis

10.5.1 Keratoconjunctivitis

	Microsporidia	Adenoviral	Thygeson's SPK
Laterality	Usually unilateral	Bilateral in 70% cases	Asymmetrically bilateral
Lesions	Multifocal, elevated, coarse, round-oval lesions, "stuck-on" appearance	Multifocal, fine punctate subepithelial infiltrates as a result of cellular reaction against viral antigens	Coarse, oval shaped, slightly raised lesions
Appearance of lesions	Appears in one phase	Gradually appear	Evanescent pattern
Location	Epithelial, subepithelial, anterior stromal	Subepithelial	Classically intraepithelial, but can be subepithelial and anterior stromal
Staining pattern (fluorescein)	Stains positively and negatively	Stains positively	Stains minimally
Duration	Mean duration of symptoms was 7.7 ± 6.2 (range: 1–60) days	1–2 weeks but may persist for longer duration	2 months to 41 years
Conjunctival involvement	Papillary and or follicular reaction	Follicular conjunctivitis	Rarely involved
Treatment	Lubricants	Lubricants and topical steroids, PTK	Topical steroids, tacrolimus, cyclosporine, BCL, PTK
Scarring	Rarely scars only if subepithelial	Usually subepithelial haze and scarring noticed	Scars when Bowman's membrane and anterior stroma involved
Systemic associations	None	Pharyngoconjunctival fever	Viral associations- *Varicella zoster*, HSV, HLADR3

10.5.2 Stromal Keratitis

Microsporidial stromal keratitis presents as multifocal, dense grayish infiltrates with surrounding edema, endoexudates, and keratic precipitates with or without vascularization. The abovementioned clinical features along with prolong history of recurrent redness with partial and no response to steroids should create a high index of suspicion for microsporidial etiology [26].

10.5.2.1 HSV Stromal Keratitis

HSV stromal keratitis can present primarily in two forms: the commoner being non-necrotizing variant and the less common necrotizing one. Microsporidial stromal keratitis is often misdiagnosed as non-necrotizing variant due to its indolent nature and early response to steroids. It present as a focal, multifocal, or diffuse infiltration associated with scarring, thinning, and vascularization.

10.5.3 Acanthamoeba Keratitis

Acanthamoeba keratitis patients present with severe pain out of proportion to the clinical signs. Few typical features seen in the early stage are punctate keratopathy, pseudodendrites, epithelial and subepithelial infiltrates, and classic perineural infiltrates. Later may develop anterior uveitis, hypopyon, and occasionally lead to endothelial plaque and disciform like stromal edema. History of previous contact lens wear may be helpful in clinching towards the diagnosis. However, microbiological workup is necessary to confirm the diagnosis [27].

10.6   Diagnosis

There are several methods to detect microsporidia. Ocular specimens are submitted as corneal scrapings and corneal biopsy. Formalin (5–10%) fixation is required for routine histopathology, glutaraldehyde for electron microscopy, and fresh specimens for molecular methods and cell cultures [28].

10.6.1 Smears and Stains

Staining techniques that have been recommended for the detection of microsporidial spores include Gram, Giemsa, 10% potassium hydroxide with calcofluor white (KOH + CFW) wet mount, modified Ziehl–Neelsen, modified trichrome, and immunofluorescence tests. In a retrospective analysis of the relative performance of four standard techniques for detection of Microsporidia included Gram, Giemsa, 10% KOH + CFW, and Ziehl–Neelsen staining. Ziehl–Neelsen and 10% KOH + CFW were found to be most sensitive in the identification of the spores followed by Gram and Giemsa. Giemsa was reported to have the least efficacious among the four techniques [29].

10.6.2 Histopathology and Tissue Stains

Numerous stains have been described for detection of spores in histopathology specimens comprising biopsy and scrapings. Tissue gram stain (Brown-Hopps and Brown-Brenn) show birefringence of the spores that distinguishes them from intracytoplasmic granules, debris, etc. Spores appear as oval nonbudding intracellular or extracellular structures. Gram stain, Giemsa, calcofluor white, modified Ziehl–Neelsen (1% H_2SO_4), and Warthin-Starry (silver stain) are most effective in detecting spores. Hematoxylin and Eosin stains the spores as refractile gold bodies and is not reliable in routine formalin-fixed specimens [20, 28].

10.6.3 Transmission Electron Microscopy (TEM)

TEM remains the gold standard for detection and species identification of microsporidial spores. Microsporidial spores have a characteristic polar tubule that is required to inject contents of the sporoplasm intracellularly. However, TEM is not easily accessible to most laboratories, and species-level identification may need additional molecular or cell culture techniques [28, 30].

10.6.4 Confocal Microscopy

Confocal microscopy is a useful method to scan the cornea in vivo and an useful noninvasive adjunct for the diagnosis of infective keratitis [31]. Tiny intraepithelial opacities were seen in epithelial keratitis that were corroborated to be microsporidia in chromatrope stains of conjunctival scraping [32]. Microsporidia appear as hyperreflective dots in between keratocytes against a dark background of the confocal image in deep stromal keratitis. The spores are aligned along the corneal lamella in microsporidial stromal disease [33]. The hyperreflective dots suggestive of spores disappeared on treatment. Thus, confocal microscopy assists in imaging and monitoring the progress of deep-seated corneal lesions.

10.6.5 Antigen-Based Assays

Antigen-based detection of microsporidia uses antibodies to identify species of microsporidia by immunofluorescence assay (IFA) as antibodies against particular species are available [34]. Washed spores of Encephalitazoon are injected into mice to produce antiserum which was adsorbed with formalin fixed fecal debris to remove cross reacting antibodies. Pooled antiserum was tagged with fluorescein to stain histopathology specimens. Microsporidia spores showed apple green fluorescence [34, 35]. An experiment comparing three stains—calcofluor white, modified trichrome blue, and IFA with TEM as a standard of reference—reported sensitivity of 83.3% for IFA as opposed to 100% sensitivity of calcofluor white and modified trichrome blue. Specificity was higher at 96% with IFA technique. This is important for species identification if species-specific antibodies are available [35, 36].

10.6.6 Cell Culture

Microsporidia are obligate intracellular parasites that can be cultivated in a variety of cell lines by primary cell cultures. These include monkey and rabbit kidney (vero and RK13), Madin-Darby canine kidney, human fetal lung fibroblasts (MRC-%), etc. The monolayer cell culture can help to propagate the parasite by replenishing the growth medium and allows harvesting of large number of spores. In a comparison of growth-promoting properties of three cell lines for four types of microsporidial species, Joseph et al. reported good growth in SIRC cells for *E. cuniculi* and *E. intestinalis* at an inoculum size of 1×10 [4] spores/ml compared to HeLa cell lines [37]. The technique of cultivating microsporidia from cell lines is time consuming, expensive, and with limited availability to a few laboratories. However, inclusion of cell lines whenever available improves the diagnostic yield and is an important step for developing molecular diagnostic methods.

10.6.7 PCR-Based Molecular Methods

Polymerase chain reaction (PCR) based assays have improved the sensitivity and specificity of detection of Microsporidia. Small and large subunit rRNA and intergenic sequences have highly conserved regions that may be amplified and detected as a target sequence. A sequencing and BLAST analysis helps in validating the results. Joseph et al. have reported the use of pan microsporidian 16S rRNA for identification of *E. hellum*, *E. cuniculi*, and *E. intestinalis* in ocular samples for patients with microsporidial keratitis [38]. They have reported a sensitivity of 83% and specificity of 98%. Due to limitation of PCR-based assays such as laborious and reagent consuming processes of extraction of microsporidian DNA and design of species-specific primers, an alternative technique is an oligonucleotide probe. Species-specific oligonucleotide microarray probes produced from specific 18S SSU-rRNA genes immobilized on a microchip can detect four microsporidian species. Clinical samples detected that coinfection with various species is quite common. This technique can reliably detect samples containing as less as 100 spores [39].

10.7 Treatment

Microsporidia can affect individuals irrespective of immune status. It may cause ocular manifestations such as keratoconjunctivitis or stromal keratitis. Several drugs have been described for the treatment, viz., fluoroquinolone, fumagillin, albendazole, and itraconazole. The management of microsporidia can be described under two subcategories: keratoconjunctivitis and stromal keratitis.

No definitive treatment regimen exists for microsporidial keratoconjunctivitis. While several drugs have been reported to have a therapeutic effect the condition is known to resolve on its own. A single-center double-masked randomized control trial subdivided 145 patients in two arms of 0.05% polyhexamethylene biguanide (PHMB) versus lubricants for management of microsporidial keratoconjunctivitis. The mean resolution time was 4.9 ± 2.2 and 4.6 ± 2.3 days with PHMB and lubricants, respectively. The study conclusively provided evidence of the self-limiting nature of the condition [40]. In a retrospective case series, topical fluoroquinolones, fumagillin 0.3%, and oral albendazole were administered. The study recommended topical monotherapy with fluoroquinolones as a viable first-line treatment option in microsporidial keratitis, the visual acuity was largely unaffected and associated corneal edema and limbitis needed adjuvant corticosteroid treatment [17]. Debridement of the epithelial lesions has also been reported to have beneficial effects in debulking the cornea of infective load and hastening resolution [41]. Despite a multitude of treatment options microsporidial keratoconjunctivitis remains a self-limited disease with 75% of patients regaining 20/30 vision or better with a mean resolution time of 6.0 ± 2.9 days with no specific treatment or placebo [12].

Microsporidial stromal keratitis is the possible diagnosis in chronic culture-negative stromal keratitis. Fumagillin, a methionine aminopeptidase 2 inhibitor, has been described on the management of microsporidial stromal keratitis. Topical chlorhexidine gluconate 0.02% in combination with albendazole has been described for management of stromal keratitis. It requires long-term therapy of several weeks duration [42].

The definitive treatment of microsporidial stromal keratitis remains surgical as the disease tends to smolder in the deeper stromal layers. Often the topical drugs are unable to eliminate deep stromal infection and the treatment options include deep anterior lamellar keratoplasty (DALK) or full thickness penetrating keratoplasty (PKP). Big bubble DALK with removal of all stromal tissue may lead to complete eradication of the disease without recurrences and has been described to have a favorable outcome in stromal microsporidiosis [43]. Microsporidial spores have been reported to cross the Descemet's membrane and are also found in the anterior chamber exudates [44]. Recurrences have been described post DALK for microsporidial stromal keratitis if there is insufficient removal of the stromal layers or the organism has crossed the Descemet's membrane [45].

Microsporidial stromal keratitis may present as a slow indolent deep stromal keratitis of 1 month to several years duration. There is no definitive treatment for this condition and often the disease natural history is marred by episodic inflammation, corneal thinning, and recurrences. It has also been reported to cross the Descemet's membrane. Therefore, the definitive treatment includes complete removal of the diseased cornea by performing full thickness PKP in order to eradicate the infection and achieve disease-free remission [46]. In a large case series of 34 patients of microbiologically proven microsporidial stromal keratitis, five patients responded to topical PHMB 0.02% and Chlorhexidine 0.02% with formation of a vascularized corneal scar. Twenty five patients required keratoplasty of which 21 were full thickness grafts. All the patients had control of infection post PKP. Five of 25 grafts were clear at the end of 1 year of follow-up. The only case of recurrence was noted in a patient who had DALK and seven patients were lost to follow-up. The study concluded that surgical excision is the best management option for the treatment of microsporidial stromal keratitis [47]. Post penetrating keratoplasty treatment regimen included use of topical corticosteroids as in routine PKP procedures.

References

1. Weber R, Bryan RT, Schwartz DA, Owen RL. Human microsporidial infections. Clin Microbiol Rev. 1994;7(4):426–61.
2. Friedberg DN, Ritterband DC. Ocular microsporidiosis. In: Wittner M, Weiss LM, editors. The microsporidia and microsporidiosis. Washington DC: ASM Press; 1999. p. 293–313.
3. Keeling PJ, Fast NM. Microsporidia: biology and evolution of highly reduced intracellular parasites. Annu Rev Microbiol. 2002;56:93–116.
4. Franzen C. Microsporidia: a review of 150 years of research. Open Parasitol J. 2008;2:1–34.
5. Vávra J, Larsson JIR. Structure of the microsporidia. In: Wittner M, Weiss LM, editors. The microsporidia and microsporidiosis. Washington DC: ASM Press; 1999. p. 7–84.
6. Sprague V, Becnel JJ, Hazard EI. Taxonomy of phylum microspora. Crit Rev Microbiol. 1992;18(5–6):285–395.
7. Friedberg DN, Stenson SM, Orenstein JM, Tierno PM, Charles NC. Microsporidial keratoconjunctivitis in acquired immunodeficiency syndrome. Arch Ophthalmol. 1990;108(4):504–8.
8. Lowder CY, McMahon JT, Meisler DM, Dodds EM, Calabrese LH, Didier ES, Cali A. Microsporidial keratoconjunctivitis caused by Septata intestinalis in a patient with acquired immunodeficiency syndrome. Am J Ophthalmol. 1996;121(6):715–7.
9. McCluskey PJ, Goonan PV, Marriott DJ, Field AS. Microsporidial keratoconjunctivitis in AIDS. Eye. 1993;7(1):80–3.
10. Yee RW, Tio FO, Martinez JA, Held KS, Shadduck JA, Didier ES. Resolution of microsporidial epithelial keratopathy in a patient with AIDS. Ophthalmology. 1991;98(2):196 201.
11. Chan CM, Theng JT, Li L, Tan DT. Microsporidial keratoconjunctivitis in healthy individuals: a case series. Ophthalmology. 2003;110(7):1420–5.
12. Das S, Sharma S, Sahu SK, Nayak SS, Kar S. Diagnosis, clinical features and treatment outcome of microsporidial keratoconjunctivitis. Br J Ophthalmol. 2012;96(6):793–5.
13. Joseph J, Sridhar MS, Murthy S, Sharma S. Clinical and microbiological profile of microsporidial keratoconjunctivitis in southern India. Ophthalmology. 2006;113(4):531–7.
14. Agashe R, Radhakrishnan N, Pradhan S, Srinivasan M, Prajna VN, Lalitha P. Clinical and demographic study of microsporidial keratoconjunctivitis in South India: a 3-year study (2013-2015). Br J Ophthalmol. 2017;101(10):1436–9.
15. Silverstein BE, Cunningham ET Jr, Margolis TP, Cevallos V, Wong IG. Microsporidial keratoconjunctivitis in a patient without human immunodeficiency virus infection. Am J Ophthalmol. 1997;124(3):395–6.
16. Theng J, Chan C, Ling ML, Tan D. Microsporidial keratoconjunctivitis in a healthy contact lens wearer without human immunodeficiency virus infection. Ophthalmology. 2001;108(5):976–8.
17. Loh RS, Chan CM, Ti SE, Lim L, Chan KS, Tan DT. Emerging prevalence of microsporidial keratitis in Singapore: epidemiology, clinical features, and management. Ophthalmology. 2009;116(12):2348–53.
18. Kakrania R, Joseph J, Vaddavalli PK, Gangopadhyay N, Sharma S. Microsporidia keratoconjunctivitis in a corneal graft. Eye. 2006;20(11):1314–5.

19. Didier ES, Didier PJ, Friedberg DN, Stenson SM, Orenstein JM, Yee RW, Tio FO, Davis RM, Vossbrinck C, Millichamp N, Shadduck JA. Isolation and characterization of a new human microsporidian, Encephalitozoon hellem (n. sp.), from three AIDS patients with keratoconjunctivitis. J Infect Dis. 1991;163(3):617–21.
20. Sharma S, Das S, Joseph J, Vemuganti GK, Murthy S. Microsporidial keratitis: need for increased awareness. Surv Ophthalmol. 2011;56(1):1–22.
21. Lowder CY, Meisler DM, McMahon JT, Longworth DL, Rutherford I. Microsporidia infection of the cornea in a man seropositive for human immunodeficiency virus. Am J Ophthalmol. 1990;109(2):242–4.
22. Lewis NL, Francis IC, Hawkins GS, Coroneo MT. Bilateral microsporidial keratoconjunctivitis in an immunocompetent non-contact lens wearer. Cornea. 2003;22(4):374–6.
23. Rauz S, Tuft S, Dart JKG, Bonshek R, Luthert P, Curry A. Ultrastructural examination of two cases of stromal microsporidial keratitis. J Med Microbiol. 2004;53(8):775–81.
24. Mietz H, Franzen C, Hoppe T, Bartz-Schmidt KU. Microsporidia-induced sclerouveitis with retinal detachment. Arch Ophthalmol. 2002;120(6):864–5.
25. Yoken J, Forbes B, Maguire AM, Prenner JL, Carpentieri D. Microsporidial endophthalmitis in a patient with acute myelogenous leukemia. Retina. 2002;22(1):123–5.
26. Garg P. Microsporidia infection of the cornea-a unique and challenging disease. Cornea. 2013;32(Suppl-1):S33–8.
27. Dart JK, Saw VP, Kilvington S. Acanthamoeba keratitis: diagnosis and treatment update 2009. Am J Ophthalmol. 2009;148(4):487–99.
28. Garcia LS. Laboratory identification of the microsporidia. J Clin Microbiol. 2002;40(6):1892–901.
29. Joseph J, Murthy S, Garg P, Sharma S. Use of different stains for microscopic evaluation of corneal scrapings for diagnosis of microsporidial keratitis. J Clin Microbiol. 2006;44(2):583–5.
30. Xu Y, Weiss LM. The microsporidian polar tube: a highly specialised invasion organelle. Int J Parasitol. 2005;35(9):941–53.
31. Hau SC, Dart JK, Vesaluoma M, Parmar DN, Claerhout I, Bibi K, Larkin DF. Diagnostic accuracy of microbial keratitis with in vivo scanning laser confocal microscopy. Br J Ophthalmol. 2010;94(8):982–7.
32. Shah GK, Pfister D, Probst LE, Ferrieri P, Holland E. Diagnosis of microsporidial keratitis by confocal microscopy and the chromatrope stain. Am J Ophthalmol. 1996;121(1):89–91.
33. Sagoo MS, Mehta JS, Hau S, Irion LD, Curry A, Bonshek RE, Tuft SJ. Microsporidium stromal keratitis: in vivo confocal findings. Cornea. 2007;26(7):870–3.
34. Schwartz DA, Visvesvara GS, Diesenhouse MC, Weber R, Font RL, Wilson LA, Corrent G, Serdarevic ON, Rosberger DF, Keenen PC, Grossnikiaus HE, Hewan-Lowe K, Bryan RT. Pathologic features and immunofluorescent antibody demonstration of ocular microsporidiosis (Encephalitozoon hellem) in seven patients with acquired immunodeficiency syndrome. Am J Ophthalmol. 1993;115(3):285–92.
35. Didier ES, Orenstein JM, Aldras A, Bertucci D, Rogers LB, Janney FA. Comparison of three staining methods for detecting microsporidia in fluids. J Clin Microbiol. 1995;33(12):3138–45.
36. Aldras AM, Orenstein JM, Kotler DP, Shadduck JA, Didier ES. Detection of microsporidia by indirect immunofluorescence antibody test using polyclonal and monoclonal antibodies. J Clin Microbiol. 1994;32(3):608–12.
37. Joseph J, Sharma S. In vitro culture of various species of microsporidia causing keratitis: evaluation of three immortalized cell lines. Indian J Med Microbiol. 2009;27(1):35–9.
38. Joseph J, Sharma S, Murthy SI, Krishna PV, Garg P, Nutheti R, Kenneth J, Balasubramanian D. Microsporidial keratitis in India: 16S rRNA gene-based PCR assay for diagnosis and species identification of microsporidia in clinical samples. Invest Ophthalmol Vis Sci. 2006;47(10):4468–73.
39. Wang Z, Orlandi PA, Stenger DA. Simultaneous detection of four human pathogenic microsporidian species from clinical samples by oligonucleotide microarray. J Clin Microbiol. 2005;43(8):4121–8.

40. Das S, Sahu SK, Sharma S, Nayak SS, Kar S. Clinical trial of 0.02% polyhexamethylene bigu-anide versus placebo in the treatment of microsporidial keratoconjunctivitis. Am J Ophthalmol. 2010;150(1):110–5.
41. Sridhar MS, Sharma S. Microsporidial keratoconjunctivitis in a HIV-seronegative patient treated with debridement and oral itraconazole. Am J Ophthalmol. 2003;136(4):745–6.
42. Sangit VA, Murthy SI, Garg P. Microsporidial stromal keratitis successfully treated with medi-cal therapy: a case report. Cornea. 2011;30(11):1264–6.
43. Ang M, Mehta JS, Mantoo S, Tan D. Deep anterior lamellar keratoplasty to treat microsporid-ial stromal keratitis. Cornea. 2009;28(7):832–5.
44. Murthy SI, Sangit VA, Rathi VM, Vemuganti GK. Microsporidial spores can cross the intact Descemet membrane in deep stromal infection. Middle East Afr J Ophthalmol. 2013;20(1):80–2.
45. Font RL, Samaha AN, Keener MJ, Chevez-Barrios P, Goosey JD. Corneal microspo-ridiosis. Report of case, including electron microscopic observations. Ophthalmology. 2000;107(9):1769–75.
46. Vemuganti GK, Garg P, Sharma S, Joseph J, Gopinathan U, Singh S. Is microsporidial keratitis an emerging cause of stromal keratitis? A case series study. BMC Ophthalmol. 2005;5:19.
47. Sabhapandit S, Murthy SI, Garg P, Korwar V, Vemuganti GK, Sharma S. Microsporidial stro-mal keratitis: clinical features, unique diagnostic criteria, and treatment outcomes in a large case series. Cornea. 2016;35(12):1569–74.

Fungal Keratitis

Aravind Roy, M. Srinivasan, and Sujata Das

11.1 Introduction

Microbial keratitis continues to be a leading cause of ocular morbidity and blindness worldwide [1]. Fungal keratitis accounts for 30–50% of all cases of microbial keratitis in developing countries [1–4]. In recent times, there has been an increase in awareness and recognition of the clinical signs of fungal keratitis, particularly in geographic areas where these infections are common such as tropical and subtropical parts of the world. Increased awareness coupled with improved laboratory and in vivo diagnostic techniques have led to an increase in the frequency of correct diagnosis and consequent increase in prevalence of the disease. The diagnosis and treatment of fungal keratitis can be quite challenging. However, prompt diagnosis, appropriate and timely management are required to increase the chance of cure.

11.2 Epidemiology

The epidemiological features of fungal keratitis vary among different geographic regions and climatic conditions [5]. It occurs more frequently in warm and humid climate than in temperate zones. It may vary considerably between countries and also within countries. It is essential to determine local etiology within a given region

A. Roy (✉)
Cornea & Anterior Segment Service, L V Prasad Eye Institute,
Vijayawada, Andhra Pradesh, India
e-mail: aravindroy@lvpei.org

M. Srinivasan
Cornea & Refractive Surgery Services, Aravind Eye Hospital, Madurai, Tamil Nadu, India
e-mail: m.srinivasan@aravind.org

S. Das
Cornea and Anterior Segment Service, L V Prasad Eye Institute, Bhubaneswar, Odisha, India
e-mail: sujatadas@lvpei.org

© Springer Nature Singapore Pte Ltd. 2021
S. Das, V. Jhanji (eds.), *Infections of the Cornea and Conjunctiva*,
https://doi.org/10.1007/978-981-15-8811-2_11

when planning a corneal ulcer management strategy. Several studies have investigated the epidemiology of fungal keratitis and causative microorganisms (Table 11.1). *Fusarium* spp. and *Aspergillus* spp. are the most common fungi isolated from patients of tropics, while *Candida albicans* is the most common pathogen of mycotic keratitis in temperate region.

Table 11.1 Mycotic keratitis—a review of the literature

Place	Year	Cases	% Fungi	Organism-1	Organism-2	Risk factor
Europe						
France [6]	2002	19	–	*Candida* spp., 58%	*Aspergillus* spp., 21%; *Fusarium* spp., 21%	Topical steroid treatment (42.1%), corneal graft (31.6%), trauma or foreign body (31.6%)
Britain, London [7]	2007	66	–	*Candida* spp., 60.6%	*Fusarium* spp., 18.18%	Ocular surface disease or a prior penetrating keratoplasty (97.4%) for *Candida* spp. trauma (30.8%) or cosmetic contact lens wear (30.8%) for filamentary fungal infection
North America						
Florida [8]	1994	125	–	*Fusarium* spp., 62%	*Candida* spp., 12.5%	Trauma (44%). Five patients were using extended wear contact lenses and one patient was wearing a therapeutic bandage contact lens
Philadelphia [9]	2000	24	–	*Candida albicans*, 46%	*Fusarium* spp., 25%	Chronic ocular surface disease (41.7%), contact lens wear (29.2%), atopic disease (16.7%), topical steroid use (16.7%), and ocular trauma (8.3%)
New York [10]	2006	5083	1.2%	*Candida* spp., 48%	*Fusarium solani*, 10%	Human immunodeficiency virus (HIV) seropositivity (15 eyes), chronic ocular surface disease (14 eyes), and trauma (7 eyes)
Northern California [11]	2010	29	3.4%	*Candida parapsilosis*	–	Contact lens (55%), trauma (11.9%)

Table 11.1 (continued)

Place	Year	Cases	% Fungi	Organism-1	Organism-2	Risk factor
South America						
Paraguay [12]	1991	26	58%	*Fusarium* spp., 42%	*Aspergillus* spp., 19%	–
Africa						
Ghana (Accra) [4]	1995	199	34%	*Fusarium* spp., 52%	*Aspergillus* spp., 15%	–
Tanzania [13]	1999	212	15%	*Fusarium* spp., 75%	*Aspergillus* spp., 19%	Human immunodeficiency virus (HIV) seropositivity (81.2%)
Egypt [14]	2017	110	45.5%	*Aspergillus* spp.,41%	*Fusarium* spp.,26.2%	Trauma (51.4%), diabetes mellitus (15.1%), foreign body (5.7%), local ocular pathology (4.5%), postoperative keratitis (4.5%), and contact lens (2.4%)
Australia and New Zealand						
New Zealand [15]	2003	103	4%	–	–	–
Australia [16]	2007	56	–	*Candida albicans*, 37.2%	*Aspergillus fumigatus*, 17.1%	Ocular trauma (37.1%), chronic steroid use (31.4%), and poor ocular surface (25.7%)
Asia						
Bangladesh [17]	1991	127	34%	*Aspergillus* spp., 49%	*Fusarium* spp., 28%	–
Nepal [18]	1991	405	17%	*Aspergillus* spp., 47%	*Candida* spp., 13%	–
Saudi Arabia [19]	1992	27	14%	*Aspergillus* spp., 41%	*Fusarium* spp., *Candida albicans*	–
Bangladesh [3]	1994	66	36%	*Aspergillus* spp., 40%	*Fusarium* spp., 21%	Injury due to rice grains
Sri Lanka [20]	1994	66	33%	*Aspergillus* spp., 18%	–	–
Thailand [21]	1995	145	25%	*Aspergillus* spp., 34%	*Fusarium* spp., 26%	–
India, New Delhi [22]	1997	211	10.8%	*Aspergillus* spp., 40%	*Fusarium* spp., 11%	Trauma (55.3%), associated systemic illness (11.2%), and previous ocular surgery (9.8%). Corneal injury contaminated with vegetable matter was responsible for 60.5% of traumatic cases

(continued)

Table 11.1 (continued)

Place	Year	Cases	% Fungi	Organism-1	Organism-2	Risk factor
India, Madurai [1]	1997	434	35%	*Fusarium* spp., 47%	*Aspergillus* spp., 16%	–
Singapore [23]	1997	29	–	*Fusarium* spp., 52%	*Aspergillus flavus*, 17%	Ocular trauma (>50%), antecedent topical corticosteroid therapy (25%)
Bangladesh [24]	1998	63	–	*Aspergillus* spp., 35%; *Fusarium* spp., 35%	–	–
India, Mumbai [25]	1999	367	–	*Aspergillus* spp., 60%	*Candida* spp., 10%	Antecedent corneal trauma (89.92%)
Hong Kong [26]	2001	223	2%	*Fusarium* spp., 60%	–	–
India, Hyderabad [2]	2002	3399	39.8%	*Fusarium* spp., 37.2%	*Aspergillus* spp., 30.7%	Ocular trauma (54.4%)
India, East [27]	2005	1198	62.7%	*Aspergillus* spp., 59.8%	*Fusarium* spp., 21.2%	–
China, North [28]	2006	1056	61.9%	*Fusarium* spp., 73.3%	*Aspergillus* spp., 12.1%	Corneal trauma (51.4%), especially injury from plants (25.7% in all patients)
India, Madurai [29]	2012	3028	63%	*Fusarium* spp., 42.3%	–	Seasonal variation ($p < 0.001$) with peaks in July and January
India (South) [30]	2016	117	49.5%	*Fusarium* spp., 31%	*Aspergillus* spp.,13%	Trauma (46%), diabetes mellitus (26.5%), contactlens (19%), and corticosteroid (3.5%)

11.3 Risk Factors

Fungi are a normal part of the microbial environment. Although the eye is continuously exposed to these microorganisms, the normal external ocular defenses including the eyelids and tear components provide adequate protection. Fungal infections, in the absence of a predisposing factor, are unusual in human cornea.

The importance of trauma, often trivial and frequently associated with plant material, is well documented in the initiation of fungal infection. Usually adult, rural, and agrarian population is afflicted with fungal keratitis. Adding to this problem is the unsolicited use of over the counter corticosteroids and traditional medicines. Fungi may be responsible for some cases of microbial keratitis associated with contact lens wear. It can grow within matrix of the contact lenses. Wearing contact lens may be categorized as a major cause of minor injuries where either microbes present in the atmosphere or the contaminated lens preservation solution is generally responsible for the onset of corneal ulcers. Fungal keratitis has been reported from cosmetic (phakic and aphakic) contact lens wearer and therapeutic lens user.

Prolonged use of topical broad-spectrum antibiotics and indiscriminate use of steroids has been described to be associated with fungal keratitis. This may be attributed to disturbance in the microbial flora of the eye and local immunosuppression.

Other less common risk factors include vernal or allergic keratoconjunctivitis, ocular surface disorder, penetrating keratoplasty, bullous keratopathy, and exposure keratitis. Recently, several reports of fungal keratitis after laser refractive surgery have also been published [31, 32].

11.4 Clinical Features

The onset of fungal infection of cornea is mostly insidious although it may not present as acutely as bacterial keratitis. Classical clinical features of fungal keratitis may vary considerably. A prospective study looking at the characteristic clinical features as an aid to the diagnosis concluded that no single clinical feature can be considered as absolutely pathognomonic of a particular type of etiological agent [33]. Usually there is no or minimal lid edema, no conjunctival chemosis. Overall inflammatory signs are lesser than other types of suppurative keratitis. Linear finger-like extensions and feathery borders are characteristic clinical features of early fungal keratitis. The clinical features in early stages may be confused with herpetic keratitis.

The traditional academic approach for the initial diagnosis and management of microbial keratitis considers diagnostic scraping of corneal ulcers mandatory. However, this requires a well-equipped laboratory with trained manpower to process minute samples and involves the cost of maintaining various culture media and processing samples. Furthermore, many ophthalmologists do not have access to culture media. Therefore, it is imperative to get familiar with the classical clinical features.

11.5 Classical Clinical Features

(a) Fungal keratitis classically presents as a slowly progressive disease characterized by a localized infiltrate.
(b) The infiltrate is dry and is raised above the plane of the cornea (Fig. 11.1).
(c) The infiltrate has fine branching linear extensions in the surrounding cornea.
(d) There may be satellite lesions and an immune ring associated with the main infiltrate.
(e) Some ulcers may show brown to black pigmentation on the surface of the infiltrate.
(f) Other characteristic features of fungal infection of cornea are the presence of thick fluffy endothelial exudates and a thick hypopyon (Fig. 11.2).

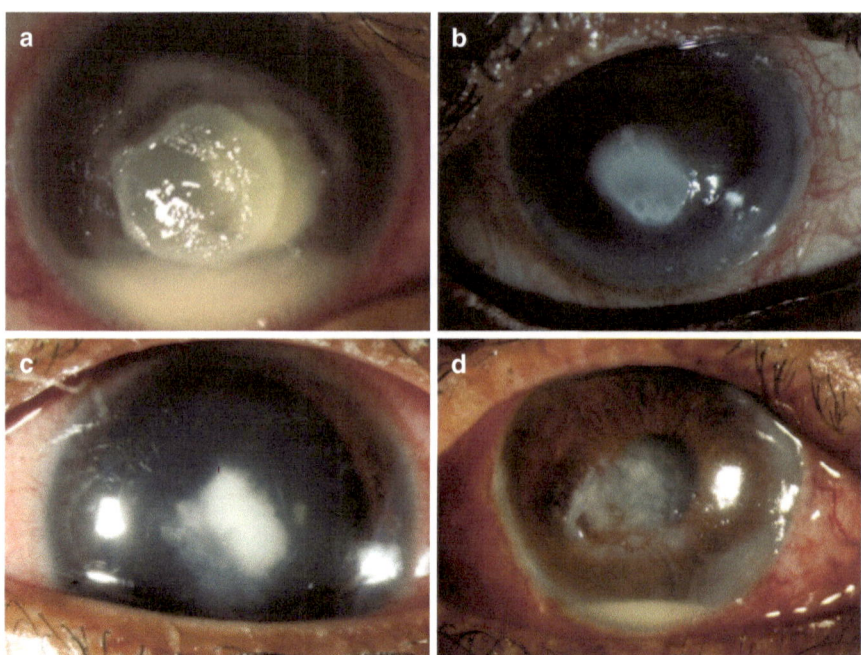

Fig. 11.1 Fungal keratitis presenting as (**a**) central dry raised plaque with hypopyon; (**b**) raised plaque with surrounding infiltrate; (**c**) deep stromal infiltrate with irregular margin; and (**d**) superficial infiltrate with hyphate edge and hypopyon

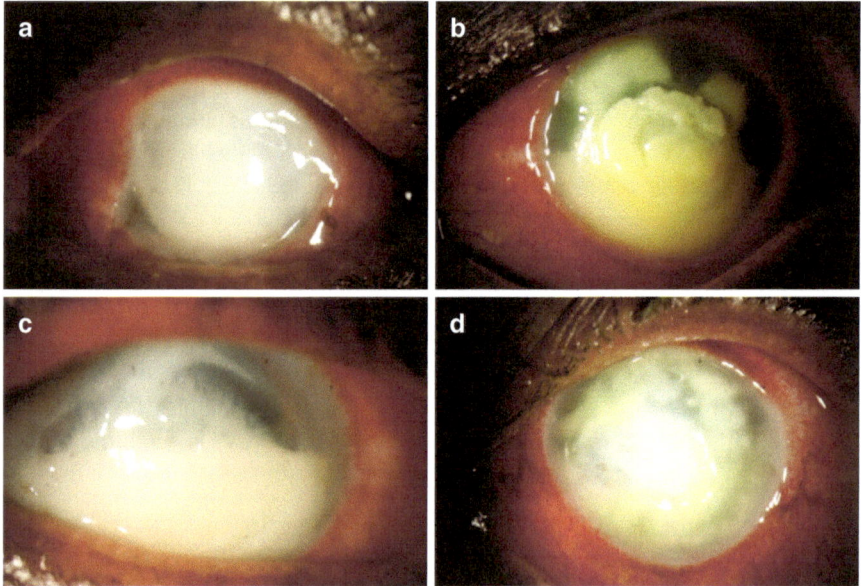

Fig. 11.2 (**a**) Fulminant fungal infection of the total cornea and melting; (**b**) Dense superficial plaque with deep stromal infiltrate approaching the limbus and hypopyon; (**c**) Extensive corneal infiltrate with irregular feathery margins and hypopyon involving half of the anterior chamber; and (**d**) Central tissue necrosis with extensive anterior chamber exudates and infiltrates approaching to involve 12'O clock limbus

11.5.1 Fungal Infection After Cataract Surgery

Cataract surgery is the most commonly performed intraocular surgery. Self-sealing wound can be either sclero-corneal or clear-corneal. Infection of the sclera corneal tunnel poses a diagnostic and therapeutic challenge. Clinical picture is atypical and varies depending on the location of involvement. It may involve sclera, cornea, or the whole sclero-corneal tunnel. Bacteria and fungi can infect the surgical wound. While only corneal involvement due to fungi present as typical features of fungal keratitis, scleral infection presents as scleritis, scleral necrosis, and wound gape [34, 35]. It may be associated with endophthalmitis. Avascular intrascleral pocket, prolonged steroid usage, enhances organism to spread diffusely to adjacent tissue (Fig. 11.2). Compared to bacterial infections fungal infections present late and are difficult to treat.

11.5.2 Fungal Infection After Laser Refractive Surgery

Fungal keratitis is an uncommon but potentially vision-threatening complication after Laser in situ keratomilcusis (LASIK) and photoretractive keratectomy (PRK). Microbial contamination may occur from eyelids, eyelashes, conjunctiva, and microkeratome. Infection from filamentous fungi and yeast has been reported after laser refractive surgery. *Aspergillus* species has been reported as the most common fungal species associated with post-LASIK infection [32, 36, 37]. It can occur within days, weeks, or even years after LASIK. It is important to understand that the typical clinical features may not be noted in post refractive fungal keratitis.

11.5.3 Fungal Infection After Lamellar Surgery

Fungal interface keratitis is a rare complication after lamellar keratoplasty. It has been reported after deep anterior lamellar keratoplasty (DALK) [38], Descemet stripping automated endothelial keratoplasty (DSAEK) [39], and Descemet membrane endothelial keratoplasty (DMEK) [40]. Lamellar surgeries provide a unique environment for infection. Typical signs of infection may remain altered due to prolonged use of steroid and slow growing organism.

11.6   Diagnosis

A rapid and accurate diagnosis of fungal keratitis ensures specific therapy and complete recovery. A systematic approach to make a quick diagnosis involves elicitation of history, meticulous slit-lamp examination, confocal microscopy, and appropriate microbiological methods.

11.6.1 Noninvasive Techniques

11.6.1.1 Confocal Microscopy

Confocal microscopy is fast emerging as a clinically important tool in the diagnosis of various corneal conditions. It offers magnifications of up to ×500 with increased image contrast and the ability to visualize details even in hazy corneas. Its noninvasive nature makes it an important modality in the rapid diagnosis of fungal keratitis. Additionally, it can be used for real-time repetitive observations, which could become important in the diagnosis, management, and the follow-up of cases of infective keratitis [41]. However, there are certain limitations in the use of this technique, including difficulty in returning to the exact area of interest for serial examination, lack of a distinctive morphology of pathogens, and limited resolution of the microscope. Detection of yeast cells may be difficult with the morphology overlapping with inflammatory cells. Few recent studies reported the sensitivity and specificity of confocal for diagnosing fungi range from 85.7–88.3% and 81.4–91.1% [42–43].

Filamentous fungus can be seen as branching filaments that are >3 μm in width. This needs to be differentiated from *Actinomycetes* and *Nocardia* spp. which are <2 μm in width. Limitations of confocal microscopy include the following: the technique is dependent on operator skill and observer's experience for interpretation of results. Patients with microbial keratitis may not be cooperative for a confocal scan. Confocal microscopes are not widely available and are not cost effective.

11.6.2 Invasive Techniques

11.6.2.1 Conventional Microbiological Investigations

Demonstration of fungus in smears or culture of corneal scrapings remains the gold standard for diagnosis of fungal keratitis. These methods continue to be employed worldwide and require a modest laboratory set-up. Although the need to perform microbiological diagnosis is still rather controversial [44], these investigations are essential in areas with high prevalence of fungal keratitis.

11.6.2.2 Sample Collection

Samples need to be collected directly from the lesion using an instrument (such as a platinum spatula, beaver blade, surgical blade #15, or blunt cataract knife) to debride material from the base and edges of the ulcerated part of the cornea. Multiple scrapings under topical anesthesia are collected and inoculated on slides and culture media. The blade or spatula may be reused if a sterile medium or sterile slide is touched. Cotton swabs are not useful but calcium alginate swabs have been used for recovery of fungus in culture.

Corneal biopsy may be useful when the corneal infiltrate is situated in deeper tissues with intact epithelium such as tunnel infiltrate. The biopsy sample should be submitted for smear, culture, and histopathologic studies. Anterior chamber exudates have also been used for the diagnosis of fungal keratitis when endothelial exudates are present [45].

11.6.2.3 Direct Microscopic Examination

Demonstration of fungal filaments or yeast in direct microscopic examination of the corneal scraping or corneal biopsy sample rapidly establishes diagnosis in a clinically presumptive case of mycotic keratitis. Several studies have documented over 85% sensitivity and specificity for fungal filaments in 10% potassium hydroxide or stained with calcofluor white or lactophenol cotton blue. Grams and Giemsa stains also show fungal filaments and may be used in addition to wet mounts for direct evaluation of the smear sample.

11.6.2.4 Culture

A culture of the corneal scraping or biopsy sample is essential to confirm the diagnosis and rule out mixed infections. Clinically, there can be considerable overlap in the clinical features of bacterial, fungal, and *Acanthamoeba* keratitis. A single protocol is therefore recommended for the culture of bacteria, fungi, and *Acanthamoeba* from corneal scrapings. Corneal scraping sample is inoculated on solid media in "C" streaks, and liquid media are inoculated by twirling the spatula or blade in the broth. The solid media that are typically used for the identification of fungal pathogens include Sabouraud dextrose agar and potato dextrose agar. These media contain chloramphenicol to prevent bacterial contamination.

A number of criteria have been described which help determine the significance of fungal growth in culture. They include: fungal growth in more than one media in the absence of fungus in smears, fungal growth in one media with presence of fungus in direct smear examination, or confluent growth of fungus on the inoculated site in a single solid media [46].

The conventional methods of fungal species identification include characteristic growth (rate of growth, texture, pigment-reverse, and obverse) and sexual and asexual spores. Recently, molecular methods have been introduced for fungal species identification. *Candida* spp. would require employment of biochemical tests for species identification. Automated methods such as API Candida (bioMérieux, France) are also available.

11.6.2.5 Molecular Methods

Polymerase chain reaction (PCR), the most versatile molecular method, offers a means to rapidly detect presence of organisms that are difficult to culture. However, PCR does not distinguish viable from nonviable organisms. In an experimental *Fusarium* keratitis study in rabbits, compared to gold standard of culture, PCR (targeting *Fusarium* cutinase gene) was 89% sensitive and 88% specific [47]. The study noted PCR positivity in ulcers that were clinically healed and culture negative, thus undermining the relevance of positive PCR results in healed or healing ulcers. Its role in diagnosis for clinical samples that may contain transient commensal fungi is also controversial [48]. Concerns regarding its specificity and false positives in such samples remain. Primers amplifying conserved regions of the 28S rDNA and 18S rDNA (with or without further separation of genus and species targeting internal transcribed spacer region) have been used in conventional as well as real-time PCR [48, 49].

11.6.2.6 Histopathology

Though microbiologic evaluation of corneal scrapings remains the mainstay of diagnosis in fungal keratitis, the pathobiology of fungal keratitis is better understood by the histopathologic examination of the excised tissues. The outcome of mycotic keratitis depends ultimately on the interplay of agent (virulence, resistance to drugs, and toxicity) and host factors (predisposing factors, inflammatory response, and hypersensitivity reactions) in addition to timely diagnosis and appropriate medical treatment. Insight into these complex pathogenic mechanisms in keratomycosis has been obtained from animal experiments, impression debridement of corneal ulcers, diagnostic corneal biopsy, or from corneal buttons removed during penetrating keratoplasty for medically uncontrolled mycotic keratitis [50–58]. Mycotic infections are almost always of ulcerative type, manifesting as:

- *Epithelial Ulceration*: These could be central or paracentral or could result in total sloughing of the epithelium.
- Destruction of Bowman's: Destruction of the Bowman's layer with fragmentation could be absent, focal or total.
- *Stromal Inflammation*: The inflammation is mostly suppurative with neutrophils. Depending on the duration of infection, treatment received, the extent of stromal thickness, inflammation and necrosis varies. In the early stages the inflammation could be in the anterior two-thirds with satellite lesions in the surrounding stroma. The posterior stroma when affected may show loss of stromal keratocytes due to apoptosis. Later these abscesses become confluent and lead to total destruction of stroma with necrosis and perforation. In a few cases there could be predominant deep-seated lesions along with anterior chamber exudates and hypopyon.
- Descemet's fragmentation/endothelial exudates.
- Anterior chamber exudates.

11.7 Medical Management

Medical management is the first line treatment for fungal keratitis, a Cochrane review [59–60] did not find evidence of superiority of any one class of drug. Natamycin remains the single best antifungal agent in the management of filamentous fungi. A combination of antifungal agents does not provide any superiority over monotherapy and neither does it predict reduced need for surgical interventions [61]. Medical management needs to be continued for 2 weeks after scarring as the fungal filaments may remain active in the deeper corneal stroma. The optimal dosing frequency of Natamycin is not determined, though initial loading dose of one drop half-hourly followed by gradual taper to eight or six times has been recommended. Patients with systemic comorbidities such as diabetes need to have good glycemic control in order to have satisfactory resolution of fungal keratitis.

Several factors influence the outcome of medical management of fungal keratitis. These include maintaining the dose of the drug to above MIC90 for the causative organism, the access to medications, need for compliance, and cost and access to optimal health care [61].

Oral ketoconazole or itraconazole has also been indicated in deep mycosis, limbal involvement, and endophthalmitis. These medications may be started under physician supervision with periodic assessment of liver function tests.

11.7.1 Role of Antifungals

It often constitutes the first line of treatment for fungal keratitis. There are several classes of antifungal drugs that have a unique mechanism of action and spectrum of activity (Table 11.2).

Table 11.2 Drugs used in the treatment of fungal keratitis

Category	Mechanistic of action	Type	Spectrum	Special considerations
Polyenes	Disrupts ergosterols in fungal cell walls	Amphotericin B: Topical (0.15–0.30%), Intracameral (7.5–30 μg/0.1 ml), Intravitreal (1-5 μg/0.1 ml), Intravenous (0.5–1 mg/kg/day)	Candida, Aspergillus, Fusarium	Needs to be reconstituted, chance of renal toxicity with systemic use along with antineoplastic agents, topical use causes corneal punctate erosions
	Disrupts fungal cell wall ergosterols	Natamycin: Topical (5%) solution	Filamentous fungi, Candida (variable action)	First line treatment of fungal keratitis, poor penetration, 2% of the drug is bioavailable. Not available in some geographic areas
Azoles (Imidazole and Triazoles)	Inhibit synthesis of ergosterol and damage fungal cell wall	Voriconazole: Oral (200 mg q12h), Topical (1%), Intracameral/intrastromal (50 μg/0.1 ml)	Aspergillus, Fusarium, Candida	Good penetration, broad spectrum of activity, less toxic
		Fluconazole: Oral (25–50 mg q12h), Topical (0.2–2%)	Candida	Deep penetration into tissues. Dose adjustment in renal insufficiency, less active against filamentous fungi

(continued)

Table 11.2 (continued)

Category	Mechanistic of action	Type	Spectrum	Special considerations
		Ketoconazole: Oral (100–200 mg q12h), Topical (1–2%) suspension	Aspergillus, Candida (good activity), Curvularia and Fusarium and Curvularia spp. (poor response)	Good tissue penetration Only oral preparations are available. Liver toxicity
		Posaconazole: Oral (200 mg q6h), Topical (10 mg/0.1 ml)	Aspergillus, Fusarium	Effective in refractory Fusarium and Aspergillus keratitis
		Itraconazole:- Oral (200–400 mg/day), Topical (1%) suspension	Candida, Aspergillus	Poor systemic and unpredictable ocular drug levels
		Miconazole: Topical (1%), Intravenous (600–1200 mg/day)	Yeast filamentous fungi	Variable tissue concentration
Pyrimidines	Inhibits thymidine synthesis	Flucytosine: Topical (1%)	Candida, Cryptococcus, Aspergillus (variable response)	Synergistic activity with azoles and amphotericin B Chance of emergence of resistance
Echinocandins	Inhibit glucan synthesis and cause cell wall lysis	Caspofungin: Topical (1.5–5 mg/ml), Micafungin (1 mg/ml)	Candida, Aspergillus (variable response)	Variable efficacy

Adapted from Ansari et al. [61], Thomas et al. [62, 63], and Maharana et al. [64]

The therapeutic agents commonly used for the first line treatment of fungal keratitis include fungistatic agents such as natamycin. There are concerns regarding its penetration into the ocular tissues and bioavailability. The availability of the drug in various regions is also a limitation. While Amphotericin B offers an alternative, its use is limited by systemic and local ocular toxicity.

Newer molecules such as the Azoles, especially voriconazole, have better ocular penetration, broad spectrum of activity, and in vitro susceptibility. However, large randomized control trials such as the Mycotic Ulcer Treatment Trial (MUTT-I) have demonstrated its poor clinical outcome [59]. The MUTT-I is a randomized, double-masked, multicenter clinical trial [59] that studied the outcomes of fungal keratitis with topical 5% natamycin versus topical 1% voriconazole. Visual acuity after

3 months was significantly better in patients who received natamycin. Patients those who received voriconazole had significantly higher chance of perforation and need for therapeutic penetrating keratoplasty. No difference was noted between time to reepithelialization and infiltrate or scar size in both the study arms. Besides, a significant proportion of patients treated with natamycin was culture negative for fungus at 6 days post-treatment compared to patients treated with voriconazole. While the in vitro susceptibility to voriconazole was found to be significantly better than natamycin, it did not translate into better in vivo efficacy.

A Cochrane review on medical interventions for the management of fungal keratitis compared the data from 12 clinical trials assessing eight antifungal agents [60]. This review studied clinical cure at 2–3 months, time to cure, best-corrected visual acuity, corneal perforation and need for penetrating keratoplasty, compliance to treatment and quality of life as the outcome measures. The trials included in the review were of variable quality and were underpowered to provide definitive evidence of superiority of one particular class of antifungals. The exception was the comparison of natamycin to voriconazole in the MUTT-I study which found good evidence of natamycin being more effective than voriconazole in the treatment of fungal keratitis, especially in Fusarium infections [59]. A reappraisal of natamycin versus voriconazole yielded similar results of no additional advantages of voriconazole in the treatment of filamentous fungal keratitis over natamycin [65].

The MUTT-II is a prospective multicentric, placebo-controlled, randomized clinical trial to assess additional benefit of adding oral voriconazole versus placebo in the management of filamentous fungal keratitis treated with topical antifungals [66]. The study did not find any difference in the rates of corneal perforation or need for therapeutic keratoplasty, best-corrected visual acuity, infiltrate or scar size at 3 weeks and 3 months, and rate of culture negativity among the study arms. A subgroup analysis suggested a possible decreased rate of perforation of Fusarium keratitis in the oral voriconazole treated group; however, the results failed to achieve statistical significance. The study emphasizes no additional benefit of adding oral voriconazole to a regimen of topical antifungal medications such as natamycin.

11.7.2 Role of In Vitro Susceptibility in the Management of Fungal Keratitis

Routine in vitro susceptibility tests for fungal isolates are not performed due to poor correlation to in vivo clinical response. There have been modifications in international standards for susceptibility testing of fungal isolates, namely the CLSI and EUCAST [67]. Sun et al. [68] reported a twofold increase in the MIC of natamycin lead to a larger 3 month infiltrate or scar size and increased chances of perforation in the mycotic ulcer treatment trial. Studies suggest a prognostic, epidemiologic, and surveillance role to studying susceptibility to antifungal isolates [68–71].

11.7.3 Role of Novel Drug Delivery Models

There has been renewed interest in modified drug formulations and drug delivery systems. In the quest for superior pharmacokinetics, tissue availability, biocompatibility and reduced toxicity, several modalities of drug delivery systems have evoked interest such as liposomal drug formulations, polymeric micelles and nano particles, cell penetrating peptides conjugated with antifungals so as to deliver optimum tissue levels of the drugs with minimal toxicity [72–75].

11.8 Surgical Management

Medical management of fungal keratitis has several challenges; these include a delayed presentation and often after using multiple topical medications including corticosteroids. There are limitations in accessing a microbiology service. Antifungal drugs are limited by lack of availability and efficacy. The drug susceptibility of antifungal drugs are unknown and not routinely done. In this scenario it is common for fungal keratitis to smolder for weeks to months, often there is corneal perforation or the imminent chance of involving the sclera or developing into a deep-seated infiltrate which might involve the anterior segment and/or the vitreous. Therefore, it is important to identify these, and, if possible, prevent further progression by opting for surgical modalities for further management of fungal keratitis.

The following conditions are those which warrant an urgent surgical approach to the management of fungal keratitis.

(a) Worsening keratitis on maximal medical management
(b) Impending or actual corneal perforation
(c) Infiltrate approaching or involving the limbus
(d) Fungal graft infiltrate, either full-thickness or lamellar graft, in the immediate postoperative period, where the donor tissue is suspected to be contaminated
(e) Miscellaneous causes such as endophthalmitis, one-eyed patient with rapid worsening, and patients requesting surgical options.

11.8.1 Superficial Keratectomy

Superficial keratectomy is an option for excising en bloc a dense plaque of fungal infiltrate restricted to the anterior stroma. In a series of dematiaceous fungi with a dry plaque-like lesion and variable infiltration of the anterior stroma, Garg et al. [58] reported successful outcomes following superficial keratectomy. This led to resolution in 9 out of 15 cases, the other 4 cases needed therapeutic keratoplasty and 2 cases had a perforation while excision of the plaque requiring tissue adhesives. Superficial keratectomy removes the dense carpet-like plaque and decreases the fungal load in the cornea. It also helps penetration of the drug thereby helping in rapid resolution of keratitis.

11.8.2 Intrastromal Antifungal Injections

Antifungal agents are limited by penetration across the intact epithelium; therefore, injecting the drug directly around the site of infection can increase bioavailability. Amphotericin B and voriconazole have been the two most commonly used agents for this modality of treatment. There have been reports of successful management of deep corneal fungal infiltrates and plaques after multiple injections of amphotericin B at a concentration of 5 µg in 0.1 ml [76].

Tu et al. reported successful resolution of deep mycosis at the interface infiltrate in lamellar keratoplasty with intracorneal injections of amphotericin B [77]. Intrastromal injection of voriconazole 50 µg/0.1 ml in divided doses encircling the corneal lesions leads to successful resolution as reported in several studies [78–81]. The studies have variability of dosing and frequency of injections. Besides, the information on fungal susceptibilities is also not available.

There is no additional benefit of intrastromal voriconazole compared to topical voriconazole in fungal keratitis being treated with topical 5% natamycin in a randomized control trial [82]. Patients randomized to either arm had similar time to healing, though ulcers treated with topical voriconazole healed on an average 5.5 days earlier. Rate of healing, scar size, and vascularization was comparable among both the groups. The BSCVA was significantly better in the topical arm possibly due to less number of central ulcers in the topical group as compared to the intrastromal arm. The study recommended additional benefit of adding topical 1% voriconazole to a regimen of 5% natamycin though there was no additional benefit of intrastromal voriconazole injections in recalcitrant fungal keratitis. A recent study by Kalaiselvi et al. [83] reported clinical cure with intrastromal voriconazole in 72% of eyes with deep fungal infections unresponsive to topical 5% natamycin and 1% voriconazole. Unlike the previously described randomized control trial, the authors recommend injecting intrastromal voriconazole in cases refractory to maximal medical treatment. They reported treatment failures with *Fusarium* spp. In addition, the study found ulcer size and height of hypopyon to be the most important indicators for treatment failure.

In a case series [84], intrastromal voriconazole injections eradicated infection with yeast, such as *Candida*; however, the efficacy was not sufficient in filamentous fungi where histopathology of corneal buttons after keratoplasty demonstrated presence of fungal filaments closer to the Descemet's membrane and higher MIC values for patients subjected to multiple injections of intrastromal voriconazole. The authors also performed an OCT-based analysis and concluded that the drug might not penetrate beyond two-thirds of the corneal stroma. Therefore, the intrastromal injections of voriconazole may not always lead to successful eradication of deep fungal infections though anecdotal reports and cases series exist on the beneficial effect in challenging clinical settings such as a DSAEK graft interface infection. Tu et al. [85] reported successful resolution of post DSAEK presumed Candida infection in the endothelial graft interface with multiple intrastromal voriconazole injections. These led to partial graft detachment that reapposed post injection. The penetration of drugs to the graft host interface is limited and intrastromal injections provide an approach to delay or avoid a keratoplasty or allow continued survival of a viable graft.

Intrastromal injections while providing access of the drug in deep mycoses are limited by pain, lack of uniformity in dosing and frequency and availability of definite evidence of clinical benefit. It is important to plan for therapeutic keratoplasty in patients not responding to repeated injections of intrastromal drugs or lesions threatening to involve the limbus.

11.8.3 Intracameral Injections

Intracameral injections deliver a therapeutic dose of antifungals in the anterior chamber. This allows the drug to act on the fungi in deep mycoses. Both Amphotericin B and Voriconazole has been used for this purpose. Several anecdotal reports suggest successful control of fungal infection with intracameral antifungals [86–89]. A study on the pharmacodynamics of Amphotericin B suggested that the drug clears from the anterior chamber abruptly on the first day though some of the drugs can be detected up to 7 days after injection [90]. A randomized control trial did not find evidence of therapeutic benefit on adding intracameral antifungal agents to a regimen of oral and topical antifungals [91].

11.8.4 Tissue Adhesives

With initial reports of Webster et al. [92] on the clinical use of N butyl cyanoacrylate glue in cases of infectious keratitis there are several publications highlighting the merits of this modality of treatment [93–95]. Tissue adhesives are relatively easy to apply, provide adequate tectonic support, and may potentially delay the need for a therapeutic keratoplasty. In a series of fungal keratitis managed with antifungals and additional tissue adhesives for tectonic support, Garg et al. [96] reported 63.3% clinical cure with application of tissue adhesives and medical management alone for microbiologically proven fungal keratitis. There has been some concern of worsening of infection underneath tissue adhesives due to lack of penetration of drugs [97]. This may seem probable due to poor penetration of the antifungal group of drugs. In contrast, Garg et al. [96] reported that in spite of 16 of their patients worsening with tissue adhesive and medical management, the corneal buttons from these patients following subsequent penetrating keratoplasty yielded fungal filaments in only two cases and cultures were negative. They concluded that tissue adhesives did not hinder the effect of antifungals.

Tissue adhesives are usually left in situ until complete resolution and epithelialization under the glue. Duration of 4–6 weeks is required before contemplating tissue adhesive removal. A study of fibrin glue versus cyanoacrylate glue for infective keratitis did not find significant difference in the rate of healing between both the modalities of treatment [98]. The duration of adherence of fibrin glue was found to be 2 weeks with a significantly faster rate of reepithelialization. The number of reapplication of glue and infectious complications was similar between both the groups. Both fibrin glue and cyanoacrylate glue was efficacious in treating corneal perforations up to 2 mm, though it was difficult to treat corneal perforations from 2–3 mm in size. The patients who had cyanoacrylate glue application had significantly more corneal vascularization and conjunctival giant papillary reaction [98].

11.8.5 Therapeutic Penetrating Keratoplasty

Penetrating keratoplasty with full thickness excision of the diseased cornea and transplanting a healthy donor is the most common surgical modality for treatment of advanced fungal keratitis. The goal of surgery is to eradicate the infection and decrease the fungal load so as to allow the antifungals to eliminate the infection. Restoration of vision is a secondary goal and may require later intervention. It is important to perform an adequate preoperative evaluation to identify the extent and depth of the lesions and involvement of the sclera and/or involvement of deep stroma, anterior chamber structures. Preoperative hyoptony is achieved by intravenous 20% Mannitol, adequate anesthesia and akinesia is important to prevent lens expulsion, posterior capsular rupture, and vitreous loss intraoperatively. General anesthesia is needed in cases with large perforation where local anesthesia will undesirably increase the intraorbital pressure and lead to extrusion of intraocular contents. Trephination is an important step of the surgery and it is desirable to trephine 1 mm of healthy appearing stroma so as to leave behind a healthy stromal bed. Thorough irrigation of the anterior chamber and excision of unhealthy or necrotic iris tissue is needed. It is important not to injure the lens capsule. As the eye is inflamed two to three large peripheral iridectomies are needed to avoid pupillary block glaucoma. In trephinations more than 10 mm which is usually required in a fulminant infection of the cornea, the donor cornea should be oversized by 0.75–1 mm. This is important in order to avoid development of peripheral anterior synechia (Fig. 11.3). Suturing with interrupted 10–0 nylon with an attempt to avoid injuring or distorting the angle is desirable. It is important to avoid incarceration of uveal tissue in the graft host junction and allow for meticulous epithelium-to-epithelium apposition. Postoperative care involves careful observation and early identification of a residual or recurrence of fungal infection (Fig. 11.4). Routinely 2 weeks of antifungal treatment is needed before starting topical corticosteroids. In cases that are suspicious, so as to recurrence of the disease, the antifungal regimen may be extended to beyond 2 weeks.

The outcomes of penetrating keratoplasty are good in terms of anatomical success so as to eradicate infection. Sharma et al. [99] reported 89% success in terms of clinical cure. Recurrence when noted in the postoperative period is limited to the recipient stromal bed in 70% of cases followed by the posterior segment (22%) and anterior chamber (7%) [100]. The final visual acuity was however better than 6/60 in only 6% of patients [99]. Therapeutic keratoplasty is associated with graft failure; this is primarily due to the surgery being performed in an inflamed eye, the donor

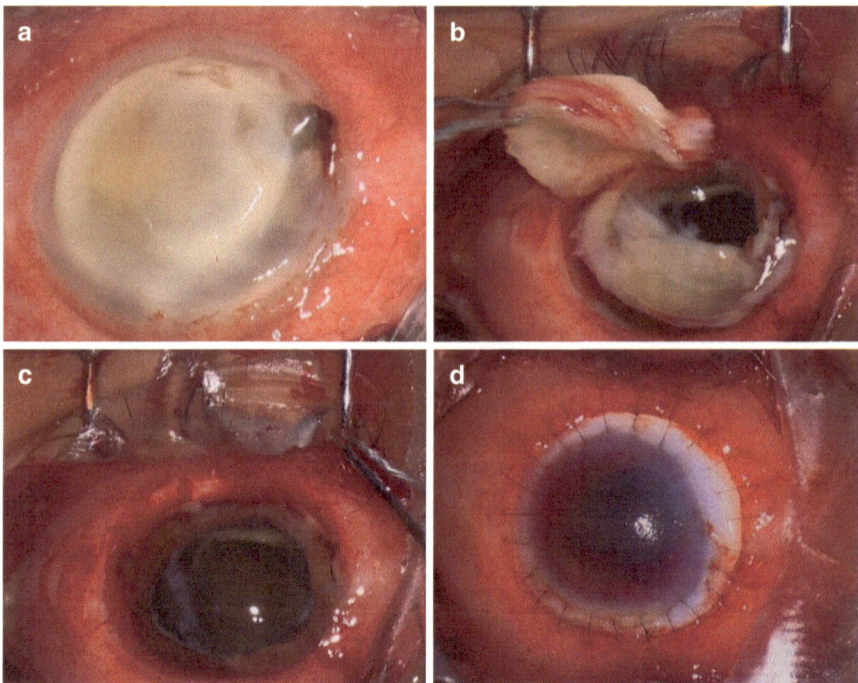

Fig. 11.3 (**a**) Advanced fungal keratitis approaching limbus with corneal perforation; (**b**) Intraoperative view post trephination, extensive intraocular exudates, aphakia due to spontaneous lens expulsion following trephination; (**c**) Exudates cleared from the Iris surface, intact posterior capsule, and few deep exudates noted behind the iris; and (**d**) Large donor graft placed in situ with 24 sutures

quality, disorganization of the anterior segment, glaucoma, and secondary surgeries such as synaechiolysis, cataract extraction, and glaucoma control surgeries.

11.8.6 Lamellar Keratoplasty

Lamellar keratoplasty is an established technique as there are several benefits associated with the procedure. It is an extraocular surgery with lesser possibility of the infection spreading to the deeper layers of the eye. The host endothelium is preserved and there are lesser chances of rejection. Optical quality tissue is not mandatory for this procedure. With these advantages, lamellar keratoplasty has been attempted in fungal keratitis. This procedure is useful when the infiltrate is superficial and the deeper layers of the stroma including the Descemet's membrane is not involved. Studies have reported 90% to total therapeutic success following lamellar keratectomy for early fungal keratitis. More than one dissection may be needed to ensure a healthy stromal bed. It is important to irrigate the host bed prior to transplanting the donor to avoid recurrences [101–103]. Histopathology studies of the excised corneal buttons for therapeutic penetrating keratoplasty suggest that there is diffuse involvement of the stroma in 49% of cases with 30% of buttons having a

Fig. 11.4 (**a**) Recurrence in anterior chamber following therapeutic penetrating keratoplasty and (**b**) Magnified image of the previous cornea showing recurrence localized to anterior chamber and superior graft host junction

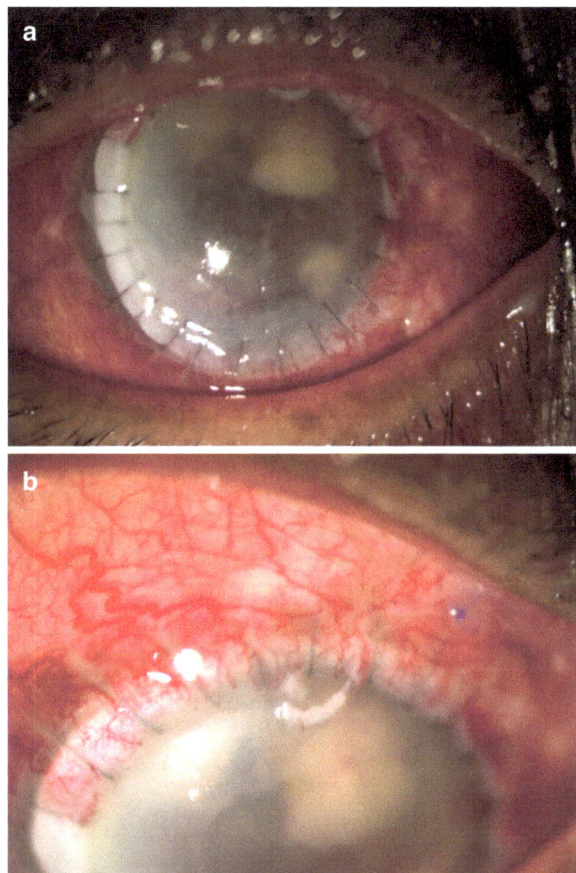

posterior stromal involvement, and 22% of cases have involvement beyond the Descemet's membrane [56, 103]. In a comparative study of therapeutic penetrating keratoplasty (TPK) versus deep anterior lamellar keratoplasty (DALK), 15.3% recurrence was noted in the DALK group as opposed to 12% in TPK [104]. There was recurrence in cases where manual stromal dissection was done without baring Descemet's membrane.

It is essential to ensure that the host bed is healthy and bare the Descemet's membrane in order to minimize chances of recurrence. In case there is complete involvement of the stroma and Descemet's membrane, it will be useful to plan for a full thickness graft.

11.8.7 Conjunctival Flaps

Conjunctival flaps are useful in the management of refractory fungal keratitis if there is no ready availability of corneal tissue or cornea subspeciality services with a refractory ulcer on maximal medical management. Conjunctival flaps provide structural support and promote healing. The flap provides a source of improved blood supply and promotes the resolution of ulcers by humoral and cellular mechanisms. Gunderson [105] described mobilizing the superior conjunctiva over the area of the ulcer. Successful outcomes are achieved on performing a lamellar keratoplasty with a thin conjunctival flap. Khodadoust et al. [106] describe mobilizing a localized pedicle of conjunctiva as this does not compromise the view of the anterior chamber and limits the vascularization thereby improving chances of a subsequent keratoplasty. Zhong et al. [107] reported successful treatment outcomes following full thickness conjunctival autograft for fungal keratitis without perforation. The authors describe dissection of a full thickness conjunctival flap from the bulbar conjunctiva with the tenon's capsule and fixation of the flap to the cornea with interrupted nylon sutures. The area of corneal abscess is surgically debrided to provide a smooth bed. Upon successful resolution, a sclerokeratoplasty is performed for restoration of vision. However, long-term follow-up would be needed to assess the viability of the grafts as the host bed would be vascularized. Abdulhalim et al. [108] reported no difference in healing rate of infected keratitis managed with either conjunctival flaps or amniotic membrane. The time to epithelialization was 26 days in flap group and 27 days in the amniotic membrane group. They performed a 360° conjunctival peritomy and mobilized the superior conjunctival bipedicle flap over the arc of the ulcer. The inferior conjunctiva was attached postoperatively to the inferior limbus thereby providing a source of limbal stem cells.

The conjunctival flap is a simple and useful technique to allow healing of recalcitrant corneal ulcerations. Most ulcers heal with acceptable cosmesis and resolution of pain and stabilization of the corneal surface with epithelialization. The drawbacks include vascularization, limited tectonic support, and chance of reduced graft survival if a penetrating keratoplasty is performed later.

11.8.8 Collagen Cross-Linking

Microbes cause an inflammatory cascade leading to collagenolysis, cell necrosis, corneal melt, and perforation. In addition to antimicrobial therapy, strategies to arrest the inflammatory reaction and control the stromal collagenolysis are needed in the management of infectious keratitis.

Since the initial reports by Tsugita et al. [109] on inactivation of Tobacco mosaic virus by application of Riboflavin and Ultraviolet A light and the report from Wollensak et al. [110] on the increase in stiffness of corneal collagen after exposure to Riboflavin and Ultraviolet A light, collagen cross-linking has captured the attention of researchers as a modality of treatment for control of corneal infections.

Collagen cross-linking would be ideal to control the collagenolysis due to the inflammatory cascade accompanying microbial keratitis as well also provide antimicrobial action by deactivating the disease-causing organisms. In vivo experiments [111] on three groups of fungi: *Fusarium*, Aspergillus, and *Candida* showed an increase in the growth inhibition zone if they were PrEP treated with Amphotericin B and exposed to Riboflavin and Ultraviolet A radiation. The damaged fungal cell wall following collagen cross-linking allows greater access to Amphotericin B thereby having a synergistic effect. Cell morphology of *Candida* and *Fusarium* spp. showed significant alteration of fungal viability after exposure to Riboflavin and Ultraviolet A light [112]. Rose bengal as a photosensitizing agent has also been found to be effective against *Fusarium*, *Aspergillus*, and *Candida* [113]. Collagen cross-linking increases the number of covalent bonds between collagen fibrils thereby increasing its mechanical strength. The cross-linked cornea has increased diameter of the collagen fibrils and altered biomechanical properties and stiffness [114–116]. Cross-linking also increases the resistance of collagen to enzymatic degradation [117]. The additional anti-inflammatory effects of cross-linking also cause decrease in pain sensitivity and provide significant pain relief in nonhealing refractory ulcers [118].

Experience in clinical cases of cross-linking has mixed response. Li et al. [119] and Said et al. [120] reported complete healing of keratitis and disappearance of hypopyon with cross-linking. There were no perforations or need for corneal transplantation. However, in a randomized clinical trial, Uddaraju et al. [121] did not find additional benefit of collagen cross-linking in deep recalcitrant fungal keratitis. The healing time and final visual acuity were not found to be different in cases managed with collagen cross-linking as compared to medical management alone. The cross-linked corneas experienced more perforations as compared to conservative management. The authors attributed no additional benefit to collagen cross-linking in deep fungal keratitis. In a review of literature on cross-linking in infectious keratitis [122], we recommended that the evidence in favor of cross-linking for infectious keratitis be limited mostly to case reports and case series. The disease definition as well as variability in the disease severity makes interpretation of results difficult. Treatment failure and stromal melt is not a uniformly agreed-upon entity in most papers on crosslinking; therefore the inclusion of patients for crosslinking becomes subjective. In light of the evidence that is currently available, collagen crosslinking serves as an adjunctive treatment modality especially in cases with a superficial infiltrate.

11.9 Conclusions

Fungal keratitis is a relatively common cause of corneal ulceration in the hot humid climate of the tropics. Most of the population is engaged in agriculture-based activities and predisposition to vegetative trauma is common. Contact lens solution related fungal keratitis has also triggered a lot of attention to this entity in the previous decade. Fungal keratitis is slowly progressive with a delayed presentation often limited by lack of access to adequate treatment. Pretreatment with multiple over the counter topical medications including corticosteroids confuse the clinical picture. The increased prevalence of diabetes mellitus is a significant comorbidity. The diagnosis is fairly simple with a smear positivity of close to 90%. Treatment is challenging due to delayed presentation, lack of penetration of drugs into the corneal stroma, and most of the antifungals being of a fungistatic nature. The recently conducted randomized control trials have found natamycin to be the single best drug in the management of fungal keratitis. Surgical management is mostly limited to cases refractory to maximal medical treatment, development of a corneal perforation, or impending spread of the disease to the limbus and sclera. While eradication of the focus of infection and preservation of the structural integrity of the globe is the primary goal of surgery, vision restoration often needs endothelial keratoplasty or a repeat penetrating keratoplasty in the setting of a failed graft. Fungal keratitis being a common entity in the tropics, a strong clinical suspicion, early identification, and timely management will help achieving adequate control of this disease entity.

References

1. Srinivasan M, Gonzales CA, George C, Cevallos V, Mascarenhas JM, Asokan B, Wilkins J, Smolin G, Whitcher JP. Epidemiology and aetiological diagnosis of corneal ulceration in Madurai, South India. Br J Ophthalmol. 1997;81(11):965–71.
2. Gopinathan U, Sharma S, Garg P, Rao GN. Review of epidemiological features, microbiological diagnosis and treatment outcome of microbial keratitis: experience of over a decade. Indian J Ophthalmol. 2009;57(4):273–9.
3. Dunlop AA, Wright ED, Howlader SA, Nazrul I, Husain R, McClellan K, Billson FA. Suppurative corneal ulceration in Bangladesh. A study of 142 cases examining the microbiological diagnosis, clinical and epidemiological features of bacterial and fungal keratitis. Aust N Z J Ophthalmol. 1994;22(2):105–10.
4. Hagan M, Wright E, Newman M, Dolin P, Johnson G. Causes of suppurative keratitis in Ghana. Br J Ophthalmol. 1995;79(11):1024–8.
5. Leck AK, Thomas PA, Hagan M, Kaliamurthy J, Ackuaku E, John M, Newman MJ, Codjoe FS, Opintan JA, Kalavathy CM, Essuman V, Jesudasan CA, Johnson GJ. Aetiology of suppurative corneal ulcers in Ghana and South India, and epidemiology of fungal keratitis. Br J Ophthalmol. 2002;86(11):1211–5.
6. Rondeau N, Bourcier T, Chaumeil C, Borderie V, Touzeau O, Scat Y, Thomas F, Baudouin C, Nordmann JP, Laroche L. [Fungal keratitis at the Centre Hospitalier National d'Ophtalmologie des Quinze-Vingts: retrospective study of 19 cases]. J Fr Ophtalmol. 2002;25(9):890–6.
7. Galarreta DJ, Tuft SJ, Ramsay A, Dart JK. Fungal keratitis in London: microbiological and clinical evaluation. Cornea. 2007;26(9):1082–6.
8. Rosa RH Jr, Miller D, Alfonso EC. The changing spectrum of fungal keratitis in South Florida. Ophthalmology. 1994;101(6):1005–13.
9. Tanure MA, Cohen EJ, Sudesh S, Rapuano CJ, Laibson PR. Spectrum of fungal keratitis at Wills Eye Hospital, Philadelphia, Pennsylvania. Cornea. 2000;19(3):307–12.
10. Ritterband DC, Seedor JA, Shah MK, Koplin RS, McCormick SA. Fungal keratitis at the New York eye and ear infirmary. Cornea. 2006;25(3):264–7.
11. Jeng BH, Gritz DC, Kumar AB, Holsclaw DS, Porco TC, Smith SD, Whitcher JP, Margolis TP, Wong IG. Epidemiology of ulcerative keratitis in Northern California. Arch Ophthalmol. 2010;128(8):1022–8.
12. Miño de Kaspar H, Zoulek G, Paredes ME, Alborno R, Medina D, Centurion de Morinigo M, Ortiz de Fresco M, Aguero F. Mycotic keratitis in Paraguay. Mycoses. 1991;34(5–6):251–4.
13. Mselle J. Fungal keratitis as an indicator of HIV infection in Africa. Trop Dr. 1999;29(3):133–5.
14. Badawi AE, Moemen D, El-Tantawy NL. Epidemiological, clinical and laboratory findings of infectious keratitis at Mansoura Ophthalmic Center, Egypt. Int J Ophthalmol. 2017;10(1):61–7.
15. Wong T, Ormonde S, Gamble G, McGhee CN. Severe infective keratitis leading to hospital admission in New Zealand. Br J Ophthalmol. 2003;87(9):1103–8.

16. Bhartiya P, Daniell M, Constantinou M, Islam FM, Taylor HR. Fungal keratitis in Melbourne. Clin Exp Ophthalmol. 2007;35(2):124–30.
17. Williams G, McClellan K, Billson F. Suppurative keratitis in rural Bangladesh: the value of gram stain in planning management. Int Ophthalmol. 1991;15(2):131–5.
18. Upadhyay MP, Karmacharya PC, Koirala S, Tuladhar NR, Bryan LE, Smolin G, Whitcher JP. Epidemiologic characteristics, predisposing factors, and etiologic diagnosis of corneal ulceration in Nepal. Am J Ophthalmol. 1991;111(1):92–9.
19. Khairallah SH, Byrne KA, Tabbara KF. Fungal keratitis in Saudi Arabia. Doc Ophthalmol. 1992;79(3):269–76.
20. Gonawardena SA, Ranasinghe KP, Arseculeratne SN, Seimon CR, Ajello L. Survey of mycotic and bacterial keratitis in Sri Lanka. Mycopathologia. 1994;127(2):77–81.
21. Imwidthaya P. Mycotic keratitis in Thailand. J Med Vet Mycol. 1995;33(1):81–2.
22. Panda A, Sharma N, Das G, Kumar N, Satpathy G. Mycotic keratitis in children: epidemiologic and microbiologic evaluation. Cornea. 1997;16(3):295–9.
23. Wong TY, Fong KS, Tan DT. Clinical and microbial spectrum of fungal keratitis in Singapore: a 5-year retrospective study. Int Ophthalmol. 1997;21(3):127–30.
24. Rahman MR, Johnson GJ, Husain R, Howlader SA, Minassian DC. Randomised trial of 0.2% chlorhexidine gluconate and 2.5% natamycin for fungal keratitis in Bangladesh. Br J Ophthalmol. 1998;82(8):919–25.
25. Deshpande SD, Koppikar GV. A study of mycotic keratitis in Mumbai. Indian J Pathol Microbiol. 1999;42(1):81–7.
26. Houang E, Lam D, Fan D, Seal D. Microbial keratitis in Hong Kong: relationship to climate, environment and contact-lens disinfection. Trans R Soc Trop Med Hyg. 2001;95(4):361–7.
27. Basak SK, Basak S, Mohanta A, Bhowmick A. Epidemiological and microbiological diagnosis of suppurative keratitis in Gangetic West Bengal, eastern India. Indian J Ophthalmol. 2005;53(1):17–22.
28. Xie L, Zhong W, Shi W, Sun S. Spectrum of fungal keratitis in North China. Ophthalmology. 2006;113(11):1943–8.
29. Lin CC, Lalitha P, Srinivasan M, Prajna NV, McLeod SD, Acharya NR, Lietman TM, Porco TC. Seasonal trends of microbial keratitis in South India. Cornea. 2012;31(10):1123–7.
30. Ranjini CY, Waddepally VV. Microbial profile of corneal ulcers in a Tertiary Care Hospital in South India. J Ophthalmic Vis Res. 2016;11(4):363–7.
31. Alfonso JF, Baamonde MB, Santos MJ, Astudillo A, Fernández-Vega L. Acremonium fungal infection in 4 patients after laser in situ keratomileusis. J Cataract Refract Surg. 2004;30(1):262–7.
32. Sun Y, Jain A, Ta CN. Aspergillus fumigatus keratitis following laser in situ keratomileusis. J Cataract Refract Surg. 2007;33(10):1806–7.
33. Thomas PA, Leck AK, Myatt M. Characteristic clinical features as an aid to the diagnosis of suppurative keratitis caused by filamentous fungi. Br J Ophthalmol. 2005;89(12):1554–8.
34. Garg P, Mahesh S, Bansal AK, Gopinathan U, Rao GN. Fungal infection of sutureless self-sealing incision for cataract surgery. Ophthalmology. 2003;110(11):2173–7.
35. Roy A, Sahu SK, Padhi TR, Das S, Sharma S. Clinicomicrobiological characteristics and treatment outcome of sclerocorneal tunnel infection. Cornea. 2012;31(7):780–5.
36. Kuo IC, Margolis TP, Cevallos V, Hwang DG. Aspergillus fumigatus keratitis after laser in situ keratomileusis. Cornea. 2001;20(3):342–4.
37. Foster CS. Fungal keratitis. Infect Dis Clin N Am. 1992;6(4):851–7.
38. Wessel JM, Bachmann BO, Meiller R, Kruse FE. Fungal interface keratitis by Candida orthopsilosis following deep anterior lamellar keratoplasty. BMJ Case Rep. 2013;2013.
39. McElnea E, Power B, Murphy C. Interface fungal keratitis after descemet stripping automated endothelial keratoplasty: a review of the literature with a focus on outcomes. Cornea. 2018;37(9):1204–11.
40. Augustin VA, Weller JM, Kruse FE, Tourtas T. Fungal interface keratitis after descemet membrane endothelial keratoplasty. Cornea. 2018;37(11):1366–9.

41. Kaufman SC, Musch DC, Belin MW, Cohen EJ, Meisler DM, Reinhart WJ, Udell IJ, Van Meter WS. Confocal microscopy: a report by the American Academy of Ophthalmology. Ophthalmology. 2004;111(2):396–406.

42. Chidambaram JD, Prajna NV, Larke NL, Palepu S, Lanjewar S, Shah M, Elakkiya S, Lalitha P, Carnt N, Vesaluoma MH, Mason M, Hau S, Burton MJ. Prospective study of the diagnostic accuracy of the in vivo laser scanning confocal microscope for severe microbial keratitis. Ophthalmology. 2016;123(11):2285–93.

43. Vaddavalli PK, Garg P, Sharma S, Sangwan VS, Rao GN, Thomas R. Role of confocal microscopy in the diagnosis of fungal and acanthamoeba keratitis. Ophthalmology. 2011;118(1):29–35.

44. McLeod SD. The role of cultures in the management of ulcerative keratitis. Cornea. 1997;16(4):381–2.

45. Sridhar MS, Sharma S, Gopinathan U, Rao GN. Anterior chamber tap: diagnostic and therapeutic indications in the management of ocular infections. Cornea. 2002;21(7):718–22.

46. Gopinathan U, Garg P, Fernandes M, Sharma S, Athmanathan S, Rao GN. The epidemiological features and laboratory results of fungal keratitis: a 10-year review at a referral eye care center in South India. Cornea. 2002;21(6):555–9.

47. Alexandrakis G, Jalali S, Gloor P. Diagnosis of Fusarium keratitis in an animal model using the polymerase chain reaction. Br J Ophthalmol. 1998;82(3):306–11.

48. Gaudio PA, Gopinathan U, Sangwan V, Hughes TE. Polymerase chain reaction based detection of fungi in infected corneas. Br J Ophthalmol. 2002;86(7):755–60.

49. Halliday C, Wu QX, James G, Sorrell T. Development of a nested qualitative real-time PCR assay to detect Aspergillus species DNA in clinical specimens. J Clin Microbiol. 2005;43(10):5366–8.

50. Badenoch PR, Coster DJ, Wetherall BL, Brettig HT, Rozenbilds MA, Drenth A, Wagels G. Pythium insidiosum keratitis confirmed by DNA sequence analysis. Br J Ophthalmol. 2001;85(4):502–3.

51. Hamilton HI, McLaughlin SA, Whitley EM, Gilger BC, Whitley RD. Histological findings in corneal stromal abscesses of 11 horses: correlation with cultures and cytology. Equine Vet J. 1994;26(6):448–53.

52. Panda A, Mohan M, Mukherjee G. Mycotic keratitis in Indian patients (a histopathological study of corneal buttons). Indian J Ophthalmol. 1984;32(5):311–5.

53. Naumann G, Green WR, Zimmerman LE. A histopathologic study of 73 cases. Am J Ophthalmol. 1967;64(4):668–82.

54. Ishibashi Y, Kaufman HE. Corneal biopsy in the diagnosis of keratomycosis. Am J Ophthalmol. 1986;101(3):288–93.

55. Ishibashi Y, Hommura S, Matsumoto Y. Direct examination vs culture of biopsy specimens for the diagnosis of keratomycosis. Am J Ophthalmol. 1987;103(5):636–40.

56. Vemuganti GK, Garg P, Gopinathan U, Naduvilath TJ, John RK, Buddi R, Rao GN. Evaluation of agent and host factors in progression of mycotic keratitis: a histologic and microbiologic study of 167 corneal buttons. Ophthalmology. 2002;109(8):1538–46.

57. Thomas PA. Mycotic keratitis-an underestimated mycosis. J Med Vet Mycol. 1994;32(4):235–56.

58. Garg P, Vemuganti GK, Chatarjee S, Gopinathan U, Rao GN. Pigmented plaque presentation of dematiaceous fungal keratitis: a clinicopathologic correlation. Cornea. 2004;23(6):571–6.

59. Prajna NV, Krishnan T, Mascarenhas J, Rajaraman R, Prajna L, Srinivasan M, Raghavan A, Oldenburg CE, Ray KJ, Zegans ME, McLeod SD, Porco TC, Acharya NR, Lietman TM, Mycotic Ulcer Treatment Trial Group. The mycotic ulcer treatment trial: a randomized trial comparing natamycin vs voriconazole. JAMA Ophthalmol. 2013;131(4):422–9.

60. FlorCruz NV, Peczon IV, Evans JR. Medical interventions for fungal keratitis. Cochrane Database Syst Rev. 2012;2:CD004241.

61. Ansari Z, Miller D, Galor A. Current thoughts in fungal keratitis: diagnosis and treatment. Curr Fungal Infect Rep. 2013;7(3):209–18.

62. Thomas PA. Current perspectives on ophthalmic mycoses. Clin Microbiol Rev. 2003;16(4):730–97.
63. Thomas PA, Kaliamurthy J. Mycotic keratitis: epidemiology, diagnosis and management. Clin Microbiol Infect. 2013;19(3):210–20.
64. Maharana PK, Sharma N, Nagpal R, Jhanji V, Das S, Vajpayee RB. Recent advances in diagnosis and management of Mycotic keratitis. Indian J Ophthalmol. 2016;64(5):346–57.
65. Sharma S, Das S, Virdi A, Fernandes M, Sahu SK, Kumar Koday N, Ali MH, Garg P, Motukupally SR. Re-appraisal of topical 1% voriconazole and 5% natamycin in the treatment of fungal keratitis in a randomised trial. Br J Ophthalmol. 2015;99(9):1190–5.
66. Prajna NV, Krishnan T, Rajaraman R, Patel S, Srinivasan M, Das M, Ray KJ, O'Brien KS, Oldenburg CE, McLeod SD, Zegans ME, Porco TC, Acharya NR, Lietman TM, Rose-Nussbaumer J, Mycotic Ulcer Treatment Trial II Group. Effect of oral voriconazole on fungal keratitis in the Mycotic Ulcer Treatment Trial II (MUTT II): a randomized clinical trial. JAMA Ophthalmol. 2016;134(12):1365–72.
67. Alastruey-Izquierdo A, Melhem MS, Bonfietti LX, Rodriguez-Tudela JL. Susceptibility test for fungi: clinical and laboratorial correlations in medical mycology. Rev Inst Med Trop Sao Paulo. 2015;57(Suppl-19):57–64.
68. Sun CQ, Lalitha P, Prajna NV, Karpagam R, Geetha M, O'Brien KS, Oldenburg CE, Ray KJ, McLeod SD, Acharya NR, Lietman TM, Mycotic Ulcer Treatment Trial Group. Association between in vitro susceptibility to natamycin and voriconazole and clinical outcomes in fungal keratitis. Ophthalmology. 2014;121(8):1495–500.
69. Shapiro BL, Lalitha P, Loh AR, Fothergill AW, Prajna NV, Srinivasan M, Kabra A, Chidambaram J, Acharya NR, Lietman TM. Susceptibility testing and clinical outcome in fungal keratitis. Br J Ophthalmol. 2010;94(3):384–5.
70. Lalitha P, Prajna NV, Oldenburg CE, Srinivasan M, Krishnan T, Mascarenhas J, Vaitilingam CM, McLeod SD, Zegans ME, Porco TC, Acharya NR, Lietman TM. Organism, minimum inhibitory concentration, and outcome in a fungal corneal ulcer clinical trial. Cornea. 2012;31(6):662–7.
71. Garg P, Roy A, Roy S. Update on fungal keratitis. Curr Opin Ophthalmol. 2016;27(4):333–9.
72. de Sá FA, Taveira SF, Gelfuso GM, Lima EM, Gratieri T. Liposomal voriconazole (VOR) formulation for improved ocular delivery. Colloids Surf B Biointerfaces. 2015;133:331–8.
73. Leal AF, Leite MC, Medeiros CS, Cavalcanti IM, Wanderley AG, Magalhães NS, Neves RP. Antifungal activity of a liposomal itraconazole formulation in experimental Aspergillus flavus keratitis with endophthalmitis. Mycopathologia. 2015;179(3–4):225–9.
74. Jaiswal M, Kumar M, Pathak K. Zero order delivery of itraconazole via polymeric micelles incorporated in situ ocular gel for the management of fungal keratitis. Colloids Surf B Biointerfaces. 2015;130:23–30.
75. Jain A, Shah SG, Chugh A. Cell penetrating peptides as efficient nanocarriers for delivery of antifungal compound, natamycin for the treatment of fungal keratitis. Pharm Res. 2015;32(6):1920–30.
76. Garcia-Valenzuela E, Song CD. Intracorneal injection of amphotericin B for recurrent fungal keratitis and endophthalmitis. Arch Ophthalmol. 2005;123(12):1721–3.
77. Tu EY, Majmudar PA. Adjuvant stromal amphotericin B injection for late-onset DMEK infection. Cornea. 2017;36(12):1556–8.
78. Prakash G, Sharma N, Goel M, Titiyal JS, Vajpayee RB. Evaluation of intrastromal injection of voriconazole as a therapeutic adjunctive for the management of deep recalcitrant fungal keratitis. Am J Ophthalmol. 2008;146(1):56–9.
79. Sharma N, Agarwal P, Sinha R, Titiyal JS, Velpandian T, Vajpayee RB. Evaluation of intrastromal voriconazole injection in recalcitrant deep fungal keratitis: case series. Br J Ophthalmol. 2011;95(12):1735–7.
80. Siatiri H, Daneshgar F, Siatiri N, Khodabande A. The effects of intrastromal voriconazole injection and topical voriconazole in the treatment of recalcitrant Fusarium keratitis. Cornea. 2011;30(8):872–5.

81. Tu EY. Alternaria keratitis: clinical presentation and resolution with topical fluconazole or intrastromal voriconazole and topical caspofungin. Cornea. 2009;28(1):116–9.
82. Sharma N, Chacko J, Velpandian T, Titiyal JS, Sinha R, Satpathy G, Tandon R, Vajpayee RB. Comparative evaluation of topical versus intrastromal voriconazole as an adjunct to natamycin in recalcitrant fungal keratitis. Ophthalmology. 2013;120(4):677–81.
83. Kalaiselvi G, Narayana S, Krishnan T, Sengupta S. Intrastromal voriconazole for deep recalcitrant fungal keratitis: a case series. Br J Ophthalmol. 2015;99(2):195–8.
84. Niki M, Eguchi H, Hayashi Y, Miyamoto T, Hotta F, Mitamura Y. Ineffectiveness of intrastromal voriconazole for filamentous fungal keratitis. Clin Ophthalmol. 2014;8:1075–9.
85. Tu EY, Hou J. Intrastromal antifungal injection with secondary lamellar interface infusion for late-onset infectious keratitis after DSAEK. Cornea. 2014;33(9):990–3.
86. Yilmaz S, Ture M, Maden A. Efficacy of intracameral amphotericin B injection in the management of refractory keratomycosis and endophthalmitis. Cornea. 2007;26(4):398–402.
87. Sharma B, Kataria P, Anand R, Gupta R, Kumar K, Kumar S, Gupta R. Efficacy profile of intracameral amphotericin B. The often forgotten step. Asia Pac J Ophthalmol. 2015;4(6):360–6.
88. Yoon KC, Jeong IY, Im SK, Chae HJ, Yang SY. Therapeutic effect of intracameral amphotericin B injection in the treatment of fungal keratitis. Cornea. 2007;26(7):814–8.
89. Shen YC, Wang CY, Tsai HY, Lee HN. Intracameral voriconazole injection in the treatment of fungal endophthalmitis resulting from keratitis. Am J Ophthalmol. 2010;149(6):916–21.
90. Qu L, Li L, Xie H. Corneal and aqueous humor concentrations of amphotericin B using three different routes of administration in a rabbit model. Ophthalmic Res. 2010;43(3):153–8.
91. Sharma N, Sankaran P, Agarwal T, Arora T, Chawla B, Titiyal JS, Tandon R, Satapathy G, Vajpayee RB. Evaluation of intracameral amphotericin B in the management of fungal keratitis: randomized controlled trial. Ocul Immunol Inflamm. 2016;24(5):493–7.
92. Webster RG Jr, Slansky HH, Refojo MF, Boruchoff SA, Dohlman CH. The use of adhesive for the closure of corneal perforations. Report of two cases. Arch Ophthalmol. 1968;80(6):705–9.
93. Hirst LW, Smiddy WE, Stark WJ. Corneal perforations. Changing methods of treatment, 1960–1980. Ophthalmology. 1982;89(6):630–5.
94. Weiss JL, Williams P, Lindstrom RL, Doughman DJ. The use of tissue adhesive in corneal perforations. Ophthalmology. 1983;90(6):610–5.
95. Leahey AB, Gottsch JD, Stark WJ. Clinical experience with N-butyl cyanoacrylate (Nexacryl) tissue adhesive. Ophthalmology. 1993;100(2):173–80.
96. Garg P, Gopinathan U, Nutheti R, Rao GN. Clinical experience with N-butyl cyanoacrylate tissue adhesive in fungal keratitis. Cornea. 2003;22(5):405–8.
97. Cavanaugh TB, Gottsch JD. Infectious keratitis and cyanoacrylate adhesive. Am J Ophthalmol. 1991;111(4):466–72.
98. Sharma A, Kaur R, Kumar S, Gupta P, Pandav S, Patnaik B, Gupta A. Fibrin glue versus N-butyl-2-cyanoacrylate in corneal perforations. Ophthalmology. 2003;110(2):291–8.
99. Sharma N, Jain M, Sehra SV, Maharana P, Agarwal T, Satpathy G, Vajpayee RB. Outcomes of therapeutic penetrating keratoplasty from a Tertiary Eye Care Centre in Northern India. Cornea. 2014;33(2):114–8.
100. Shi W, Wang T, Xie L, Li S, Gao H, Liu J, Li H. Risk factors, clinical features, and outcomes of recurrent fungal keratitis after corneal transplantation. Ophthalmology. 2010;117(5):890–6.
101. Sabatino F, Sarnicola E, Sarnicola C, Tosi GM, Perri P, Sarnicola V. Early deep anterior lamellar keratoplasty for fungal keratitis poorly responsive to medical treatment. Eye. 2017;31(12):1639–46.
102. Gao H, Song P, Echegaray JJ, Jia Y, Li S, Du M, Perez VL, Shi W. Big bubble deep anterior lamellar keratoplasty for management of deep fungal keratitis. J Ophthalmol. 2014;2014:209759.
103. Xie L, Shi W, Liu Z, Li S. Lamellar keratoplasty for the treatment of fungal keratitis. Cornea. 2002;21(1):33–7.
104. Anshu A, Parthasarathy A, Mehta JS, Htoon HM, Tan DT. Outcomes of therapeutic deep lamellar keratoplasty and penetrating keratoplasty for advanced infectious keratitis: a comparative study. Ophthalmology. 2009;116(4):615–23.

105. Gundersen T. Conjunctival flaps in the treatment of corneal disease with reference to a new technique of application. AMA Arch Ophthalmol. 1958;60(5):880–8.
106. Khodadoust A, Quinter AP. Microsurgical approach to the conjunctival flap. Arch Ophthalmol. 2003;121(8):1189–93.
107. Zhong J, Wang B, Li S, Deng Y, Huang H, Chen L, Yuan J. Full-thickness conjunctival flap covering surgery combined with amniotic membrane transplantation for severe fungal keratitis. Exp Ther Med. 2018;15(3):2711–8.
108. Abdulhalim BE, Wagih MM, Gad AA, Boghdadi G, Nagy RR. Amniotic membrane graft to conjunctival flap in treatment of non-viral resistant infectious keratitis: a randomised clinical study. Br J Ophthalmol. 2015;99(1):59–63.
109. Tsugita A, Okada Y, Uehara K. Photosensitized inactivation of ribonucleic acids in the presence of riboflavin. Biochim Biophys Acta. 1965;103(2):360–3.
110. Wollensak G, Spoerl E, Seiler T. Riboflavin/ultraviolet-a-induced collagen crosslinking for the treatment of keratoconus. Am J Ophthalmol. 2003;135(5):620–7.
111. Sauer A, Letscher-Bru V, Speeg-Schatz C, Touboul D, Colin J, Candolfi E, Bourcier T. In vitro efficacy of antifungal treatment using riboflavin/UV-A (365 nm) combination and amphotericin B. Invest Ophthalmol Vis Sci. 2010;51(8):3950–3.
112. Kashiwabuchi RT, Carvalho FR, Khan YA, Hirai F, Campos MS, McDonnell PJ. Assessment of fungal viability after long-wave ultraviolet light irradiation combined with riboflavin administration. Graefes Arch Clin Exp Ophthalmol. 2013;251(2):521–7.
113. Arboleda A, Miller D, Cabot F, Taneja M, Aguilar MC, Alawa K, Amescua G, Yoo SH, Parel JM. Assessment of rose Bengal versus riboflavin photodynamic therapy for inhibition of fungal keratitis isolates. Am J Ophthalmol. 2014;158(1):64–70.
114. Wollensak G, Wilsch M, Spoerl E, Seiler T. Collagen fiber diameter in the rabbit cornea after collagen crosslinking by riboflavin/UVA. Cornea. 2004;23(5):503–7.
115. He X, Spoerl E, Tang J, Liu J. Measurement of corneal changes after collagen crosslinking using a noninvasive ultrasound system. J Cataract Refract Surg. 2010;36(7):1207–12.
116. Spoerl E, Terai N, Scholz F, Raiskup F, Pillunat LE. Detection of biomechanical changes after corneal cross-linking using Ocular Response Analyzer software. J Refract Surg. 2011;27(6):452–7.
117. Spoerl E, Wollensak G, Seiler T. Increased resistance of crosslinked cornea against enzymatic digestion. Curr Eye Res. 2004;29(1):35–40.
118. Shetty R, Nagaraja H, Jayadev C, Shivanna Y, Kugar T. Collagen crosslinking in the management of advanced non-resolving microbial keratitis. Br J Ophthalmol. 2014;98(8):1033–5.
119. Li Z, Jhanji V, Tao X, Yu H, Chen W, Mu G. Riboflavin/ultravioilet light-mediated crosslinking for fungal keratitis. Br J Ophthalmol. 2013;97(5):669–71.
120. Said DG, Elalfy MS, Gatzioufas Z, El-Zakzouk ES, Hassan MA, Saif MY, Zaki AA, Dua HS, Hafezi F. Collagen cross-linking with photoactivated riboflavin (PACK-CXL) for the treatment of advanced infectious keratitis with corneal melting. Ophthalmology. 2014;121(7):1377–82.
121. Uddaraju M, Mascarenhas J, Das MR, Radhakrishnan N, Keenan JD, Prajna L, Prajna VN. Corneal cross-linking as an adjuvant therapy in the management of recalcitrant deep stromal fungal keratitis: a randomized trial. Am J Ophthalmol. 2015;160(1):131–4.
122. Garg P, Das S, Roy A. Collagen cross-linking for microbial keratitis. Middle East Afr J Ophthalmol. 2017;24(1):18–23.

Pythium Keratitis

Bhupesh Bagga and Maneesha M. Bellala

12.1 Introduction

Human pythiosis is fatal, and an emerging disease of the tropical [1], subtropical, and temperate region. Although more commonly reported from southeast Asia [1, 2] (i.e., India, Indonesia, Japan, Korea, New Guinea, and Thailand), it has also been reported from the eastern coast of Australia and New Zealand, South America (Argentina, Brazil, Colombia, Venezuela), Costa Rica, Guatemala, Haiti, Panama and Nicaragua, and North America (Mexico, the United States, and Gulf coast states) [1, 3]. It is caused by a fungus like, oomycete *Pythium insidiosum* [4]. Human pythiosis [1] can be divided into four various clinical groups depending on their presentations: cutaneous/subcutaneous (5%), vascular (59%), ocular (33%), and disseminated cases (3%). Among the risk factors, Thalassemia-hemoglobinopathy syndrome [5] was found to be associated in most of the cases with cutaneous/subcutaneous, vascular, and disseminated pythiosis (85%). Ocular pythiosis is common during rainy season [2, 6], and the risk factors [1] include exposure to farming, direct contact with water resource (i.e., lake, river, lagoon, swamp, or even swimming pool), and contact lens wear [7–9]. Systemic immunosuppressants [10] used for chronic diseases like Crohn's disease have also been reported to predispose to such serious infections. Among the ocular involvement, corneal involvement was first reported by Vergille et al. in 1993 [11].

B. Bagga (✉) · M. M. Bellala
Cornea & Anterior Segment Service, L V Prasad Eye Institute, Hyderabad, Telangana, India
e-mail: bhupesh@lvpei.org

© Springer Nature Singapore Pte Ltd. 2021

177

S. Das, V. Jhanji (eds.), *Infections of the Cornea and Conjunctiva*,
https://doi.org/10.1007/978-981-15-8811-2_12

12.2   The Organism

Pythium is an oomycete which closely mimics fungus in its morphological features. It belongs to the genus of parasitic oomycetes. Previously they were classified under the fungi. It is primarily a plant pathogen but can cause pythiosis in animals. This was described as fungus in 1884 by Smith et al. [12] Due to lack of sporulation, it could not be identified until 1961, when it was first recognized as Hyphomycosis destruens by Bridges et al. [13] Later in 1974, Austwick and Copland [14] observed zoospore formation during transfer of colonies from Sabouraud's dextrose medium to aqueous medium. It has coenocytic hyphae [4] without septations. The term coenocytic refers to multinucleated cells without cytokinesis; this is caused by divisions of nucleus. Phylogenetically, it resembles more with algae than fungi. *Pythium* species belong to the kingdom *Stramenopila*, the class Oomycetes, the order *Pythiales*, and the family *Pythiacae*. It is not a true fungus. The cell wall [4] of *Pythium* lacks chitin, and has cellulose instead. The Cell membrane does not contain ergosterol. Production of zoospores is responsible for infection. Zoospores are single nucleated cells and biflagellate without a cell wall. It is considered to be an infective propagule which can swim and has chemotactic properties. When in contact with injured plants, zoospores encyst themselves and attaches to the plant via glycoprotein. It does not need any mammalian host for its survival as it can remain alive in its natural location. The life cycle as proposed by Mendoza et al., based on the light and electron microscopic features [15], is different in humans and plants. After colonization of plants, differentiation and maturation of sporangium occur with the release of zoospores which can swim and infect other plants. In humans or other animals after contact, zoospores lose their flagella and attach to the tissue with the help of a sticky substance followed by encystment, germination, and invasion resulting in pythiosis.

12.3   Clinical Features

The onset is usually 6–7 days with a history of exposure of any of the mentioned risk factors. The clinical features [6, 16, 17] at presentation usually include central white infiltration with tentacles like extension and pinhead lesions into the surrounding stroma (Figs. 12.1, 12.2, and 12.3). The infiltrate may be associated with

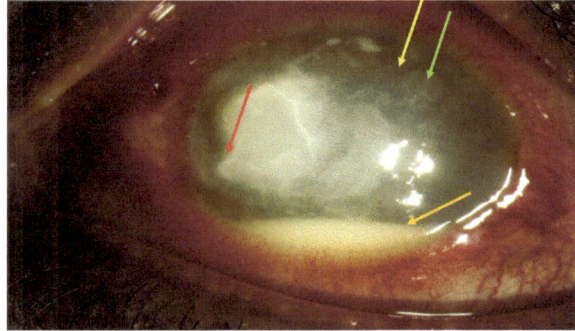

Fig. 12.1 Raised whitish infiltrate like a plaque (red arrow), tentacles (yellow arrow), pinhead lesions (green arrow), and hypopyon (orange arrow)

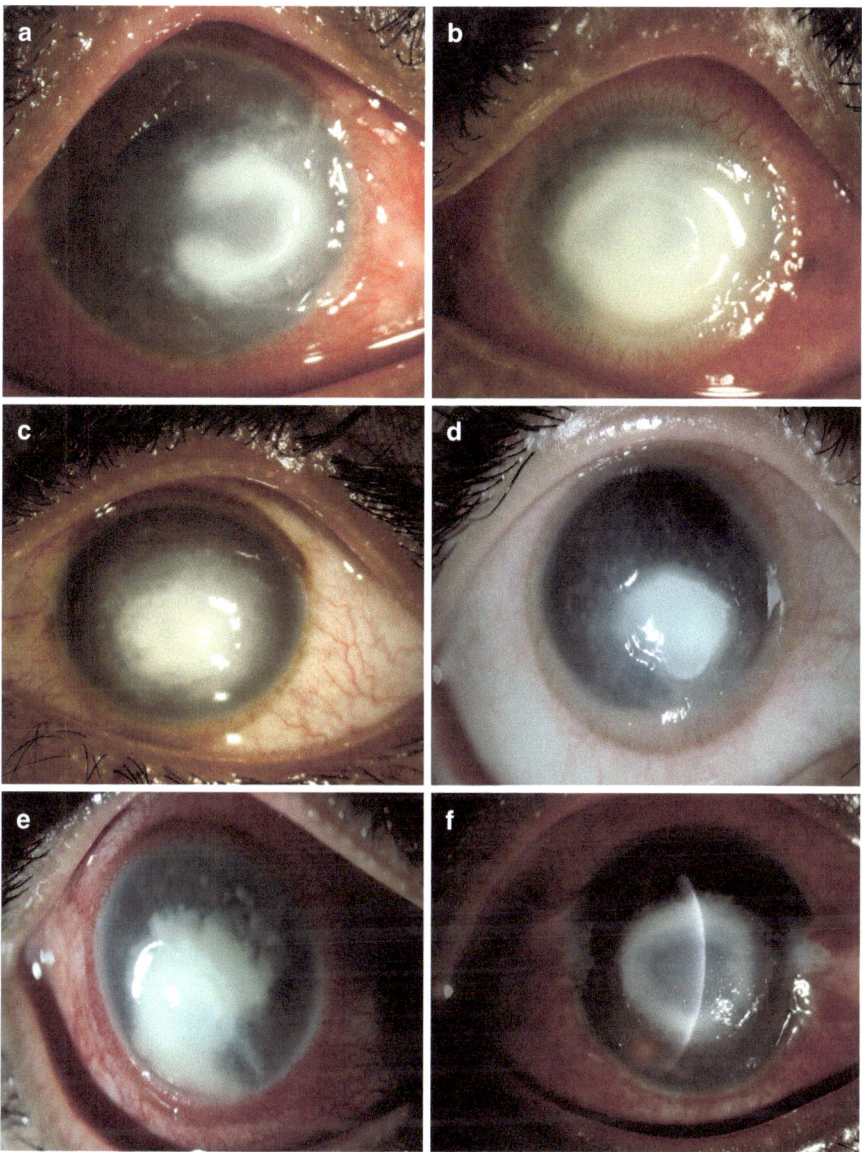

Fig. 12.2 Different presentations of *Pythium* keratitis: (**a**) peripheral ring shaped infiltrate with extension, (**b**) diffuse anterior to midstromal infiltrate, (**c**) central yellowish infiltrate with deep stromal extension, (**d**) raised whitish plaque with tentacular extension, (**e**) aggressive posterior stromal extension, and (**f**) ring shaped infiltrate with tentacle like extension

peripheral furrowing along with raised edges. Stromal thinning and deep vessels increase as the disease progresses. The frequency of each clinical sign at the time of presentation to clinic is shown in Table 12.1 [18]. The most important and frequent clinical sign associated is the presence of fine radiating tentacles along the margin of the infiltrate. However, there can be typical and atypical presentations (Fig. 12.2).

Fig. 12.3 Peripheral guttering (red arrow) with raised central plaque (yellow arrow) along with peripheral radiating tentacles (orange arrow) is uniformly present

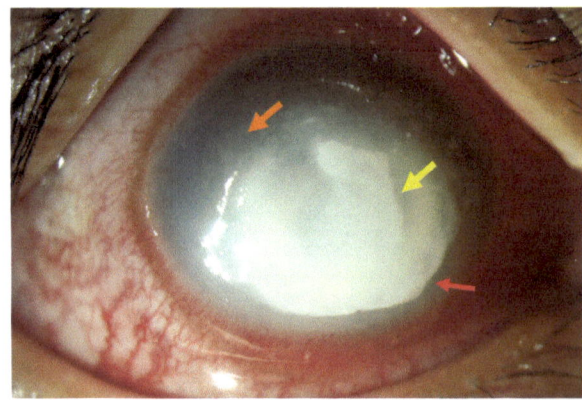

Table 12.1 Clinical signs in cases of *Pythium* keratitis (some patients have more than one clinical sign)

Sl. #	Characteristics	%
(a)	Tentacles	86.96%
(b)	Pinhead lesions	82.61%
(c)	Guttering	46.38%
(d)	Hypopyon	46.38%
(e)	Plaque	20.29%
(f)	Central thinning	13%
(g)	Endoexudates	10.14%
(h)	Endothelial ring	2.90%
(i)	Perforated ulcer	1.45%

12.4 Diagnosis

Microbiological workup to confirm the clinical diagnosis includes corneal scraping of the infiltrate for direct microscopic examination of the *Pythium* filaments and/or its growth on culture media. These filaments are classically aseptate or sparsely septate, relatively broad, ribbon-like filaments as observed under direct microscopy on 10% potassium hydroxide with 0.1% calcofluor white or Gram stain. As illustrated by Mittal [19] et al., these filaments can be differentiated from fungal filaments with the help of potassium iodide–sulfuric acid (IKI-H_2SO_4). Growth on blood agar is flat, feathery edged, appressed, glabrous, colorless, or light brown radiating colonies (Fig. 12.4).

Formation of characteristic zoospores in aqueous medium, as described by Mendoza [15] et al., has been one of the measures to confirm the diagnosis [16, 20, 21] for *Pythium insidiosum*. Among oomycetes, formation of zoospores is also seen in *Phytophthora* and *Lagenidium*.

Other ways to diagnose are molecular methods such as PCR-based DNA sequencing [20, 22, 23] which have been used to confirm the species. Confocal microscopy has been used for in vivo diagnosis but could not differentiate conclusively from fungal keratitis [24].

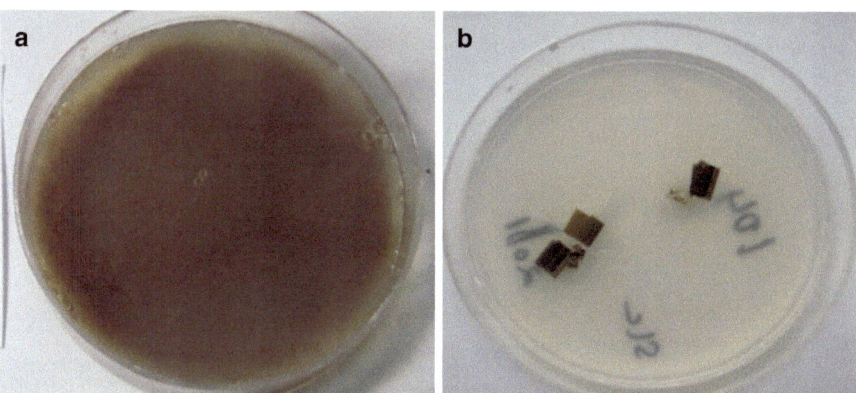

Fig. 12.4 Greyish, translucent, flat, and appressed growth with feathery edges on chocolate agar: (**a**) carnation leaves in an induction medium and (**b**) used for zoospore induction

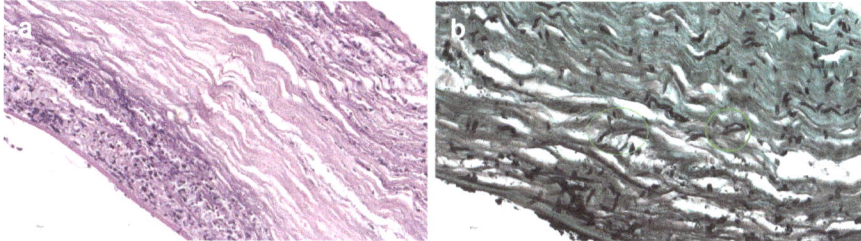

Fig. 12.5 Corneal histopathology of a corneal button of *Pythium* keratitis retrieved after therapeutic keratoplasty (**a**) Hematoxylin-Eosin stain (10×) and (**b**) GMS stain (20×). (Courtesy: Saumya Jakati)

On histopathological examination [19] of the corneal button obtained after keratoplasty, an inverse correlation was observed between the degree of inflammatory infiltrates and load of *Pythium* filaments (Fig. 12.5). Granulomatous inflammation was found in 30% of corneal tissue from therapeutic keratoplasty (TPK) specimens of *Pythium*. Other important findings were a relatively rare invasion of Descemet's membrane in contrast to fungal keratitis where DM perforation by fungal filaments are more commonly observed. Involvement of other ocular structures has been found to be less common. On electron microscopy, these hyphae were found to have a layered zone separating cell wall and membrane, but the most important finding was the presence of vesicles, which were either empty or filled with homogenous material [25].

12.5 Treatment

Medical treatment of *Pythium* keratitis alone may not be sufficient to manage the keratitis. Therapeutic keratoplasty may be required in some cases. Some of the causes include delayed or inaccurate diagnosis due to close similarity with fungal

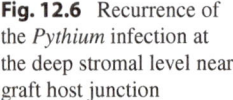
Fig. 12.6 Recurrence of the *Pythium* infection at the deep stromal level near graft host junction

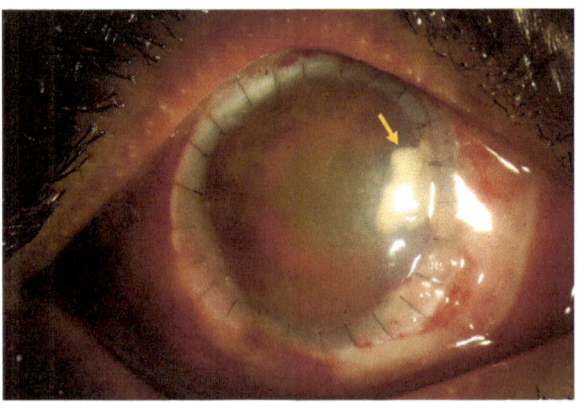

filaments. In the recently published prospective trial by Permpalung [26] et al., nearly half the number of patients had undergone enucleation due to worsening of infection and suggested early surgical intervention in terms of therapeutic keratoplasty. Similarly, Agarwal [17] et al. also reported the role of surgical management, as in their experience, medical treatment alone is not successful. They have also mentioned high risk of recurrences of *Pythium* keratitis after TPK (Fig. 12.6) and recommended adjuvant treatment in the form of cryotherapy to decrease the recurrence. There has been recent evidence related to the antipythium efficacy of alcohol [27].

Early diagnosis by keen observation of salient clinical and microbiological features can lead to proper diagnosis, and thereby modifying the prognosis. Based on in vitro susceptibility testing for antibiotics, and a pilot trial [28], the efficacy of combination of linezolid and azithromycin has been found to be effective in the treatment of *Pythium* keratitis. The Recommended regimen is to use topical linezolid 0.2% (prepared from IV preparation) and azithromycin eye ointment 1% along with oral azithromycin 500 mg once a day for nearly 2 weeks. Use of oral azithromycin needs preevaluation by a general physician to rule out any associated cardiac contraindication or possible interaction with any of the drug which may cause QT-interval prolongation in ECG. Based on this trial, it is advisable to initiate treatment in a strategic manner [18]. Firstly, it should be diagnosed with the help of clinical and microbiological examination. Then it should be confirmed by the formation of zoospores or PCR-assisted diagnosis. Cases who are not in very advanced stage of keratitis should be managed initially with combination of antibiotics with minimum of 2 weeks of treatment to ascertain the clinical response. Patients who show poor response with medical treatment manifesting as extension of the infiltrate either peripherally or posteriorly should be subjected to therapeutic penetrating keratoplasty with 1 mm of clear cornea as safe margin. Response to medical treatment is noted by blunting of the tentacles and clearing of the surrounding stroma (Fig. 12.7). On follow-up, a formation of peripheral thinning surrounding the infiltrate can be observed (Fig. 12.3). In cases with significant corneal thinning, cyanoacrylate glue application should be planned to avoid corneal perforation. In general,

Fig. 12.7 (**a**) Whitish ring shaped infiltrate: (a) with surrounding tentacular extension with stromal edema which responded and (**b**) infiltrate responded to combination of antibiotics

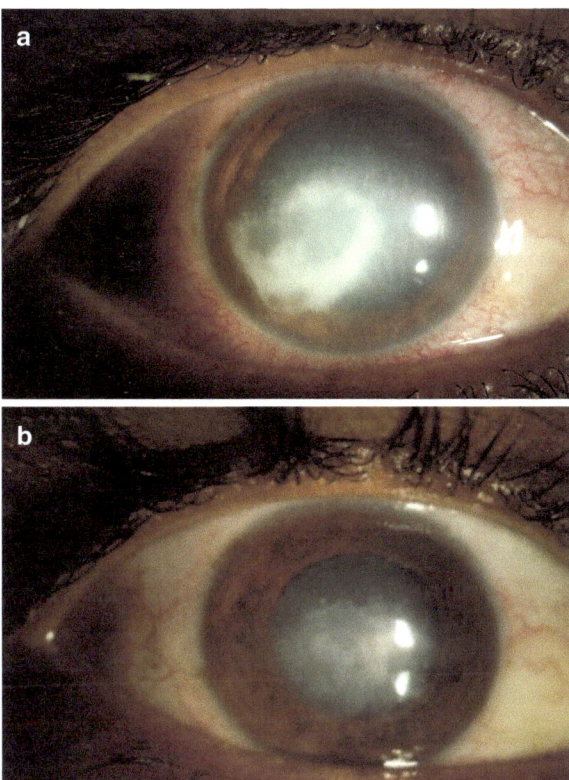

infection resolves with increase in stromal vascularization associated with decrease in the size of infiltrate (Fig. 12.4). Medical treatment results in the resolution of infection in nearly 50–60% cases, provided early diagnosis of infection is made. Median duration of resolution is 3 months. The outcome of penetrating keratoplasty for corneal scar after resolution of keratitis is shown to be better as compared to active keratitis (Fig. 12.8).

12.6   Prognosis

The prognosis of infection depends on the early diagnosis. On reevaluations of the cases being managed by medical and surgical treatment, few prognostic factors have been noted. Factors associated with better prognosis are younger age at presentation without associated comorbid conditions, early confirmation of the diagnosis along with <6 mm size of the infiltrate, and limited to the anterior stroma. Cases with corneal Infiltrate extending to posterior stromal involvement with associated endo-exudates are usually associated with bad prognosis and need early surgical intervention. The tell-tale signs mentioned can help in providing strategic approach towards the management of *Pythium* keratitis.

Fig. 12.8 Severe *Pythium* keratitis: (**a**) with lesions extending both posteriorly as well as till the limbus, (**b**) showing the complete resolution of infection following medical treatment, and (**c**) followed by optical keratoplasty along with cataract surgery with PCIOL placement

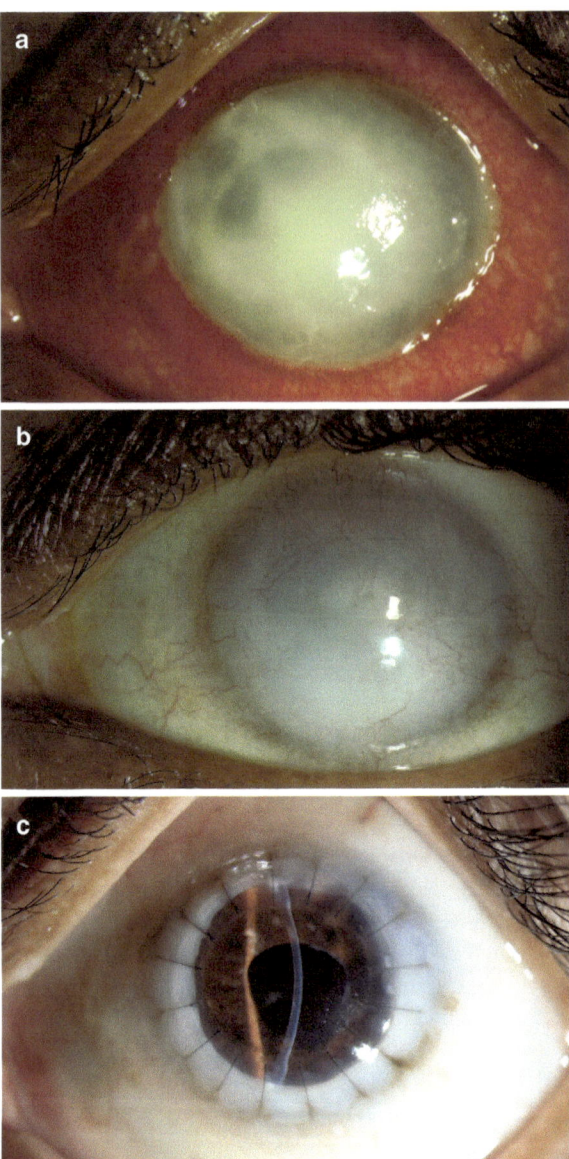

References

1. Krajaejun T, Sathapatayavongs B, Pracharktam R, Nitiyanant P, Leelachaikul P, Wanachiwanawin W, Chaiprasert A, Assanasen P, Saipetch M, Mootsikapun P, Chetchotisakd P, Lekhakula A, Mitarnun W, Kalnauwakul S, Supparatpinyo K, Chaiwarith R, Chiewchanvit S, Tananuvat N, Srisiri S, Suankratay C, Kulwichit W, Wongsaisuwan M, Somkaew S. Clinical and epidemiological analyses of human pythiosis in Thailand. Clin Infect Dis. 2006;43(5):569–76.

2. Thanathanee O, Enkvetchakul O, Rangsin R, Waraasawapati S, Samerpitak K, Suwan-apichon O. Outbreak of Pythium keratitis during rainy season: a case series. Cornea. 2013;32(2):199–204.
3. Presser JW, Goss EM. Environmental sampling reveals that Pythium insidiosum is ubiquitous and genetically diverse in North Central Florida. Med Mycol. 2015;53(7):674–83.
4. De Cock AW, Mendoza L, Padhye AA, Ajello L, Kaufman L. Pythium insidiosum sp. nov., the etiologic agent of pythiosis. J Clin Microbiol. 1987;25(2):344–9.
5. Chitasombat MN, Jongkhajornpong P, Lekhanont K, Krajaejun T. Recent update in diagnosis and treatment of human pythiosis. Peer J. 2020;8:e8555.
6. Hasika R, Lalitha P, Radhakrishnan N, Rameshkumar G, Prajna NV, Srinivasan M. Pythium keratitis in South India: incidence, clinical profile, management, and treatment recommendation. Indian J Ophthalmol. 2019;67(1):42–7.
7. Lekhanont K, Chuckpaiwong V, Chongtrakool P, Aroonroch R, Vongthongsri A. Pythium insidiosum keratitis in contact lens wear: a case report. Cornea. 2009;28(10):1173–7.
8. Tanhehco TY, Stacy RC, Mendoza L, Durand ML, Jakobiec FA, Colby KA. Pythium insidiosum keratitis in Israel. Eye Contact Lens. 2011;37(2):96–8.
9. Raghavan A, Bellamkonda P, Mendoza L, Rammohan R. Pythium insidiosum and Acanthamoeba keratitis in a contact lens user. BMJ Case Rep. 2018;11(1).
10. Hung C, Leddin D. Keratitis caused by Pythium insidiosum in an immunosuppressed patient with Crohn's disease. Clin Gastroenterol Hepatol. 2014;12(10):A21–2.
11. Virgile R, Perry HD, Pardanani B, Szabo K, Rahn EK, Stone J, Salkin I, Dixon DM. Human infectious corneal ulcer caused by Pythium insidiosum. Cornea. 1993;12(1):81–3.
12. Smith F. The pathology of bursattee. Vet J. 1884;19:16 7.
13. Bridges CH, Emmons CW. A phycomycosis of horses caused by Hyphomyces destruens. J Am Vet Med Assoc. 1961;138:579–89.
14. Austwick PK, Copland JW. Swamp cancer. Nature. 1974;250(461):84.
15. Mendoza L, Hernandez F, Ajello L. Life cycle of the human and animal oomycete pathogen Pythium insidiosum. J Clin Microbiol. 1993;31(11):2967–73.
16. Sharma S, Balne PK, Motukupally SR, Das S, Garg P, Sahu SK, Arunasri K, Manjulatha K, Mishra DK, Shivaji S. Pythium insidiosum keratitis: clinical profile and role of DNA sequencing and zoospore formation in diagnosis. Cornea. 2015;34(4):438–42.
17. Agarwal S, Iyer G, Srinivasan B, Agarwal M, Panchalam Sampath Kumar S, Therese LK. Clinical profile of Pythium keratitis: perioperative measures to reduce risk of recurrence. Br J Ophthalmol. 2018;102(2):153–7.
18. Bagga B, Kate A, Mohamed A, Sharma S, Das S, Mitra S. Successful strategic management of Pythium insidiosum keratitis with antibiotics. Ophthalmology 2020; Published online ahead of print.
19. Mittal R, Jena SK, Desai A, Agarwal S. Pythium insidiosum keratitis: histopathology and rapid novel diagnostic staining technique. Cornea. 2017;36(9):1124–32.
20. Badenoch PR, Coster DJ, Wetherall BL, Brettig HT, Rozenbilds MA, Drenth A, Wagels G. Pythium insidiosum keratitis confirmed by DNA sequence analysis. Br J Ophthalmol. 2001;85(4):502–3.
21. Thongsri Y, Wonglakorn L, Chaiprasert A, Svobodova L, Hamal P, Pakarasang M, Prariyachatigul C. Evaluation for the clinical diagnosis of Pythium insidiosum using a single-tube nested PCR. Mycopathologia. 2013;176(5-6):369–76.
22. Kosrirukvongs P, Chaiprasert A, Uiprasertkul M, Chongcharoen M, Banyong R, Krajaejun T, Wanachiwanawin W. Evaluation of nested pcr technique for detection of Pythium insidiosum in pathological specimens from patients with suspected fungal keratitis. Southeast Asian J Trop Med Public Health. 2014;45(1):167–73.
23. Kosrirukvongs P, Chaiprasert A, Canyuk C, Wanachiwanawin W. Comparison of nested PCR and culture identification of Pythium insidiosum in patients with Pythium keratitis. J Med Assoc Thail. 2016;99(9):1033–8.
24. Anutarapongpan O, Thanathanee O, Worrawitchawong J, Suwan-Apichon O. Role of confocal microscopy in the diagnosis of Pythium insidiosum keratitis. Cornea. 2018;37(2):156–61.

25. Badenoch PR, Mills RA, Chang JH, Sadlon TA, Klebe S, Coster DJ. Pythium insidiosum keratitis in an Australian child. Clin Exp Ophthalmol. 2009;37(8):806–9.
26. Permpalung N, Worasilchai N, Manothummetha K, Torvorapanit P, Ratanawongphaibul K, Chuleerarux N, Plongla R, Chindamporn A. Clinical outcomes in ocular Pythiosis patients treated with a combination therapy protocol in Thailand: a prospective study. Med Mycol. 2019;57(8):923–8.
27. Agarwal S, Srinivasan B, Janakiraman N, Therese LK, Kumar SK, Patel N, Thenmozhi V, Iyer G. Role of topical ethanol in the treatment of Pythium insidiosum keratitis—a proof of concept. Cornea 2020; Published online ahead of print.
28. Bagga B, Sharma S, Madhuri Guda SJ, Nagpal R, Joseph J, Manjulatha K, Mohamed A, Garg P. Leap forward in the treatment of Pythium insidiosum keratitis. Br J Ophthalmol. 2018;102(12):1629–33.

Herpes Simplex Virus (HSV) Keratitis

Zeba A. Syed, Beeran B. Meghpara,
and Christopher J. Rapuano

13.1 Background

Herpes simplex virus (HSV) is a ubiquitous double-stranded DNA virus that is a member of the human herpesvirus family. Humans are the only known natural reservoir for the virus. HSV is the etiology for several systemic infections including orolabial herpes, herpes gladiatorum, and herpes encephalitis [1]. When involving the ocular and periocular tissue, HSV can manifest as blepharitis, conjunctivitis, keratitis, iritis, trabeculitis, or retinitis. HSV keratitis is the most common etiology for infectious corneal blindness in developed countries [2]. The annual cost of treatment for this infectious condition reaches the tens of millions of dollars in the United States alone [3].

Disease may either occur as a primary infection or as a recurrence of latent disease. Primary infection with HSV typically occurs secondary to HSV spread through direct contact of infected lesions or secretions, such as tears or saliva, with mucous membranes of the host [4]. Asymptomatic individuals may shed HSV into their saliva, and one study found that 92% of asymptomatic HSV-infected subjects shed HSV-1 DNA from tears at least once during a 30-day period [5]. Interestingly, only 74% of subjects from this study were IgG positive for HSV-1, indicating that individuals who are seronegative can still harbor and shed HSV [5]. Many patients experience symptoms during primary infection; however, approximately two-thirds of primary HSV infections are unrecognized or asymptomatic.

Ocular HSV infection typically occurs secondary to the HSV-1 virus, although HSV-2 can also be responsible for HSV keratitis [1]. While HSV-2 is classically responsible for most genital herpes infections, HSV-1 and HSV-2 have been identified in similar numbers in the trigeminal and sacral ganglia at autopsy [6]. Therefore, host cell factors are the likely reason for the preference of HSV-1 for the facial area

Z. A. Syed · B. B. Meghpara · C. J. Rapuano (✉)
Wills Eye Hospital, Thomas Jefferson University, Philadelphia, PA, USA
e-mail: cjrapuano@willseye.org

© Springer Nature Singapore Pte Ltd. 2021
S. Das, V. Jhanji (eds.), *Infections of the Cornea and Conjunctiva*,
https://doi.org/10.1007/978-981-15-8811-2_13

and HSV-2 for the genital area. In the United States, approximately 50% of the population harbors HSV-1 by 30 years of age, while at least 90% is infected by age 60 years [7, 8]. Studies from across different countries estimate the incidence of new cases of ocular HSV to range from 5 to 15 new cases per 100,000 individuals per year [4, 9–12]. This rate appears to be slowly trending upwards [4, 13].

13.2   Manifestations of HSV Keratitis

13.2.1 Epithelial Keratitis

Epithelial keratitis is the most common subtype of HSV keratitis [14]. Typical symptoms include redness, discharge, pain, and photophobia. With recurrent disease, chronic neurotrophic changes may result in fewer ocular pain symptoms. The differential diagnosis of HSV epithelial keratitis includes Acanthamoeba keratitis, varicella zoster virus (VZV) keratitis, Epstein-Barr virus keratitis, and epithelial regeneration lines.

The classic features of HSV epithelial keratitis are coarse, granular epithelial lesions that coalesce to form corneal dendrites [15]. A corneal dendrite is linear, branching, and exhibits terminal bulbs (Fig. 13.1). These dendrites are ulcerated and feature fluorescein staining at their base (Fig. 13.2) with rose bengal or lissamine green staining of the surrounding devitalized epithelial cells. Upon healing, a "ghost dendrite" can appear, characterized by subepithelial haze in a dendritic pattern. Dendrites present less frequently during recurrent disease. Other features of HSV epithelial keratitis include larger geographic ulcers (Fig. 13.3) or peripheral ulcers. The presence of a peripheral ulcer may result in misdiagnosis as an autoimmune-related keratitis.

Epithelial keratitis typically resolves without treatment in 2 weeks, but early initiation of antiviral therapy can reduce disease severity and hasten recovery [1]. Although epithelial debridement is a long-standing practice, there is strong evidence that debridement alone is insufficient therapy for HSV epithelial keratitis

Fig. 13.1 Dendrite in HSV epithelial keratitis

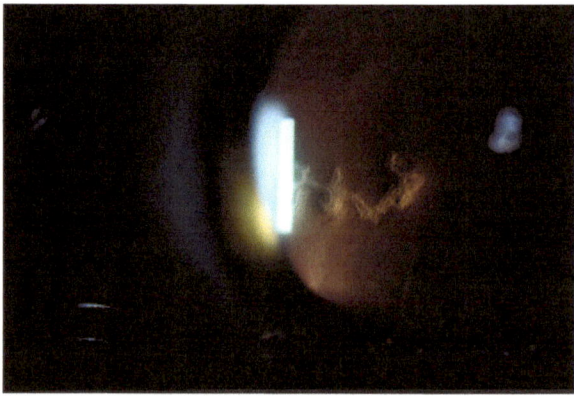

Fig. 13.2 Fluorescein staining of multiple dendrites in HSV epithelial keratitis

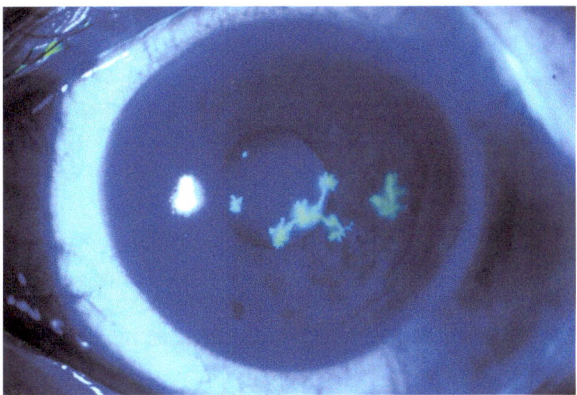

Fig. 13.3 Fluorescein staining of geographic HSV epithelial keratitis in an eye after penetrating keratoplasty for HSV scarring

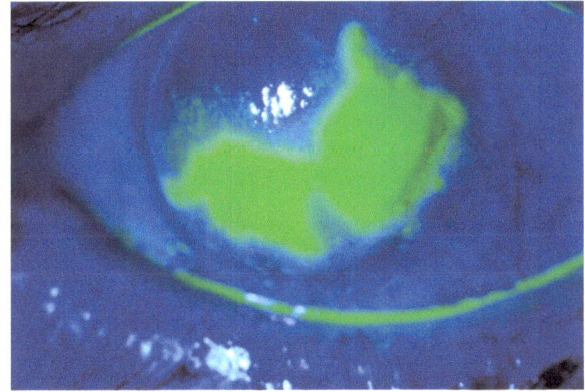

[16]. Several studies suggest that treatment with a combination of antiviral therapy and debridement results in faster healing than treatment with antiviral therapy alone [17, 18]. Debridement may be followed by amniotic membrane placement to potentially hasten recovery [19].

Medication options include systemic agents and topical therapy, with overall equal effectiveness between oral and ophthalmic options. In general, it is advisable to avoid or minimize topical corticosteroids in cases of HSV epithelial keratitis. Many cornea specialists prefer systemic over topical antiviral therapy due to its higher bioavailability, ease of administration, and the surface toxicity associated with many topical agents. Acyclovir and its derivatives contain nucleoside analogs that are selectively phosphorylated by viral and not host enzymes, therefore exhibiting few side effects. The analog is incorporated into viral DNA and results in chain termination, preventing further viral replication [20, 21]. Oral acyclovir reaches therapeutic levels in both tears and aqueous humor [22].

Oral treatment regimens include a 7–10 day course of acyclovir 400 mg three to five times daily, valacyclovir 500 mg two to three times daily, or famciclovir 250 mg two to three times daily. In cases of geographic ulcers, practitioners may extend treatment for 14–21 days and increase dosing to acyclovir 800 mg five times daily, valacyclovir 1 g three times daily, or famciclovir 500 mg two to three times daily. Compared with oral acyclovir, valacyclovir is better absorbed from the gastrointestinal tract with a threefold to fourfold higher circulating drug level, requiring a reduced frequency of administration and possibly improved patient adherence [23, 24]. Side effects of these medications include nausea, vomiting, diarrhea, or other gastrointestinal disturbances [24]. Oral antiviral agents should be employed with caution in elderly patients or in those with renal disease, as they have the potential to induce nephrotoxicity. In refractory cases, systemic valganciclovir has also shown successful results [25].

Although many clinicians prefer systemic to topical antiviral therapy, some cases of HSV keratitis may not respond to oral therapy alone, and can benefit from the addition of topical treatment [26]. While such selected cases exist, no large-scale study has demonstrated a benefit to dual topical and oral therapy for HSV keratitis compared to treatment with a single antiviral medication [27]. For decades, topical regimens for HSV epithelial keratitis included idoxuridine, vidarabine, and trifluridine 1%. These agents are limited primarily by toxicity, resulting in keratoconjunctivitis, allergic conjunctivitis, and punctal stenosis [28]. Overall, topical antiviral medications result in an allergic or toxic blepharoconjunctivitis or corneal epitheliopathy in 5–10% of patients [29].

Current topical regimens available in the United States for HSV epithelial keratitis include trifluridine 1% ophthalmic solution nine times daily for 7 days or ganciclovir 0.15% ophthalmic gel five times daily until the epithelium closes, followed by three times daily for 7 days. Many practitioners avoid using trifluridine 1% for more than 14–21 days due to toxicity. Acyclovir 3% ophthalmic ointment, which was approved by the United States Food and Drug Administration (FDA) in 2019, is better tolerated than trifluridine 1%, even with long-term use, but can cause blurred vision [30]. Ganciclovir 0.15% ophthalmic gel causes less visual disturbances and toxicity as compared to acyclovir 3% ointment with equivalent efficacy [31]. Despite having fewer side effects, ganciclovir 0.15% gel can also result in blurred vision and punctate keratitis [32].

Importantly, most topical antiviral medications fail to reach therapeutic levels in the aqueous humor, with the exception of acyclovir 3% ointment, and should not be used as monotherapy in cases of HSV keratouveitis [33]. Adequate aqueous concentrations of trifluridine 1% can be attained after epithelial debridement [34, 35]. Furthermore, topical therapy does not prevent reactivation of the virus from the sensory ganglia [30].

Long-term treatment with any of these medications can uncommonly result in the emergence of resistance due to viral mutations [36, 37]. Resistance to acyclovir has been shown to present more frequently in immunocompromised individuals those with recurrent ocular HSV infections [38]. Mutations in thymidine kinase are responsible for most cases of acyclovir resistance, and these strains are also resistant to valacyclovir, ganciclovir, and famciclovir [39, 40]. In these cases, other antiviral agents such as foscarnet, cidofovir, and trifluridine should be considered [40–42]. There is some evidence for corneal collagen cross-linking in the management of refractory cases of HSV keratitis, although recurrences may occur [43].

13.2.2 Stromal Keratitis

HSV stromal keratitis develops secondary to retained HSV antigens that initiate an antigen-antibody complement cascade, triggering an immune reaction [1]. The condition may exist with or without epithelial ulceration. The differential diagnosis of HSV stromal keratitis includes any other cause of interstitial keratitis including VZV keratitis, syphilis, Cogan's syndrome, measles keratitis, and mumps keratitis.

The pathogenesis of HSV stromal keratitis has been shown to involve T-cell activation and cytokine release [44, 45]. The condition may occur primarily or may present secondary to epithelial or endothelial disease. Findings on examination for stromal keratitis without epithelial ulceration include unifocal, multifocal (Fig. 13.4), or diffuse stromal infiltrates. Stromal edema or thinning may variably be present, and slit lamp examination may demonstrate an immune ring or neovascularization. Although these vessels may recede with time to form "ghost vessels," persistent active vessels may result in lipid keratopathy and visually significant scarring (Fig. 13.5).

HSV stromal keratitis without epithelial ulceration is treated with prophylactic oral antiviral therapy and the addition of a topical corticosteroid, usually prednisolone acetate 1% ophthalmic suspension six to eight times daily. Corticosteroid

Fig. 13.4 Multifocal stromal infiltrates in HSV stromal keratitis

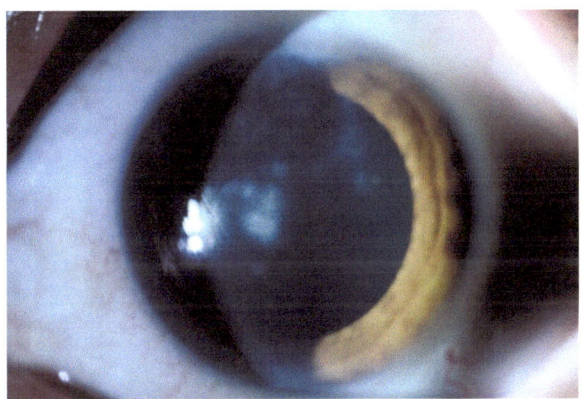

Fig. 13.5 HSV scar with neovascularization and lipid keratopathy

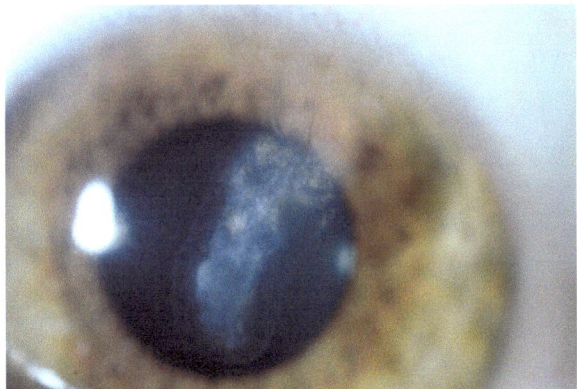

alternatives include fluorometholone 0.1–0.25% suspension and difluprednate 0.05% emulsion. Prophylactic oral antiviral options include acyclovir 400 mg twice daily, valacyclovir 500 mg once or twice daily, or famciclovir 250 mg once or twice daily. Oral antiviral medications should be continued for at least as long as corticosteroids are in use.

The Herpetic Eye Disease Study (HEDS) established the importance of topical corticosteroids in the treatment of HSV stromal keratitis and demonstrated a decrease in persistent or progressive stromal keratitis as well as a shortened duration of keratitis with initiation of topical corticosteroids [46]. The corticosteroid should be tapered very slowly, often over at least 10 weeks, to the lowest dose required to control inflammation. Long-term corticosteroid maintenance therapy may be required in addition to oral antiviral prophylaxis. Topical cyclosporine 2% has shown comparable results to topical prednisolone 1% in best-corrected visual acuity and corneal densitometry after stromal keratitis [47]. There is some evidence that topical cyclosporine ranging in concentration from 0.05 to 2% may replace or reduce the need for topical corticosteroids in HSV stromal keratitis cases with steroid-induced glaucoma [48–50].

A more severe form of stromal keratitis, often referred to as necrotizing stromal keratitis, involves concomitant epithelial ulceration and stromal loss (Fig. 13.6). This less frequent manifestation is thought to be secondary to viral invasion of the corneal stroma. The differential diagnosis includes microbial keratitis, keratolysis from chemical injuries and autoimmune conditions, and neurotrophic keratopathy. This aggressive condition is typically more resistant to therapy and involves significant keratolysis, ulceration, thinning (Fig. 13.7), and possibly corneal perforation. Since this condition shares features of bacterial keratitis, cultures should be performed to rule out other sources of infection.

Many physicians will treat stromal keratitis with epithelial ulceration with acyclovir 400–800 mg three to five times daily, valacyclovir 500 mg to 1 g three times daily, or famciclovir 250–500 mg two to three times daily. Topical trifluridine 1% and ganciclovir 0.15% demonstrate insufficient penetration of the corneal stroma, and therefore oral agents are preferred [35]. Judicious topical corticosteroids, often

Fig. 13.6 Stromal melt in HSV stromal keratitis with epithelial ulceration

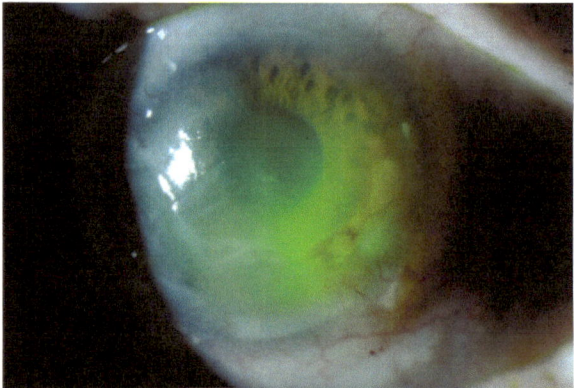

Fig. 13.7 Significant stromal thinning demonstrated using slit beam in the eye with HSV stromal keratitis with epithelial ulceration seen in Fig. 13.6

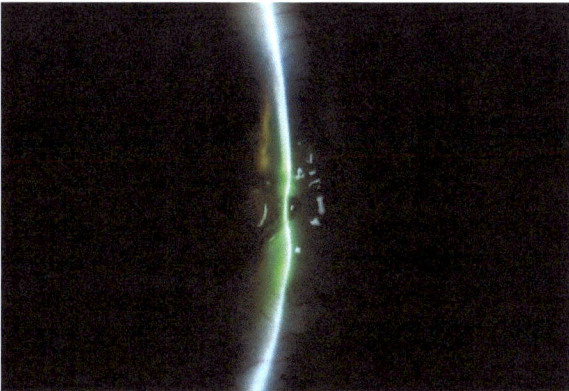

Fig. 13.8 Pattern of disciform endothelitis associated with keratic precipitates in HSV endothelial keratitis

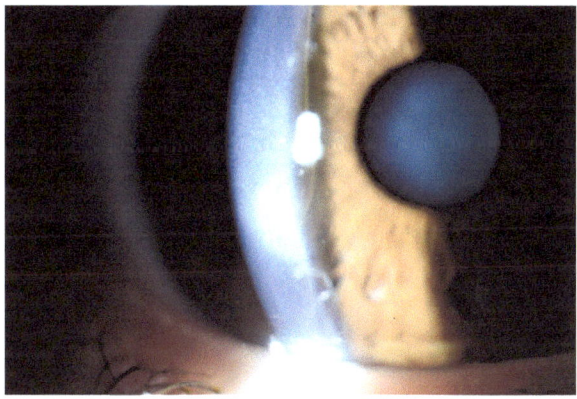

prednisolone 1% one to four times daily, may also be employed. Combining amniotic membrane grafting with medical therapy may help, but definitive data for the success of this approach has not been demonstrated [51]. Once the infection is controlled, oral antiviral therapy is reduced to a prophylactic dose and continued for as long as topical corticosteroids are used.

13.2.3 Endothelial Keratitis

HSV endothelial keratitis, also known as HSV endotheliitis, results from virus in the anterior chamber. Clinical findings include keratic precipitates, iritis, and stromal edema. The differential diagnosis of HSV endotheliitis includes any etiology of keratouveitis, Posner-Schlossman syndrome, and cytomegalovirus endothelial keratitis. In many cases, there is no prior known history of HSV epithelial or stromal keratitis. Endotheliitis may be subdivided based on the pattern of involvement as disciform, diffuse, or linear. Disciform endotheliitis is the most common form (Fig. 13.8), featuring a focal round area of stromal edema associated with underlying keratic precipitates and anterior uveitis [52]. Diffuse endotheliitis occurs less frequently, demonstrating keratic precipitates distributed throughout the endothelium. Diffuse endotheliitis may sometimes involve a retrocorneal plaque or a hypopyon, therefore potentially resembling a fungal infection. Finally, linear endotheliitis is characterized by a well-defined linear or serpiginous arrangement of keratic precipitates that demarcates edematous cornea from uninvolved and clear cornea.

The treatment regimen of HSV endotheliitis varies across practitioners, but active HSV in the anterior chamber necessitates systemic antiviral therapy instead of topical agents. Antiviral therapy is acyclovir 400 mg five times daily, valacyclovir 500 mg two to three times daily, or famciclovir 250 mg two to three times daily. Topical corticosteroids are typically initiated as well, usually prednisolone 1% six to eight times daily. Oral antiviral medication is continued until resolution of keratitis, and reduced to a prophylactic dose for as long as topical corticosteroids are being used. Linear endotheliitis may be more difficult to treat than the other patterns, and higher dosing of oral antivirals and corticosteroids may be indicated [1]. This would include acyclovir 400–800 mg five times daily, valacyclovir 500 mg to 1 g three times daily, or famciclovir 250–500 mg three times daily.

13.2.4 Keratouveitis

HSV keratouveitis may occur in association with epithelial, stromal, or endothelial disease. Anterior chamber inflammation occurs in up to 10% of patients with HSV keratitis [53]. Although the recognition of herpetic anterior uveitis is typically straightforward in the context of obvious herpetic lesions such as dendrites, it can be more challenging to identify the diagnosis in the absence of these findings. Clues pointing to the diagnosis of HSV keratouveitis include the presence of corneal scars or edema, decreased corneal sensation, geographically or diffusely distributed keratic precipitates, acutely elevated intraocular pressure, unilateral findings, and iris atrophy which can produce pupillary distortion and transillumination defects (Fig. 13.9) [30].

Fig. 13.9 Iris atrophy demonstrated using slit lamp transillumination in a patient with previous HSV keratouveitis and penetrating keratoplasty

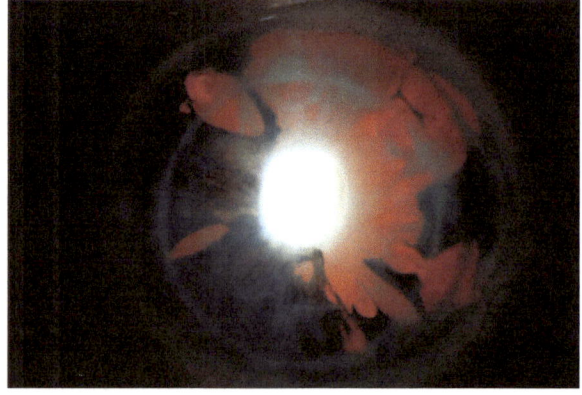

It is critical to distinguish HSV keratouveitis from VZV keratouveitis [54]. Typical concurrent or prior cutaneous lesions may provide strong support for VZV-related iritis, although these findings are not always present. Dendritic keratitis may help differentiate between the two, although it may be challenging to distinguish between HSV dendrites and VZV pseudodendrites, which are slightly elevated, polymorphous, exhibit less regular branching, demonstrate few terminal dilations, and have central rose bengal staining [30].

The treatment of HSV keratouveitis typically includes acyclovir 400–800 mg five times daily, valacyclovir 500 mg to 1 g three times daily, or famciclovir 250–500 mg three times daily. HEDS examined the effect of oral acyclovir in cases of herpetic keratitis on the duration and recurrence of anterior uveitis, and failed to identify a statistically significant treatment effect [55]. However, this arm of HEDS was relatively small and potentially underpowered [30]. Furthermore, patients were initially treated with both oral acyclovir and topical trifluridine, and therefore it may have been more difficult to identify a treatment effect of the oral acyclovir [30]. Hence, many practitioners will treat herpetic keratouveitis with high dose oral anti-viral medication until resolution of infection, and continued maintenance therapy with oral antiviral medication is typically employed to decrease recurrences [56]. Patients are started on topical corticosteroids and a cycloplegic agent to prevent posterior synechiae development and for improved comfort.

13.3   Diagnosis

Early diagnosis of HSV keratitis enables immediate treatment initiation to reduce viral replication and hasten healing. Furthermore, inappropriate treatment can aggravate corneal inflammation and lead to visually debilitating results.

The diagnosis of HSV keratitis is primarily clinical, with classic features as described above. However, the diagnosis can be confounded by factors such as duration of disease, systemic illnesses, prior therapy, and previous keratoplasty, all of which can distort the appearance of HSV lesions [57]. In one study, 8% of HSV cases diagnosed based on clinical appearance were identified using polymerase chain reaction (PCR) as secondary to VZV [58]. When using PCR to confirm a clinical diagnosis of HSV epithelial keratitis, only a moderate correlation was detected, which was even poorer with atypical HSV lesions [57, 59]. Corneal lesions caused by cytomegalovirus, adenovirus, and fungal infections also share features with HSV keratitis and may cause misdiagnosis [7].

Viral culture and antigen detection methods [e.g., enzyme-linked immunosorbent assay (ELISA)] are available to detect HSV; however, the sensitivity of these techniques is inferior to nucleic acid amplification tests [60]. PCR can be used to identify HSV in cases of active viral replication, as is the case in epithelial keratitis [61]. Viral PCR has the advantages of rapid results and a higher sensitivity as compared to other methods [61]. Previous studies have demonstrated that PCR detects anywhere from 29.2 to 76% more cases of HSV as compared to viral culture [62]. Using tear collections of clinically suspected HSV keratitis cases, one study found a sensitivity of ELISA to be 49.2% and specificity to be 82.6%, whereas sensitivity of PCR was 55.8% and specificity 100% [63]. There is significant variation in studies comparing the rates of HSV detection by PCR and clinical diagnosis [59].

One advantage of PCR is that specimens may be obtained from the corneal surface or the anterior chamber, allowing for detection of epithelial or endothelial infection. Unfortunately, PCR has shown less utility for the identification of immune-mediated stromal keratitis, given that viral infection does not directly cause this condition [59]. In cases of endotheliitis in post-keratoplasty eyes, the findings may clinically mimic graft rejection; PCR analysis of aqueous humor can be particularly useful in this setting [64, 65].

One major limitation of PCR is that it may produce false negatives in patients with atypical herpetic lesions or in patients actively using antiviral therapy [66]. One report identified an 80% decrease in detectable virus among individuals who had been treated with acyclovir 400 mg twice daily [67]. In addition, several compounds utilized during clinical evaluation can also affect PCR results. For example, oxybuprocaine, a topical anesthetic used in combination with fluorescein to enhance visualization of HSV lesions, can decrease PCR yield by more than 2 logs (DNA copies/sample) [68]. Rose bengal and lissamine green may also interfere with the detection of HSV-DNA using PCR [69].

An alternative means of diagnosis is in vivo confocal microscopy (IVCM), in which viral keratitis is suggested by a lack of atypical organisms, presence of dendritic cells in the basal epithelial and subepithelial nerve plexus regions, decrease in the subepithelial nerve plexus, and hyperreflective keratocytes in the anterior stroma [70]. Although highly operator-dependent, one study demonstrated a sensitivity and specificity of IVCM in identifying HSV keratitis as 100% and 93.2%, respectively [71].

Newer techniques include tear film analyses, for which a combined assay for HSV immunoglobulins and HSV-DNA demonstrated a 98% positive predictive value for stromal keratitis [72]. Tear samples have also been employed to detect HSV epithelial keratitis, with PCR testing as well as evaluation for HSV-1 antigens by indirect immunofluorescence assays [73]. Tear collection analysis has been shown to yield lower detection rates for HSV endotheliitis compared to HSV epithelial keratitis [63]. Furthermore, viral loads in tear collections diminish after 11 days of illness, which could contribute to false negatives [63]. Other technologies include gene sequencing of intraocular samples [74].

13.4 Special Circumstances

13.4.1 Pediatric Disease

In infants, primary HSV keratitis typically occurs secondary to HSV-2, which is transmitted through antenatal, intrapartum, or postnatal exposures. Due to a weaker immune system, HSV infection in this population may have a severe course. Immediate and aggressive treatment is crucial to prevent amblyopia and poor visual results [75, 76].

Older children with HSV keratitis also tend to experience more severe infection than adults, increased frequency of recurrences, and worse corneal scarring and astigmatism, resulting in poorer visual outcomes and amblyopia [77–79]. Similarly, episodes of HSV stromal keratitis in children tend to be more severe [79]. Pediatric HSV keratitis is compounded by the difficulty in examining this population, and as a result the condition may be commonly misdiagnosed resulting in delayed treatment [79]. In addition, pediatric cases of HSV keratitis are more likely to present bilaterally, with rates of 3.4–26%, as compared to 1.3–12% in adults [7, 77, 78, 80–83]. Furthermore, children are more likely to experience HSV keratitis recurrences within the first year of an initial episode as compared to adults (45–50% vs. 18%, respectively) [77, 80, 84].

The treatment of pediatric HSV keratitis differs from adults. Topical trifluridine 1% is only FDA approved for children age six and above, whereas ganciclovir 0.15% is FDA approved in children over the age of 2 years. Acyclovir is safe in neonates, however valacyclovir is indicated in children age two years or above. Famciclovir, on the other hand, is only indicated in patients older than 18 years of age. Acyclovir dosing may vary based on experience of the physician, and one study advised a treatment dose of 12–80 mg/kg/day in divided doses, and a prophylactic dose of 12–20 mg/kg/day [85].

13.4.2 Bilateral Disease

Although most cases of HSV keratitis are unilateral, in approximately 1.3–12% of adult cases, bilateral infections occur. This presentation may occur in immunocompromised individuals [59, 81]. Additionally, bilateral HSV keratitis is more common in cases of primary as compared to recurrent HSV keratitis [12]. As described above, bilateral HSV keratitis is more prevalent in the pediatric age group.

In addition, patients with atopy are also more likely to suffer from bilateral HSV keratitis [86]. Atopic describes patients with a personal or family history of hay fever, asthma, or eczema. In general, patients with atopy exhibit an exaggerated reactivity to common environmental antigens that typically cause no response in other individuals; these antigens stimulate the production and activation of eosinophils. These individuals experience altered cell-mediated immunity and are therefore susceptible to HSV keratitis [87–89]. One study documented a 2.0–4.8-fold increased odds of developing ocular HSV in individuals with atopic disease compared to those without atopy [86]. Patients with atopy and HSV keratitis often have severe cases of infection with a poorer therapeutic response to topical antiviral agents as compared to oral therapy [87]. These patients may necessitate relatively higher doses of oral antivirals.

13.4.3 Recurrent Disease

Oftentimes, primary infection of the cornea is detected on clinical exam. However, initial disease may be subclinical and still establish latent infection. After primary infection, the virus can be subsequently transported in a retrograde fashion via sensory neurons, establishing latency in the trigeminal ganglia [90]. The virus remains asymptomatic in the sensory ganglia until reactivation, resulting in secondary or recurrent HSV infection. Each episode of recurrent keratitis increases the risk of subsequent episodes [12]. Recurrence rates of HSV keratitis are approximately 25% in the first year after initial disease and 33% by the second year [91]. Evidence indicates that short intervals between previous episodes of HSV keratitis are associated with similarly short intervals between future episodes [92]. Seroprevalence is affected by the level of exposure to the source of infection, and therefore is influenced by factors such as crowding, poor hygiene, and age [7].

The severity and probability of recurrent HSV keratitis is dependent on the virulence of the viral strain and the susceptibility of the host to this particular strain. The underlying mechanism of reactivation or recurrence remains largely unknown; however, several hypotheses have been proposed. One possible explanation is that a high quantity of latent viral copies and the number of latently infected neurons may overwhelm the cellular defense mechanisms against viral infection [93].

Local stressors are well-known triggers for reactivation of HSV keratitis, and infection has been documented to occur more frequently following intravitreal injections [94], after cataract surgery [95], and after corneal transplantation [96]. HSV keratitis has also been reported after laser-assisted in situ keratomileusis (LASIK) [97, 98], laser iridotomy [99], argon laser trabeculoplasty [100], phototherapeutic keratectomy (PTK) [101], and photorefractive keratectomy (PRK) [102].

Certain topical medications also result in a predisposition of the cornea to HSV recurrence. For example, topical prostaglandin analogs, used for the treatment of elevated intraocular pressure, have been shown to be associated with HSV epithelial keratitis [103, 104]. Prostaglandins are therefore best avoided in patients with a known history of HSV keratitis. Additionally, several forms of corticosteroids, including topical, intravitreal, or systemic formulations, can predispose to HSV epithelial keratitis [105–107].

HEDS found no association of ocular HSV recurrence with psychological stress, systemic infection, ultraviolet light exposure, menstruation, contact lens wear, or eye injury [46]. However, other individual studies have identified possible associations of recurrent HSV infection with systemic fever [108], menstruation [109], psychological stress [110], and upper respiratory tract infections [111].

13.4.4 Prophylaxis

HEDS investigated the benefit of acyclovir 400 mg twice daily for the prevention of recurrent ocular HSV over a 12 month period and found that this regimen reduced the recurrence of ocular disease by approximately 50% [46]. This finding established the recommendation for long-term prophylaxis. Additionally, 12 months of oral antiviral prophylaxis reduces episodes of both HSV epithelial and stromal keratitis, the latter of which was only significant in individuals with a known history of HSV stromal keratitis [112]. Given the degree of morbidity associated with HSV stromal keratitis, long-term oral antiviral prophylaxis is beneficial for individuals with a history of this condition.

Importantly, antiviral agents may not prevent the development of new stromal keratitis, which is immunomediated; however, by reducing viral load, the magnitude of the inflammatory response may be suppressed [7]. HEDS included patients treated for HSV epithelial keratitis with topical trifluridine and evaluated whether oral acyclovir 400 mg five times daily for 3 weeks reduced future episodes of HSV stromal keratitis. The study found no benefit of short-term systemic antivirals in preventing stromal keratitis [29].

Prophylaxis options include acyclovir 400 mg twice daily, valacyclovir 500 mg once or twice daily, or famciclovir 250 mg once or twice daily. A trial of patients with a history of recurrent ocular HSV found no difference between the efficacy of oral acyclovir 400 mg twice daily and valacyclovir 500 mg once daily in the prevention of recurrences [113]. A study comparing systemic and topical acyclovir 3% ointment for the prevention of HSV keratitis recurrence following corneal transplant found significantly better results in those treated with oral acyclovir [114]. Prophylaxis is typically continued for at least 1 year, but often for many years, and permanently after corneal transplantation.

Indications for prophylaxis include, but are not limited to, cases of multiple recurrences of any form of HSV keratitis, postoperatively in patients with a history of HSV ocular disease, and a history of ocular HSV in patients undergoing immunosuppressive therapy. Additional populations that may benefit from prophylaxis include immunosuppressed, monocular, and atopic individuals.

The host immune system plays a central role in dictating general susceptibility to ocular HSV infections and prevention of HSV recurrences. For example, patients with prior organ transplants are often immunocompromised due to systemic immunosuppressive medications. These patients face an increased risk of HSV infection and reactivation [115–117]. Other predisposing conditions for HSV infection and recurrence include long-standing diabetes mellitus, especially with poor glycemic control [118–120]. HIV positive patients have been shown to have a higher recurrence rate of HSV keratitis [121].

Finally, a study of patients with a history of recurrent HSV keratitis identified that recurrences were more likely in patients with ocular surgery within the prior 6 weeks. Among those with recurrences following ocular surgery, individuals on higher doses of oral acyclovir (average 1321 mg/day) faced fewer recurrences compared to those on lower doses (average 1000 mg/day) [122]. Hence, a higher dosing of prophylactic acyclovir may be appropriate in the perioperative period for patients with a history of HSV keratitis. This may include acyclovir 400 mg four or five times daily for a week preceding surgery until 1–2 weeks after surgery, although the regimen may vary based on the practitioner.

13.5 Management of Sequelae

13.5.1 Neurotrophic Keratopathy

The cornea is the most densely innervated tissue in the human body [123]. Corneal nerves are responsible for several reflexive, sensory, and trophic processes involving the ocular surface, and play a central role in the blink reflex, tear production, tear secretion, epithelial integrity, epithelial proliferation, and wound healing [124–126]. Prior episodes of herpetic keratitis may result in damage to corneal nerves, leading to neurotrophic keratopathy and corneal hypoesthesia. As the number of previous episodes of HSV keratitis increases, corneal sensitivity decreases [127]. A decrease in subbasal nerve corneal nerve fiber length and nerve branch density correlate with this decreased sensitivity [123].

Neurotrophic keratopathy may range in severity from mild epitheliopathy to oval-shaped ulceration. Patients often experience decreased corneal sensation, recurrent epithelial defects, or in more advanced cases, corneal ulceration, melting, and possibly perforation [128, 129]. Progressive corneal thinning and perforation may be managed with amniotic membrane grafting, corneal glue, tarsorrhaphy, conjunctival flap, patch grafting, or tectonic keratoplasty [130].

Corneal nerves have been demonstrated to regenerate in other instances of acute neuronal damage, such as after corneal refractive surgery [131, 132]. However, confocal microscopy studies of corneas previously infected by HSV found that nerves regenerate to a limited extent, which is often not clinically significant [123, 133, 134]. In one study, over an average follow-up of over 3 years, there was no significant change in corneal sensation compared to the initial visit as measured by Cochet-Bonnet esthesiometry (Luneau Ophthalmologie, Chartres, France), despite a small but statistically significant increase in central total corneal nerve density [133]. Another study showed that corneal sensation increased significantly at 6 months of follow-up, but did not reach normal levels [134].

Interestingly, subbasal nerve parameters of seemingly uninvolved contralateral eyes in patients with HSV keratitis have also been shown to be lower than controls [135–137]. The precise pathophysiology of contralateral eye changes remains unknown, although several hypotheses have been postulated. One possible explanation is that the central nervous system may regulate contralateral neuronal effects. Alternatively, there may exist subclinical viral expansion to the contralateral side [123].

Management of neurotrophic keratopathy typically begins with lubrication, bandage soft contact lens, serum tears, tarsorrhaphy, and amniotic membrane placement. Systemic antiviral prophylaxis should be continued indefinitely. Topical steroids may be employed judiciously if there is suspicion that inflammation is inhibiting reepithelialization. Recombinant human nerve growth factor (rhNGF) agents are being used increasingly in the management of neurotrophic keratopathy. The REPARO trial evaluated the efficacy of rhNGF agents in promoting corneal epithelialization in moderate-to-severe neurotrophic keratopathy [138]. Eyes treated with rhNGF agents achieved higher rates of healing at 4 and 8 weeks [138]. This effect appears to last for at least 1 year. The commercially available rhNGF agent, Oxervate (cenegermin-bkbj, Dompé, Milan, Italy), entered the United States market in January 2019 and is administered six times a day for 8 weeks. A scleral lens may also be a valuable therapeutic tool in treating neurotrophic keratopathy as it provides continuous hydration, protects the corneal epithelium, and optimizes vision [139]. Finally, surgical management is an option, with corneal neurotization demonstrating improved corneal sensation [140]. Confocal microscopy after neurotization has identified reinnervation at the level of the subbasal nerve plexus [141].

Fig. 13.10 Corneal neovascularization and band keratopathy in an eye with a history of HSV keratitis

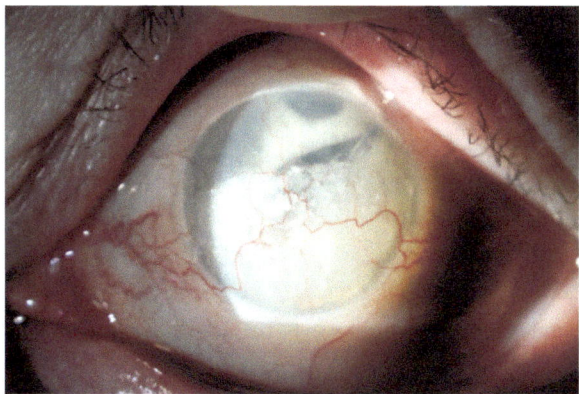

13.5.2 Corneal Opacification

Repeated epithelial, stromal, and endothelial disease increases the risk of fibrosis and neovascularization, with resulting visual loss [90]. Common findings include corneal edema, scarring, opacification, neovascularization, lipid keratopathy, band keratopathy, and irregular astigmatism (Fig. 13.10). In cases of stable, visually significant corneal scarring, surgical options may include deep anterior lamellar keratoplasty or penetrating keratoplasty. Ocular HSV is responsible for about 10% of all corneal transplants in the United Kingdom [142].

Penetrating keratoplasty in patients with a history of HSV keratitis involves several special considerations. Graft failure following penetrating keratoplasty for these patients may occur due to severe ocular surface disease, viral reactivation in the graft, or allograft rejection [143]. Many surgeons will perform a temporary tarsorrhaphy at the time of keratoplasty in eyes with a history of HSV ocular disease. HSV recurrences increase the risk of subsequent graft failure, and patients with a history of ocular HSV have a higher incidence of graft rejection compared to those with no history of HSV [144]. There are rare reports of transmission of HSV from the donor cornea [145].

Recurrences of HSV keratitis following penetrating keratoplasty may be reduced with oral antiviral prophylaxis; various reports have demonstrated that keratoplasty patients with a history of HSV keratitis treated with prophylactic acyclovir experience fewer recurrences of infection [146–148]. The recurrence rate of HSV keratitis after penetrating keratoplasty may be related to treatment length with oral acyclovir, and patients treated with oral acyclovir for 1 year after keratoplasty experienced a recurrence rate of 5% at 2 years [149]. On the other hand, individuals not treated with antiviral prophylaxis after penetrating keratoplasty experienced a 27–50% recurrence rate for HSV after 2 years [146, 150]. Many practitioners will continue antiviral systemic prophylaxis for as long as a patient is on topical corticosteroids, if not forever.

13.6   Future Directions

With continued research into HSV pathophysiology, potential new avenues for therapeutic agents have arisen. One area of active investigation is the development of a HSV vaccine, which has shown promising results for HSV keratitis in a murine model [151, 152]. While there are no FDA approved vaccines for the prevention of HSV keratitis infection or recurrence, many research trials are underway in this arena.

References

1. Valerio GS, Lin CC. Ocular manifestations of herpes simplex virus. Curr Opin Ophthalmol. 2019;30(6):525–31.
2. Farooq AV, Shah A, Shukla D. The role of herpesviruses in ocular infections. Virus Adapt Treat. 2010;2:115–23.
3. Lairson DR, Begley CE, Reynolds TF, Wilhelmus KR. Prevention of herpes simplex virus eye disease: a cost-effectiveness analysis. Arch Ophthalmol. 2003;121(1):108–12.
4. Liesegang TJ, Melton LJ 3rd, Daly PJ, Ilstrup DM. Epidemiology of ocular herpes simplex. Incidence in Rochester, Minn, 1950 through 1982. Arch Ophthalmol. 1989;107(8):1155–9.
5. Kaufman HE, Azcuy AM, Varnell ED, Sloop GD, Thompson HW, Hill JM. HSV-1 DNA in tears and saliva of normal adults. Invest Ophthalmol Vis Sci. 2005;46(1):241–7.
6. Obara Y, Furuta Y, Takasu T, Suzuki S, Suzuki H, Matsukawa S, Fujioka Y, Takahashi H, Kurata T, Nagashima K. Distribution of herpes simplex virus types 1 and 2 genomes in human spinal ganglia studied by PCR and in situ hybridization. J Med Virol. 1997;52(2):136–42.
7. Liesegang TJ. Herpes simplex virus epidemiology and ocular importance. Cornea. 2001;20(1):1–13.
8. Cohrs RJ, Randall J, Smith J, Gilden DH, Dabrowski C, van Der Keyl H, Tal-Singer R. Analysis of individual human trigeminal ganglia for latent herpes simplex virus type 1 and varicella-zoster virus nucleic acids using real-time PCR. J Virol. 2000;74(24):11464–71.
9. Labetoulle M, Auquier P, Conrad H, Crochard A, Daniloski M, Bouée S, El Hasnaoui A, Colin J. Incidence of herpes simplex virus keratitis in France. Ophthalmology. 2005;112(5):888–95.
10. Mortensen KK, Sjølie AK. Keratitis dendritica. An epidemiological investigation. Acta Ophthalmol. 1979;57(5):750–4.
11. Ribarić V. The incidence of herpetic keratitis among population. Ophthalmologica. 1976;173(1):19–22.
12. Darougar S, Wishart MS, Viswalingam ND. Epidemiological and clinical features of primary herpes simplex virus ocular infection. Br J Ophthalmol. 1985;69(1):2–6.
13. Young RC, Hodge DO, Liesegang TJ, Baratz KH. Incidence, recurrence, and outcomes of herpes simplex virus eye disease in Olmsted County, Minnesota, 1976-2007: the effect of oral antiviral prophylaxis. Arch Ophthalmol. 2010;128(9):1178–83.
14. Wilhelmus KR. Antiviral treatment and other therapeutic interventions for herpes simplex virus epithelial keratitis. Cochrane Database Syst Rev. 2015;1:CD002898.
15. Chang EJ, Dreyer EB. Herpesvirus infections of the anterior segment. Int Ophthalmol Clin. 1996;36(3):17–28.
16. Parlato CJ, Cohen EJ, Sakauye CM, Dreizen NG, Galentine PG, Laibson PR. Role of débridement and trifluridine (trifluorothymidine) in herpes simplex dendritic keratitis. Arch Ophthalmol. 1985;103(5):673–5.
17. Herbort CP, Buechi ER, Matter M. Blunt spatula debridement and trifluorothymidine in epithelial herpetic keratitis. Curr Eye Res. 1987;6(1):225–9.
18. Wilhelmus KR, Coster DJ, Jones BR. Acyclovir and debridement in the treatment of ulcerative herpetic keratitis. Am J Ophthalmol. 1981;91(3):323–7.

19. Cheng AMS, Tseng SCG. Self-retained amniotic membrane combined with antiviral therapy for herpetic epithelial keratitis. Cornea. 2017;36(11):1383–6.
20. Lisco A, Vanpouille C, Tchesnokov EP, Grivel JC, Biancotto A, Brichacek B, Elliott J, Fromentin E, Shattock R, Anton P, Gorelick R, Balzarini J, McGuigan C, Derudas M, Götte M, Schinazi RF, Margolis L. Acyclovir is activated into a HIV-1 reverse transcriptase inhibitor in herpesvirus-infected human tissues. Cell Host Microbe. 2008;4(3):260–70.
21. Tyring SK, Baker D, Snowden W. Valacyclovir for herpes simplex virus infection: long-term safety and sustained efficacy after 20 years' experience with acyclovir. J Infect Dis. 2002;186(Suppl-1):S40–6.
22. Hung SO, Patterson A, Rees PJ. Pharmacokinetics of oral acyclovir (Zovirax) in the eye. Br J Ophthalmol. 1984;68(3):192–5.
23. Dias C, Nashed Y, Atluri H, Mitra A. Ocular penetration of acyclovir and its peptide prodrugs valacyclovir and val-valacyclovir following systemic administration in rabbits: an evaluation using ocular microdialysis and LC-MS. Curr Eye Res. 2002;25(4):243–52.
24. Perry CM, Faulds D. Valaciclovir. A review of its antiviral activity, pharmacokinetic properties and therapeutic efficacy in herpesvirus infections. Drugs. 1996;52(5):754–72.
25. Koseoglu ND, Strauss BR, Hamrah P. Successful management of herpes simplex keratitis with oral valganciclovir in patients unresponsive or allergic to conventional antiviral therapy. Cornea. 2019;38(6):663–7.
26. Carter SB, Cohen EJ. Development of herpes simplex virus infectious epithelial keratitis during oral acyclovir therapy and response to topical antivirals. Cornea. 2016;35(5):692–5.
27. Colin J, Chastel C, Kaufman HE, Kissling GE. Combination therapy for dendritic keratitis with acyclovir and vidarabine. J Ocul Pharmacol. 1987;3(1):39–42.
28. Naito T, Shiota H, Mimura Y. Side effects in the treatment of herpetic keratitis. Curr Eye Res. 1987;6(1):237–9.
29. Herpetic Eye Disease Study Group. A controlled trial of oral acyclovir for the prevention of stromal keratitis or iritis in patients with herpes simplex virus epithelial keratitis. The Epithelial Keratitis Trial. Arch Ophthalmol. 1997;115(6):703–12.
30. Cunningham ET Jr. Diagnosing and treating herpetic anterior uveitis. Ophthalmology. 2000;107(12):2129–30.
31. Wilhelmus KR. Therapeutic interventions for herpes simplex virus epithelial keratitis. Cochrane Database Syst Rev. 2008;1:CD002898.
32. Kaufman HE, Haw WH. Ganciclovir ophthalmic gel 0.15%: safety and efficacy of a new treatment for herpes simplex keratitis. Curr Eye Res. 2012;37(7):654–60.
33. Wilhelmus KR, Falcon MG, Jones BR. Herpetic iridocyclitis. Int Ophthalmol. 1982;4(3):143–50.
34. Pavan-Langston D, Nelson DJ. Intraocular penetration of trifluridine. Am J Ophthalmol. 1979;87(6):814–8.
35. Poirier RH, Kingham JD, de Miranda P, Annel M. Intraocular antiviral penetration. Arch Ophthalmol. 1982;100(12):1964–7.
36. Sauerbrei A, Deinhardt S, Zell R, Wutzler P. Testing of herpes simplex virus for resistance to antiviral drugs. Virulence. 2010;1(6):555–7.
37. Kudo E, Shiota H, Naito T, Satake K, Itakura M. Polymorphisms of thymidine kinase gene in herpes simplex virus type 1: analysis of clinical isolates from herpetic keratitis patients and laboratory strains. J Med Virol. 1998;56(2):151–8.
38. Frobert E, Cortay JC, Ooka T, Najioullah F, Thouvenot D, Lina B, Morfin F. Genotypic detection of acyclovir-resistant HSV-1: characterization of 67 ACV-sensitive and 14 ACV-resistant viruses. Antivir Res. 2008;79(1):28–36.
39. Duan R, de Vries RD, Osterhaus AD, Remeijer L, Verjans GM. Acyclovir-resistant corneal HSV-1 isolates from patients with herpetic keratitis. J Infect Dis. 2008;198(5):659–63.
40. Morfin F, Thouvenot D. Herpes simplex virus resistance to antiviral drugs. J Clin Virol. 2003;26(1):29–37.
41. Castelo-Soccio L, Bernardin R, Stern J, Goldstein SA, Kovarik C. Successful treatment of acyclovir-resistant herpes simplex virus with intralesional cidofovir. Arch Dermatol. 2010;146(2):124–6.

42. Kessler HA, Hurwitz S, Farthing C, Benson CA, Feinberg J, Kuritzkes DR, Bailey TC, Safrin S, Steigbigel RT, Cheeseman SH, McKinley GF, Wettlaufer B, Owens S, Nevin T, Korvick JA. Pilot study of topical trifluridine for the treatment of acyclovir-resistant mucocutaneous herpes simplex disease in patients with AIDS (ACTG 172). AIDS Clinical Trials Group. J Acquir Immune Defic Syndr Hum Retrovirol. 1996;12(2):147–52.

43. Khalili MR, Jahadi HR, Karimi M, Yasemi M. Corneal collagen cross-linking for treatment of bacterial and herpetic keratitis. J Clin Diagn Res. 2017;11(7):NC12–6.

44. Tang Q, Chen W, Hendricks RL. Proinflammatory functions of IL-2 in herpes simplex virus corneal infection. J Immunol. 1997;158(3):1275–83.

45. Rao P, Suvas S. Development of inflammatory hypoxia and prevalence of glycolytic metabolism in progressing herpes stromal keratitis lesions. J Immunol. 2019;202(2):514–26.

46. Kalezic T, Mazen M, Kuklinski E, Asbell P. Herpetic eye disease study: lessons learned. Curr Opin Ophthalmol. 2018;29(4):340–6.

47. Peyman A, Nayebzadeh M, Peyman M, Afshari NA, Pourazizi M. Topical cyclosporine-A versus prednisolone for herpetic stromal keratitis: a randomized controlled trial. Acta Ophthalmol. 2019;97(2):e194–8.

48. Gündüz K, Ozdemir O. Topical cyclosporin as an adjunct to topical acyclovir treatment in herpetic stromal keratitis. Ophthalmic Res. 1997;29(6):405–8.

49. Heiligenhaus A, Steuhl KP. Treatment of HSV-1 stromal keratitis with topical cyclosporin A: a pilot study. Graefes Arch Clin Exp Ophthalmol. 1999;237(5):435–8.

50. Rao SN. Treatment of herpes simplex virus stromal keratitis unresponsive to topical prednisolone 1% with topical cyclosporine 0.05%. Am J Ophthalmol. 2006;141(4):771–2.

51. Shi W, Chen M, Xie L. Amniotic membrane transplantation combined with antiviral and steroid therapy for herpes necrotizing stromal keratitis. Ophthalmology. 2007;114(8):1476–81.

52. Knickelbein JE, Hendricks RL, Charukamnoetkanok P. Management of herpes simplex virus stromal keratitis: an evidence-based review. Surv Ophthalmol. 2009;54(2):226–34.

53. Gaynor BD, Margolis TP, Cunningham ET Jr. Advances in diagnosis and management of herpetic uveitis. Int Ophthalmol Clin. 2000;40(2):85–109.

54. Liesegang TJ. Classification of herpes simplex virus keratitis and anterior uveitis. Cornea. 1999;18(2):127–43.

55. Herpetic Eye Disease Study Group. A controlled trial of oral acyclovir for iridocyclitis caused by herpes simplex virus. Arch Ophthalmol. 1996;114(9):1065–72.

56. Sudesh S, Laibson PR. The impact of the herpetic eye disease studies on the management of herpes simplex virus ocular infections. Curr Opin Ophthalmol. 1999;10(4):230–3.

57. Koizumi N, Nishida K, Adachi W, Tei M, Honma Y, Dota A, Sotozono C, Yokoi N, Yamamoto S, Kinoshita S. Detection of herpes simplex virus DNA in atypical epithelial keratitis using polymerase chain reaction. Br J Ophthalmol. 1999;83(8):957–60.

58. Rübben A, Baron JM, Grussendorf-Conen EI. Routine detection of herpes simplex virus and varicella zoster virus by polymerase chain reaction reveals that initial herpes zoster is frequently misdiagnosed as herpes simplex. Br J Dermatol. 1997;137(2):259–61.

59. Azher TN, Yin XT, Tajfirouz D, Huang AJ, Stuart PM. Herpes simplex keratitis: challenges in diagnosis and clinical management. Clin Ophthalmol. 2017;11:185–91.

60. Burrows J, Nitsche A, Bayly B, Walker E, Higgins G, Kok T. Detection and subtyping of Herpes simplex virus in clinical samples by LightCycler PCR, enzyme immunoassay and cell culture. BMC Microbiol. 2002;2:12.

61. Espy MJ, Ross TK, Teo R, Svien KA, Wold AD, Uhl JR, Smith TF. Evaluation of LightCycler PCR for implementation of laboratory diagnosis of herpes simplex virus infections. J Clin Microbiol. 2000;38(8):3116–8.

62. El-Aal AM, El Sayed M, Mohammed E, Ahmed M, Fathy M. Evaluation of herpes simplex detection in corneal scrapings by three molecular methods. Curr Microbiol. 2006;52(5):379–82.

63. Shoji J, Sakimoto T, Inada N, Kamei Y, Matsubara M, Takamura E, Sawa M. A diagnostic method for herpes simplex keratitis by simultaneous measurement of viral DNA and virus-specific secretory IgA in tears: an evaluation. Jpn J Ophthalmol. 2016;60(4):294–301.

64. Shin J, Ra H, Rho CR. Herpes simplex virus linear endotheliitis in a post-keratoplasty patient: a case report. Medicine (Baltimore). 2019;98(3):e14191.
65. Basak SK, Basak S. Recurrence of herpes simplex virus endotheliitis in a Descemet membrane endothelial keratoplasty graft: mimicking fungal interface infection. BMJ Case Rep. 2019;12(5):e229441.
66. Kowalski RP, Gordon YJ, Romanowski EG, Araullo-Cruz T, Kinchington PR. A comparison of enzyme immunoassay and polymerase chain reaction with the clinical examination for diagnosing ocular herpetic disease. Ophthalmology. 1993;100(4):530–3.
67. Wald A, Corey L, Cone R, Hobson A, Davis G, Zeh J. Frequent genital herpes simplex virus 2 shedding in immunocompetent women. Effect of acyclovir treatment. J Clin Invest. 1997;99(5):1092–7.
68. Goldschmidt P, Rostane H, Saint-Jean C, Batellier L, Alouch C, Zito E, Bourcier T, Laroche L, Chaumeil C. Effects of topical anaesthetics and fluorescein on the real-time PCR used for the diagnosis of Herpesviruses and Acanthamoeba keratitis. Br J Ophthalmol. 2006;90(11):1354–6.
69. Seitzman GD, Cevallos V, Margolis TP. Rose bengal and lissamine green inhibit detection of herpes simplex virus by PCR. Am J Ophthalmol. 2006;141(4):756–8.
70. Rosenberg ME, Tervo TM, Müller LJ, Moilanen JA, Vesaluoma MH. In vivo confocal microscopy after herpes keratitis. Cornea. 2002;21(3):265–9.
71. Wang YE, Tepelus TC, Vickers LA, Baghdasaryan E, Gui W, Huang P, Irvine JA, Sadda S, Hsu HY, Lee OL. Role of in vivo confocal microscopy in the diagnosis of infectious keratitis. Int Ophthalmol. 2019;39(12):2865–74.
72. Qiu J, Huang F, Wang Z, Xu J, Zhang C. The evaluation of diagnostic efficiency for stromal herpes simplex keratitis by the combination of tear HSV-sIgA and HSV-DNA. Graefes Arch Clin Exp Ophthalmol. 2017;255(7):1409–15.
73. Satpathy G, Mishra AK, Tandon R, Sharma MK, Sharma A, Nayak N, Titiyal JS, Sharma N. Evaluation of tear samples for Herpes Simplex Virus 1 (HSV) detection in suspected cases of viral keratitis using PCR assay and conventional laboratory diagnostic tools. Br J Ophthalmol. 2011;95(3):415–8.
74. Doan T, Pinsky BA. Current and future molecular diagnostics for ocular infectious diseases. Curr Opin Ophthalmol. 2016;27(6):561–7.
75. Vadoothker S, Andrews L, Jeng BH, Levin MR. Management of herpes simplex virus keratitis in the pediatric population. Pediatr Infect Dis J. 2018;37(9):949–51.
76. Matos RJC, Pires JMS, Cortesão D. Management of neonatal herpes simplex infection: a rare case of blepharoconjunctivitis and concurrent epithelial and stromal keratitis. Ocul Immunol Inflamm. 2018;26(4):625–7.
77. Chong EM, Wilhelmus KR, Matoba AY, Jones DB, Coats DK, Paysse EA. Herpes simplex virus keratitis in children. Am J Ophthalmol. 2004;138(3):474–5.
78. Beigi B, Algawi K, Foley-Nolan A, O'Keefe M. Herpes simplex keratitis in children. Br J Ophthalmol. 1994;78(6):458–60.
79. Liu S, Pavan-Langston D, Colby KA. Pediatric herpes simplex of the anterior segment: characteristics, treatment, and outcomes. Ophthalmology. 2012;119(10):2003–8.
80. Hsiao CH, Yeung L, Yeh LK, Kao LY, Tan HY, Wang NK, Lin KK, Ma DH. Pediatric herpes simplex virus keratitis. Cornea. 2009;28(3):249–53.
81. Souza PM, Holland EJ, Huang AJ. Bilateral herpetic keratoconjunctivitis. Ophthalmology. 2003;110(3):493–6.
82. Wilhelmus KR, Falcon MG, Jones BR. Bilateral herpetic keratitis. Br J Ophthalmol. 1981;65(6):385–7.
83. Uchio E, Hatano H, Mitsui K, Sugita M, Okada K, Goto K, Kagiya M, Enomoto Y, Ohno S. A retrospective study of herpes simplex keratitis over the last 30 years. Jpn J Ophthalmol. 1994;38(2):196–201.
84. Poirier RH. Herpetic ocular infections of childhood. Arch Ophthalmol. 1980;98(4):704–6.
85. Schwartz GS, Holland EJ. Oral acyclovir for the management of herpes simplex virus keratitis in children. Ophthalmology. 2000;107(2):278–82.

86. Prabriputaloong T, Margolis TP, Lietman TM, Wong IG, Mather R, Gritz DC. Atopic disease and herpes simplex eye disease: a population-based case-control study. Am J Ophthalmol. 2006;142(5):745–9.
87. Easty D, Entwistle C, Funk A, Witcher J. Herpes simplex keratitis and keratoconus in the atopic patient. A clinical and immunological study. Trans Ophthalmol Soc UK. 1975;95(2):267–76.
88. Garrity JA, Liesegang TJ. Ocular complications of atopic dermatitis. Can J Ophthalmol. 1984;19(1):21–4.
89. Rezende RA, Hammersmith K, Bisol T, Lima AL, Webster GF, Freitas JF, Rapuano CJ, Laibson PR, Cohen EJ. Comparative study of ocular herpes simplex virus in patients with and without self-reported atopy. Am J Ophthalmol. 2006;141(6):1120–5.
90. Tsatsos M, MacGregor C, Athanasiadis I, Moschos MM, Hossain P, Anderson D. Herpes simplex virus keratitis: an update of the pathogenesis and current treatment with oral and topical antiviral agents. Clin Exp Ophthalmol. 2016;44(9):824–37.
91. Herpetic Eye Disease Study Group. Acyclovir for the prevention of recurrent herpes simplex virus eye disease. N Engl J Med. 1998;339(5):300–6.
92. Shuster JJ, Kaufman HE, Nesburn AB. Statistical analysis of the rate of recurrence of herpesvirus ocular epithelial disease. Am J Ophthalmol. 1981;91(3):328–31.
93. Sawtell NM. Comprehensive quantification of herpes simplex virus latency at the single-cell level. J Virol. 1997;71(7):5423–31.
94. Derham AM, Chen E, Bunya VY, O'Malley RE. Bilateral herpetic keratitis after bilateral intravitreal bevacizumab for exudative macular degeneration. Cornea. 2017;36(7):878–9.
95. Cho YK, Kwon JW, Konda S, Ambati BK. Epithelial keratitis after cataract surgery. Cornea. 2018;37(6):755–9.
96. Qi X, Wang M, Li X, Jia Y, Li S, Shi W, Gao H. Characteristics of new onset herpes simplex keratitis after keratoplasty. J Ophthalmol. 2018;2018:4351460.
97. Kamburoglu G, Ertan A. Peripheral herpes simplex keratitis following LASIK. J Refract Surg. 2007;23(8):742–3.
98. Jain V, Pineda R. Reactivated herpetic keratitis following laser in situ keratomileusis. J Cataract Refract Surg. 2009;35(5):946–8.
99. Hou YC, Chen CC, Wang IJ, Hu FR. Recurrent herpetic keratouveitis following YAG laser peripheral iridotomy. Cornea. 2004;23(6):641–2.
100. Reed SY, Shin DH, Birt CM, Rhee RK. Herpes simplex keratitis following argon laser trabeculoplasty. Ophthalmic Surg. 1994;25(9):640.
101. Vrabec MP, Durrie DS, Chase DS. Recurrence of herpes simplex after excimer laser keratectomy. Am J Ophthalmol. 1992;114(1):96–7.
102. Wulff K, Fechner PU. Herpes simplex keratitis after photorefractive keratectomy. J Refract Surg. 1997;13(7):613.
103. Wand M, Gilbert CM, Liesegang TJ. Latanoprost and herpes simplex keratitis. Am J Ophthalmol. 1999;127(5):602–4.
104. Ekatomatis P. Herpes simplex dendritic keratitis after treatment with latanoprost for primary open angle glaucoma. Br J Ophthalmol. 2001;85(8):1008–9.
105. Takeshita T. Bilateral herpes simplex virus keratitis in a patient with pemphigus vulgaris. Clin Exp Dermatol. 1996;21(4):291–2.
106. Gulkilik G, Demirci G, Ozdamar AM, Muftuoglu GI. A case of herpetic keratitis after intravitreal triamcinolone injection. Cornea. 2007;26(8):1000–1.
107. el-Antably SA, Atia HE. Ocular complications of corticosteroids. Bull Ophthalmol Soc Egypt. 1976;69(73):635–41.
108. Warren SL, Carpenter CM, Boak RA. Symptomatic Herpes, a sequela of artificially induced fever: incidence and C aspects; recovery of A virus from Herpetic vesicles, and comparison with a K strain of Herpes virus. J Exp Med. 1940;71(2):155–68.
109. Guinan ME, MacCalman J, Kern ER, Overall JC Jr, Spruance SL. The course of untreated recurrent genital herpes simplex infection in 27 women. N Engl J Med. 1981;304(13):759–63.
110. Dalkvist J, Wahlin TB, Bartsch E, Forsbeck M. Herpes simplex and mood: a prospective study. Psychosom Med. 1995;57(2):127–37.

111. Friedman E, Katcher AH, Brightman VJ. Incidence of recurrent herpes labialis and upper respiratory infection: a prospective study of the influence of biologic, social and psychologic predictors. Oral Surg Oral Med Oral Pathol. 1977;43(6):873–8.
112. Herpetic Eye Disease Study Group. Oral acyclovir for herpes simplex virus eye disease: effect on prevention of epithelial keratitis and stromal keratitis. Arch Ophthalmol. 2000;118(8):1030–6.
113. Miserocchi E, Modorati G, Galli L, Rama P. Efficacy of valacyclovir vs acyclovir for the prevention of recurrent herpes simplex virus eye disease: a pilot study. Am J Ophthalmol. 2007;144(4):547–51.
114. Ghosh S, Jhanji V, Lamoureux E, Taylor HR, Vajpayee RB. Acyclovir therapy in prevention of recurrent herpetic keratitis following penetrating keratoplasty. Am J Ophthalmol. 2008;145(2):198–202.
115. Papanicolaou GA, Meyers BR, Fuchs WS, Guillory SL, Mendelson MH, Sheiner P, Emre S, Miller C. Infectious ocular complications in orthotopic liver transplant patients. Clin Infect Dis. 1997;24(6):1172–7.
116. Korsager B, Spencer ES, Mordhorst CH, Andersen HK. Herpesvirus hominis infections in renal transplant recipients. Scand J Infect Dis. 1975;7(1):11–9.
117. Howcroft MJ, Breslin CW. Herpes simplex keratitis in renal transplant recipients. Can Med Assoc J. 1981;124(3):292–4.
118. Geerlings SE, Hoepelman AI. Immune dysfunction in patients with diabetes mellitus (DM). FEMS Immunol Med Microbiol. 1999;26(3-4):259–65.
119. Eliashiv A, Olumide F, Norton L, Eiseman B. Depression of cell-mediated immunity in diabetes. Arch Surg. 1978;113(10):1180–3.
120. Kaiserman I, Kaiserman N, Nakar S, Vinker S. Herpetic eye disease in diabetic patients. Ophthalmology. 2005;112(12):2184–8.
121. Hodge WG, Margolis TP. Herpes simplex virus keratitis among patients who are positive or negative for human immunodeficiency virus: an epidemiologic study. Ophthalmology. 1997;104(1):120–4.
122. Simon AL, Pavan-Langston D. Long-term oral acyclovir therapy. Effect on recurrent infectious herpes simplex keratitis in patients with and without grafts. Ophthalmology. 1996;103(9):1399–405.
123. Danileviciene V, Zemaitiene R, Gintauskiene VM, Nedzelskiene I, Zaliuniene D. Corneal sub basal nerve changes in patients with herpetic keratitis during acute phase and after 6 months. Medicina (Kaunas). 2019;55(5):E214.
124. Oliveira-Soto L, Efron N. Morphology of corneal nerves using confocal microscopy. Cornea. 2001;20(4):374–84.
125. Guthoff RF, Wienss H, Hahnel C, Wree A. Epithelial innervation of human cornea: a three-dimensional study using confocal laser scanning fluorescence microscopy. Cornea. 2005;24(5):608–13.
126. Tavakoli M, Ferdousi M, Petropoulos IN, Morris J, Pritchard N, Zhivov A, Ziegler D, Pacaud D, Romanchuk K, Perkins BA, Lovblom LE, Bril V, Singleton JR, Smith G, Boulton AJ, Efron N, Malik RA. Normative values for corneal nerve morphology assessed using corneal confocal microscopy: a multinational normative data set. Diabetes Care. 2015;38(5):838–43.
127. Gallar J, Tervo TM, Neira W, Holopainen JM, Lamberg ME, Miñana F, Acosta MC, Belmonte C. Selective changes in human corneal sensation associated with herpes simplex virus keratitis. Invest Ophthalmol Vis Sci. 2010;51(9):4516–22.
128. Bonini S, Rama P, Olzi D, Lambiase A. Neurotrophic keratitis. Eye. 2003;17(8):989–95.
129. Semeraro F, Forbice E, Romano V, Angi M, Romano MR, Filippelli ME, Di Iorio R, Costagliola C. Neurotrophic keratitis. Ophthalmologica. 2014;231(4):191–7.
130. Tuli S, Gray M, Shah A. Surgical management of herpetic keratitis. Curr Opin Ophthalmol. 2018;29(4):347–54.
131. Latvala T, Linna T, Tervo T. Corneal nerve recovery after photorefractive keratectomy and laser in situ keratomileusis. Int Ophthalmol Clin. 1996;36(4):21–7.

132. Linna TU, Pérez-Santonja JJ, Tervo KM, Sakla HF, Alió y Sanz JL, Tervo TM. Recovery of corneal nerve morphology following laser in situ keratomileusis. Exp Eye Res. 1998;66(6):755–63.

133. Moein HR, Kheirkhah A, Muller RT, Cruzat AC, Pavan-Langston D, Hamrah P. Corneal nerve regeneration after herpes simplex keratitis: a longitudinal in vivo confocal microscopy study. Ocul Surf. 2018;16(2):218–25.

134. Zemaitiene R, Rakauskiene M, Danileviciene V, Use V, Kriauciuniene L, Zaliuniene D. Corneal esthesiometry and sub-basal nerves morphological changes in herpes simplex virus keratitis/uveitis patients. Int J Ophthalmol. 2019;12(3):407–11.

135. Hamrah P, Cruzat A, Dastjerdi MH, Zheng L, Shahatit BM, Bayhan HA, Dana R, Pavan-Langston D. Corneal sensation and subbasal nerve alterations in patients with herpes simplex keratitis: an in vivo confocal microscopy study. Ophthalmology. 2010;117(10):1930–6.

136. He J, Bazan NG, Bazan HE. Mapping the entire human corneal nerve architecture. Exp Eye Res. 2010;91(4):513–23.

137. Nagasato D, Araki-Sasaki K, Kojima T, Ideta R, Dogru M. Morphological changes of corneal subepithelial nerve plexus in different types of herpetic keratitis. Jpn J Ophthalmol. 2011;55(5):444–50.

138. Bonini S, Lambiase A2, Rama P3, Sinigaglia F4, Allegretti M4, Chao W4, Mantelli F4, REPARO Study Group. Phase II randomized, double-masked, vehicle-controlled trial of recombinant human nerve growth factor for neurotrophic keratitis. Ophthalmology. 2018;125(9):1332–43.

139. Shorter E, Harthan J, Nau CB, Nau A, Barr JT, Hodge DO, Schornack MM. Scleral lenses in the management of corneal irregularity and ocular surface disease. Eye Contact Lens. 2018;44(6):372–8.

140. Catapano J, Fung SSM, Halliday W, Jobst C, Cheyne D, Ho ES, Zuker RM, Borschel GH, Ali A. Treatment of neurotrophic keratopathy with minimally invasive corneal neurotisation: long-term clinical outcomes and evidence of corneal reinnervation. Br J Ophthalmol. 2019;103(12):1724–31.

141. Giannaccare G, Bolognesi F, Biglioli F, Marchetti C, Mariani S, Weiss JS, Allevi F, Cazzola FE, Ponzin D, Lozza A, Bovone C, Scorcia V, Busin M, Campos EC. In vivo and ex vivo comprehensive evaluation of corneal reinnervation in eyes neurotized with contralateral supratrochlear and supraorbital nerves. Cornea. 2020;39(2):210–4.

142. Ficker LA, Kirkness CM, Rice NS, Steele AD. The changing management and improved prognosis for corneal grafting in herpes simplex keratitis. Ophthalmology. 1989;96(11):1587–96.

143. Cockerham GC, Krafft AE, McLean IW. Herpes simplex virus in primary graft failure. Arch Ophthalmol. 1997;115(5):586–9.

144. Epstein RJ, Seedor JA, Dreizen NG, Stulting RD, Waring GO 3rd, Wilson LA, Cavanagh HD. Penetrating keratoplasty for herpes simplex keratitis and keratoconus. Allograft rejection and survival. Ophthalmology. 1987;94(8):935–44.

145. Cleator GM, Klapper PE, Dennett C, Sullivan AL, Bonshek RE, Marcyniuk B, Tullo AB. Corneal donor infection by herpes simplex virus: herpes simplex virus DNA in donor corneas. Cornea. 1994;13(4):294–304.

146. Akova YA, Onat M, Duman S. Efficacy of low-dose and long-term oral acyclovir therapy after penetrating keratoplasty for herpes simplex heratitis. Ocul Immunol Inflamm. 1999;7(1):51–60.

147. Barney NP, Foster CS. A prospective randomized trial of oral acyclovir after penetrating keratoplasty for herpes simplex keratitis. Cornea. 1994;13(3):232–6.

148. van Rooij J, Rijneveld WJ, Remeijer LJ, Beekhuis WH. A retrospective study on the effectiveness of oral acyclovir to prevent herpes simplex recurrence in corneal grafts. Eur J Ophthalmol. 1995;5(4):214–8.

149. Mayer K, Reinhard T, Reis A, Voiculescu A, Sundmacher R. Synergistic antiherpetic effect of acyclovir and mycophenolate mofetil following keratoplasty in patients with herpetic eye disease: first results of a randomised pilot study. Graefes Arch Clin Exp Ophthalmol. 2003;241(12):1051–4.

150. van Rooij J, Rijneveld WJ, Remeijer L, Völker-Dieben HJ, Eggink CA, Geerards AJ, Mulder PG, Doornenbal P, Beekhuis WH. Effect of oral acyclovir after penetrating keratoplasty for herpetic keratitis: a placebo-controlled multicenter trial. Ophthalmology. 2003;110(10):1916–9.
151. Dong LL, Tang R, Zhai YJ, Malla T, Hu K. DNA vaccine expressing herpes simplex virus 1 glycoprotein C and D protects mice against herpes simplex keratitis. Int J Ophthalmol. 2017;10(11):1633–9.
152. Tang R, Zhai Y, Dong L, Malla T, Hu K. Immunization with dendritic cell-based DNA vaccine pRSC-NLDC145.gD-IL21 protects mice against herpes simplex virus keratitis. Immunotherapy. 2018;10(3):189–200.

Herpes Zoster Ophthalmicus (HZO) Keratitis

14

Sonal S. Tuli

14.1 Epidemiology

Herpes zoster is caused by the Varicella zoster virus (VZV) which belongs to the human herpesvirus family. All members of this family have in common a state called "latency" where the virus remains dormant in cells and periodically reactivates. Herpes zoster is neurotrophic and has an affinity for neuronal cells. VZV is a highly contagious infection that spreads through infected secretions; thus, infection with VZV is very common and most people get exposed to the virus in childhood. The initial infection with VZV is called chickenpox, or varicella, and results in a febrile illness with a characteristic itchy skin rash with blisters that heal with scabbing over but typically do not cause permanent scars. The disease is mild and self-limited in children but much more severe in adults or immunocompromised individuals in whom it can cause life-threatening complications such as pneumonitis and encephalitis. During the acute infection, the virus enters the nerve cells either via a retrograde spread from the nerve endings or due to systemic viremia [1]. The virus then becomes latent in the cranial, sensory, and autonomic ganglia in the entire nervous system and is kept from reactivating by cell-mediated immunity (CMI) that develops 1–2 weeks following the initial infection [2]. When this CMI declines with age or with immunosuppression, the latent virus can reactivate and cause recurrent disease called herpes zoster or "shingles." Antibodies to VZV develop 2–4 weeks after the initial infection and persist lifelong. They are thought to prevent the individual from getting reinfected by VZV but do not protect the individuals from reactivation of their own latent VZV [3]. In fact, high levels of antibodies after reactivation usually indicate more severe disease [4].

S. S. Tuli (✉)
Department of Ophthalmology, University of Florida Health Eye Center,
Gainesville, FL, USA
e-mail: stuli@ufl.edu

© Springer Nature Singapore Pte Ltd. 2021
S. Das, V. Jhanji (eds.), *Infections of the Cornea and Conjunctiva*,
https://doi.org/10.1007/978-981-15-8811-2_14

It is estimated that approximately one million cases of zoster occur in the US every year and that 30% of the population will develop herpes zoster at some point in their lives [2]. Herpes zoster occurring in the area supplied by the ophthalmic branch of the trigeminal nerve (CNV) is called Herpes Zoster Ophthalmicus (HZO). VZV seems to have a predilection for the trigeminal ganglion and approximately 20% of all zoster infections affect the trigeminal nerve [5]. Since the advent of a live, attenuated VZV vaccine for children, the incidence of chickenpox has decreased tremendously, especially in developed nations. However, this has resulted in unintended consequences in that the attenuated virus also becomes latent in the ganglion cells and has the potential to reactivate in the future with declining immunity to cause shingles. In addition, the lack of exposure of adults to naturally occurring chickenpox as they no longer come in contact with children with chickenpox may prevent periodic boosting of their CMI. This may be a cause of HZO occurring more commonly and at a younger age recently compared to the past [6–8].

14.2   Herpes Zoster Virus

VZV, a large double-stranded DNA virus, has an icosahedral capsid enclosed in a host nuclear membrane-derived envelope, with viral-derived glycoprotein projections (Fig. 14.1). Contact of the mucus membranes with infected secretions causes the virus to attach to the host cells using its glycoprotein projections. The viral envelope then fuses with the host cell and injects the viral capsid into the cell cytoplasm. The capsid, in turn, fuses with the nuclear membrane, and the viral DNA is injected into the nucleus of the host cell where it circularizes. It then uses the host

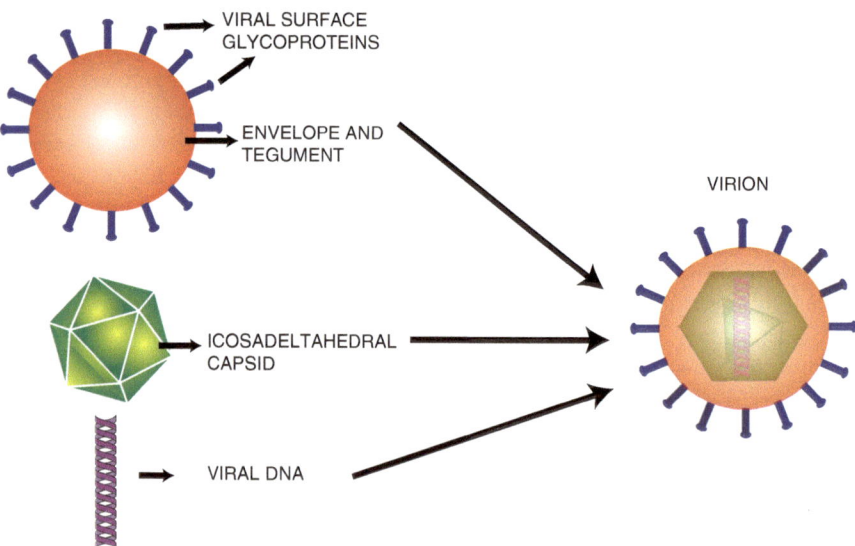

Fig. 14.1 Structure of virus consisting of a double-stranded DNA enclosed in a viral capsid and surrounded by host cell-derived envelope with protrusion of viral glycoproteins from the surface

cellular machinery to create new capsids and replicate its DNA, which is then packaged in the capsids. These capsids then bud across the nuclear membrane followed by the cellular membrane, which form the new viral envelope, thus destroying the sensory ganglion cell in the process. The destruction of the ganglion cell leads to the neurological pain (postherpetic neuralgia) as well as severe hypoesthesia, which are hallmarks of this disease, especially with HZO.

14.2.1 Ocular Involvement with Varicella

Ocular involvement with chickenpox is rare but may occur, especially in adults and immunocompromised. It is usually manifested by a mild conjunctivitis, but pseudo-dendrites, stromal keratitis, endotheliitis, and iritis may occur. These are usually self-limited and resolve without sequelae.

14.2.2 Herpes Zoster Ophthalmicus

As mentioned earlier, HZO results when there is reactivation of latent VZV in the trigeminal ganglion (TG), especially its ophthalmic branch, which supplies the forehead, upper lid, and eye. Not all episodes of HZO affect the eye and some resolve without any ophthalmic complications. Involvement of the nasociliary branch of the ophthalmic nerve leads to lesions at the tip of the nose, which is called Hutchinson sign, and indicates high likelihood of ocular involvement as it also supplies the cornea and uvea in addition to the ocular surface and eyelids. This sign is present in half to two-thirds of cases of HZO and may predict a worse outcome [9]. HZO can affect all parts of the eye and, while the most common manifestations are eyelid dermatitis, conjunctivitis, keratitis, and uveitis, it can also cause more severe ocular complications such as scleritis, extraocular muscle palsies, retinitis, and optic neuritis. In rare conditions, it may lead to vasculitis and ischemia of ocular structures, as well as cavernous sinus thrombosis [10]. There is also evidence of zoster making patients more susceptible in the future to dementia, stroke, cardiac disease, and giant cell arteritis [11, 12]. Postherpetic neuralgia (PHN) is characteristic of all zoster dermatitis but can be particularly disabling when involving the distribution of the TG.

14.2.3 HZO Dermatitis

The classic feature of HZO is a painful vesicular rash on the forehead, eyelids, and nose depending on the branches of the TG involved in the reactivation. The rash may be preceded by malaise, fever, headache, and pain over the distribution of the nerve. Classically, the rash obeys the midline though in severe cases, the edema may cross the midline and make it appear bilateral. It starts as erythema, followed by papules, vesicles, and pustules. The pustules finally crust and may form a black eschar before being shed off. There is significant variability in the appearance of the

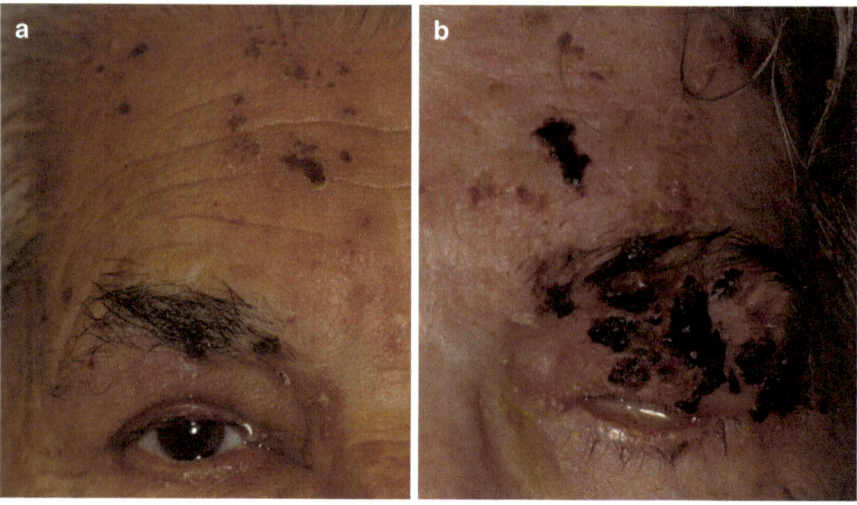

Fig. 14.2 Skin lesions of herpes zoster can vary from (**a**) a few vesicles to (**b**) extensive eschars

lesions with some patients demonstrating only a few vesicles and others with considerable inflammation and edema (Fig. 14.2). It is essential to remember that patients are infectious during this process and can transmit the virus to naïve patients who have not had chickenpox previously. In rare cases, HZO may occur without a rash and is called zoster sine herpete.

14.2.4 HZO Conjunctivitis

Follicular conjunctivitis is the most common ocular manifestation of HZO. It is usually self-limited and resolves without complications. However, vesicles may form on the conjunctival surface and subsequently ulcerate. In this case, a mucopurulent discharge may be seen. This can result in pseudo-membrane formation as well as scarring of the ulcerated surfaces resulting in symblepharon formation.

14.2.5 HZO Keratitis

Keratitis occurs in about two-thirds of HZO and may be divided into acute and chronic phases. The acute phase, which occurs within the first month after onset of the dermatitis, is thought to be due to the presence of live virus in the cornea and live VZV has been detected in the cornea for up to 34 days following the initial symptoms [13]. The late phase, which usually occurs after a month is thought to be due to an immune reaction to viral antigen in the cornea and may become chronic, lasting for years following the initial episode. VZV antigen has been found in corneas for up to 10 years following the initial zoster episode [14]. Both acute and late keratitis can affect the epithelial, stromal, or endothelial layers of the cornea.

14.2.6 Epithelial Keratitis

The initial finding is punctate epithelial keratitis or superficial punctate keratitis. These lesions are similar to the superficial punctate keratitis of Thygeson's disease; they appear opaque and stuck-on as they are composed of swollen epithelial cells that have undergone acantholysis. The lesions may coalesce to form pseudodendrites, so called because they lack the dichotomous branching, terminal bulbs, and central epithelial defect that are characteristic of the true dendrites of herpes simplex. They may stain variably or show negative staining. These may resolve spontaneously but often require treatment with gentle debridement and topical antivirals.

Late epithelial keratitis usually manifests as mucus plaques and can occur for years following the initial episode. The plaques consist of mucus that is adherent to swollen and degenerated epithelial cells [15]. The underlying epithelium, though abnormal, is usually intact. Therefore, the mucus plaques can often be gently debrided off the cornea without causing an epithelial defect. A bandage contact lens is often inserted in the eye to prevent them from recurring. Mucus plaques are often associated with underlying inflammation and steroid drops may be needed long-term to prevent recurrence of these lesions.

14.2.7 Stromal Keratitis (Interstitial Keratitis)

Stromal keratitis usually occurs between 1 and 2 weeks following the onset of zoster but may persist or reoccur for years. It is thought to be an immune-mediated response to viral antigen in the stroma. It is possible that the acute lesions are due to an immune response to live virus while chronic lesions are a response to viral capsids without the presence of live virus. The classic lesions are called nummular keratitis because of their circular coin shape (Fig. 14.3). They often appear under the previous epithelial keratitis but may be the only manifestation of keratitis. The overlying epithelium and underlying endothelium are usually

Fig. 14.3 Nummular keratitis consisting of coin-shaped inflammatory lesions in the corneal stroma

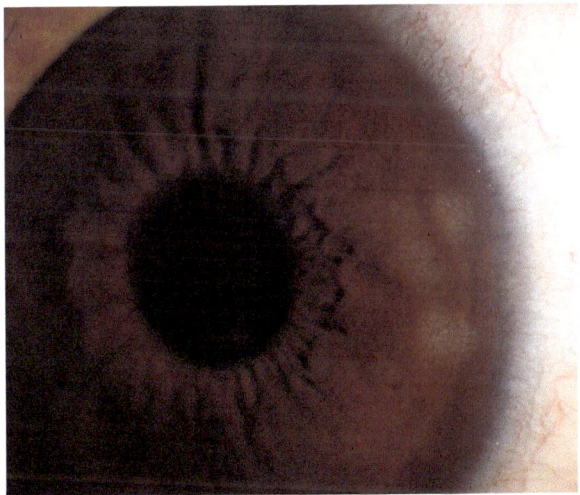

intact which is why it is called interstitial keratitis. These lesions are very sensitive to topical steroids and small doses are adequate to completely resolve the lesions without scarring. However, rapid taper of steroids can cause reappearance of the lesions and they often require chronic, low-dose steroid use to prevent recurrences. Untreated, the lesions can cause vessel growth into the cornea and permanent scarring.

14.2.8 Endotheliitis

Involvement of the endothelium results in its dysfunction and localized edema overlying the affected area. The most commonly seen form is localized endotheliitis or disciform keratitis because of it appears as a disc of edema on the cornea [16]. Careful inspection often reveals large, granulomatous (mutton fat) keratic precipitates underlying the edema but may be hard to visualize. A sharp demarcation between involved and uninvolved stroma distinguishes this from other causes of stromal edema.

Unlike autoimmune keratic precipitates in acute uveitis which result from deposition of cells that have extruded from an inflamed iris floating in the anterior chamber, these keratic precipitates are caused by a lymphocytic response directly to viral antigen in the endothelium. Therefore, the anterior chamber reaction in herpetic endotheliitis is very mild or absent compared to the amount of keratic precipitates. In acute cases, the keratic precipitates and edema respond well to topical steroids and may completely resolve without scarring. However, in chronic cases, the endothelial cells may undergo permanent damage in which case it does not respond to steroids. Long-standing stromal edema can also lead to permanent scarring and decreased vision. In these cases, surgical management is needed to clear the vision. The endotheliitis may be more diffuse in some cases and result in edema and bullae over the entire cornea. Endotheliitis, especially the diffuse kind, is often associated with trabeculitis.

14.2.9 Keratouveitis

This condition also has granulomatous keratic precipitates but, in these cases, the iris is also involved and the anterior chamber shows a fibrinoid aqueous and cells (Fig. 14.4). The uveitis is often explosive with significant inflammation and may present with a hypopyon or even a hyphema due to severe inflammation. The associated vasculitis and vascular occlusions can result in sector iris atrophy that is characteristic of zoster (Fig. 14.5) [17]. It can also lead to significant morbidity from synechiae, cataracts, and glaucoma due to associated trabeculitis.

Fig. 14.4 Granulomatous keratic precipitates

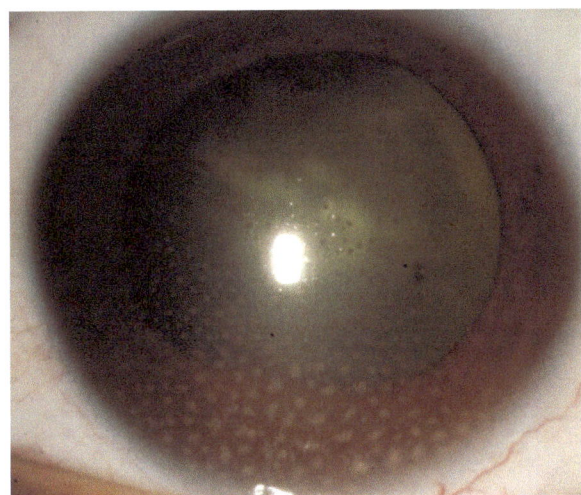

Fig. 14.5 Neurotrophic keratitis

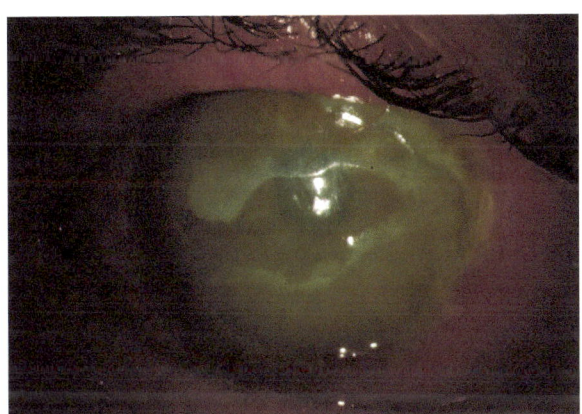

14.2.10 Trabeculitis

Inflammation of the trabecular meshwork can be associated with cases of endotheli-itis or keratouveitis. This can lead to swelling of the endothelial cells in the trabeculum or clogging of the meshwork with inflammatory cells [18]. This causes outflow obstruction resulting in acutely elevated pressures that mimic an angle closure attack due to the complete lack of outflow. The pressure responds to high dose steroids distinguishing it from steroid-induced glaucoma or other forms of open-angle glaucoma. Recurrent episodes of trabeculitis can lead to scarring of the trabecular meshwork and secondary glaucoma that behaves like chronic angle-closure glaucoma and often requires surgical management [19]. The risk of glaucomatous optic nerve damage is high due to recurrent episodes of very high intraocular pressures.

14.2.11 Neurotrophic Keratitis

HZO can result in very severe hypoesthesia due to damage to the ganglion cells in the TG as the replicating virus particles bud out of the nuclear membrane and destroy the nucleus and cells in the process. The lack of sensation leads to a relative dry eye, decreased ability to heal, and a propensity to ulcerate with minimal trauma. The causes of ulceration are multifactorial and include lack of tearing due to lack of sensation, unrecognized trauma, lack of neural-derived growth factors, and low-grade stromal inflammation. As a result, patients can present with ulcers that can be very difficult to manage (Fig. 14.6). Neurotrophic ulcers start as roughened epithelium that breaks down to produce an epithelial defect with smooth margins. The borders are grayish, elevated, and consist of multiple layers of epithelium.

14.2.12 Lipid Keratopathy

Newly formed or inflamed vessels are permeable to lipid due to the action of VEGF. Thus, this condition is seen in patients with long-standing interstitial keratitis with stromal vessels. The patient often presents with sudden loss of vision from fluid and lipid exuding from these vessels (Fig. 14.7) Once exuded, the fluid is often

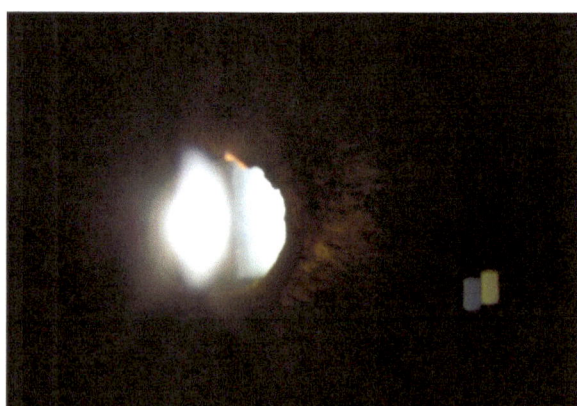

Fig. 14.6 Iris atrophy after HZO

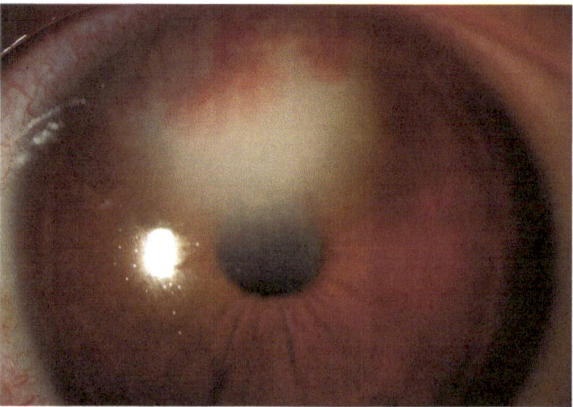

Fig. 14.7 Vascular pannus from long-standing interstitial keratitis with lipid keratopathy

reabsorbed from the cornea leaving behind a silvery-white crystalline appearance due to lipid collecting within keratocytes and intercellular matrix. Lipid keratopathy is one of the major cause of vision loss requiring corneal transplantation in patients with HZO.

14.2.13 Postherpetic Neuralgia

While a shingles outbreak is often preceded and followed by severe pain that lasts from 2 to 4 weeks, this is not considered postherpetic neuralgia (PHN). PHN is the chronic pain that persists 3 months or more following an episode of shingles and occurs in about 10% of patients with shingles. The risk of PHN increases with increasing age [20]. The characteristic of the pain varies and may be described as burning, itching, lancinating, or "electric shocks." Two features that are common are hyperalgesia (pain more severe than expected based on stimulus) and allodynia (pain associated with nonpainful stimuli). This pain is remarkably resistant to treatment and most patients are significantly physically and emotionally debilitated by the pain.

14.3   Diagnosis

Testing is seldom needed for the diagnosis of HZO as the rash is characteristic. However, in cases where the diagnosis is not certain, a swab or scraping of the rash can be sent to the laboratory for testing. Traditionally viral culture was considered the gold standard but is no longer recommended due to low sensitivity and delay in getting the results. Fluorescent antibody assay has higher sensitivity but may have false negatives. The gold standard for diagnosing viral infections currently is Polymerase chain reaction (PCR) [21]. PCR is very rapid and extremely sensitive and specific but does require specialized laboratories that can perform the test. If no laboratories that can perform these tests are available, a rapid and cheap test that can be done in any laboratory is Papanicolaou or Giemsa stains which show multinucleated giant cells and intranuclear eosinophilic inclusion bodies (Cowdry type A). However, this has very low sensitivity and specificity as it cannot distinguish between HZV and other similar viruses such as Herpes simplex. Serum antibody testing is not very helpful as it only indicates prior infection with VZV which is nearly ubiquitous [22].

14.4   Treatment of HZO

The recommended treatment of HZO is to initiate oral antiviral therapy on diagnosis. Studies have shown that oral antivirals started within 72 h of onset, and used for 7–14 days, reduce acute pain, virus shedding, rash, and acute anterior segment complications [23]. In addition, they reduce the incidence, severity, and duration of

Table 14.1 Oral antivirals used for herpes zoster

Drug (trade name)	Dose	Frequency	Adverse effects
Acycloavir (Zovirax)	800 mg	Five times a day	Headache, nausea, nephrotoxicity, neurotoxicity, diarrhea in lactose intolerant
Valacyclovir (Valtrex)	1000 mg	Three times a day	Thrombotic Thrombocytopenic Purpura (TTP) and hemolytic uremic syndrome in immunosuppressed
Famciclovir (Famvir)	500 mg	Three times a day	Similar to acyclovir

PHN. Whether antivirals have any benefit for chronic anterior segment complications is currently unknown and the currently ongoing Zoster Eye Disease Study (ZEDS) is attempting to answer that question. Interestingly, a recent survey of ZEDS investigators showed that about half of them treat HZO with prolonged antiviral use [24]. Table 14.1 shows the oral antivirals used in zoster with doses and side effects. All current antivirals are nucleoside analogs that competitively inhibit viral DNA and protein synthesis (Table 14.1). While they have a greater affinity for viral DNA polymerase, they may also interfere with host DNA synthesis which can cause toxicity. Acyclovir (ACV) is the most commonly used drug but requires high oral doses to achieve high enough serum levels to inhibit zoster. Valacyclovir is a synthetic prodrug that is converted to ACV after absorption. It is much better absorbed and reaches levels similar to IV ACV with oral use. Famciclovir is a prodrug of the antiviral penciclovir. It has high absorption and bioavailability. The drugs are typically used for 10–14 days at the doses listed in Table 14.1.

14.4.1 Epithelial Keratitis

Though epithelial keratitis may spontaneously resolve, treatment may be necessary if the lesions persist for more than a few days because of the risk of scarring. In addition, visually significant lesions may require treatment. Topical antivirals may be effective for early pseudodendrites due to the presence of live virus in the cells. Topical ganciclovir is the only medication that has shown benefit in HZO epithelial keratitis. In addition, gentle debridement removes viral antigen from the cornea and speeds up resolution as infected cells have undergone acantholysis and are poorly adherent. Steroids are usually avoided in acute keratitis due to the risk of prolonging the viral persistence in the cornea and ocular surface.

14.4.2 Stromal Keratitis and Keratouveitis

The mainstay of treatment is topical corticosteroids as they decrease inflammation and, therefore, scarring and other ocular complications. Difluprednate, Prednisolone acetate 1%, dexamethasone 0.1%, loteprednol, and fluorometholone 0.1% are the most commonly used steroid drops in order of potency from highest to lowest. Typically, these are started at 2–4 times a day, although, in severe cases, these can be instilled every 2 h. Simultaneous antiviral prophylaxis is not recommended but the ZEDS is evaluating whether it may be beneficial in select cases. Steroids, once started, should be continued without taper until resolution of the keratitis or uveitis. Once resolved completely, they should be tapered very gradually: often decreasing one drop a day every month. Too rapid a taper may result in recurrence of the inflammation. Often, a very small dose of topical steroids may be needed long-term to prevent recurrence of the inflammation. The dose to keep the eye quiescent varies and may be as low as one drop a week.

14.4.3 Neurotrophic Ulcers

The first step is surface support including elimination of any toxic medications. Punctal occlusion, artificial tear supplements, and a bandage contact lens may be used to prevent drying of the eye. Other options include autologous serum tears and amniotic membrane grafts to supply the missing growth factors. The cautious use of topical corticosteroids may be necessary if there is significant underlying inflammation. Recently, topical recombinant nerve growth factor (Oxervate™, cenegermin-bkbj, Dompé, USA) was approved for the treatment of neurotrophic keratitis. In a multicenter, randomized, double-masked, vehicle-controlled clinical trial, 8 weeks of cenegermin treatment showed statistically significant improvement in corneal healing compared to vehicle [25].

14.4.4 Postherpetic Neuralgia

PHN can be extremely difficult to manage as it is thought to occur due to chronic inflammation and degenerative changes in the TG and peripheral nerves. Prevention is definitely the best policy and vaccination to prevent HZO as well as antivirals within 72 h of the onset are the most effective methods. Once PHN develops, the treatment options are not very effective. Local application of lidocaine, capsaicin, or fentanyl patches may be used [20]. Oral medications like tricyclic antidepressants such as nortriptyline, antiepileptics like gabapentin, or serotonin uptake inhibitors such as pregabalin are often the mainstay of treatment. Opioids are often used but the chronic nature of this disease increases the risk of dependence and abuse. Other modalities that have been used are nerve blocks or stimulation, botulinum injections, and trigeminal ablation. However, the treatments do not eliminate the discomfort completely and PHN is a known risk factor for suicidal ideation.

14.5 Surgery

Corneal transplants are usually performed when corneal scarring limits vision. However, surgery also may be necessary as a therapeutic measure in patients with nonhealing ulcers or impending perforations. Corneal transplants have lower success rates due to the vascularization that usually accompanies the corneal scarring from HZO.

14.6   Herpes Zoster Vaccinations

Two VZV vaccines are commercially available for the prevention of zoster in adults. In 2006, a live, attenuated VZV vaccine (Zostavax®, Merck and Co., Inc.) was recommended by the CDC for use in patients 60 years of age or older. Although FDA approved it for use in people aged 50 years of age or older, it was not recommended for routine use in the age group 50–59 as it was thought that the immunity would decline by the age when shingles is common. It comprises a minimum of 19,400 plaque-forming units (PFU) of the attenuated Oka/Merck strain of VZV which is the same strain used in the Varicella vaccine in childhood (Varivax®, Merck and Co. Inc.), but 14 times its potency. It is given as a single subcutaneous dose and no booster doses are advised. In a phase 3 randomized, double-blind, placebo-controlled trial with nearly 40,000 participants, the vaccine efficacy was 61% overall, 67% for PHN, and 51% for incidence of zoster [26]. In addition, it was found that the median duration of pain and discomfort was significantly shorter in the vaccine group than the placebo group. They did find that the vaccine was not as efficacious in the ≥70-year-olds as it was in 60–69-year-olds.

A newer recombinant zoster vaccine (Shingrix®, GlaxoSmithKline) became commercially available in 2017 and is recommended by the CDC as the preferred shingles vaccine. It is a two-dose subunit vaccine that consists of recombinant glycoprotein E in combination with a novel adjuvant and is approved for adults ≥50 years. The two doses are administered intramuscularly 2–6 months apart. In a phase 3 randomized, placebo-controlled trial with over 16,000 participants, the vaccine was remarkably effective with 210 cases of zoster occurring in the placebo group and only 6 cases in the vaccinated group [27]. The overall vaccine efficacy was found to be over 97% and the efficacy was similar in all age groups over 50 years of age.

Zoster vaccination in patients that have already had shingles is controversial. Both vaccines are recommended for patients with previous zoster. However, there have been reports of patients with quiescent zoster keratitis who had recurrence of their keratitis approximately 2 weeks following vaccination [28, 29]. In addition, a study of individuals who developed zoster in the vaccine clinical trial showed that the CMI response to zoster was similar to that of the vaccine [4]. Therefore, patients who have had HZO probably do not need the vaccine for several years following their episode as they have developed protective CMI from their shingles and it is possible that the vaccine would reactivate their ocular inflammation so may actually be detrimental.

14.7   Summary

Herpes Zoster Ophthalmicus occurs due to reactivation of latent VZV in the Trigeminal ganglion due to declining CMI usually with advancing age. The incidence appears to be increasing recently and it is occurring at a younger age. Features of HZO include dermatitis, conjunctivitis, keratitis, and uveitis which can cause significant morbidity and loss of vision. Postherpetic neuralgia is one of the most devastating complications of HZO and is very difficult to manage. Long-term complications of this disease include glaucoma, lipid keratopathy, neurotrophic keratitis, and persistent PHN. Vaccination with the recombinant vaccine is very effective and is recommended for adults over the age of 50.

References

1. Liedtke W, Opalka B, Zimmermann CW, Lignitz E. Age distribution of latent herpes simplex virus 1 and varicella-zoster virus genome in human nervous tissue. J Neurol Sci. 1993;116(1):6–11.
2. Yawn BP, Gilden D. The global epidemiology of herpes zoster. Neurology. 2013;81(10):928–30.
3. Freer G, Pistello M. Varicella-zoster virus infection: natural history, clinical manifestations, immunity and current and future vaccination strategies. New Microbiol. 2018;41(2):95–105.
4. Weinberg A, Zhang JH, Oxman MN, Johnson GR, Hayward AR, Caulfield MJ, Irwin MR, Clair J, Smith JG, Stanley H, Marchese RD, Harbecke R, Williams HM, Chan IS, Arbeit RD, Gershon AA, Schödel F, Morrison VA, Kauffman CA, Straus SE, Schmader KE, Davis LE, Levin MJ, US Department of Veterans Affairs (VA) Cooperative Studies Program Shingles Prevention Study Investigators. Varicella-zoster virus specific immune responses to herpes zoster in elderly participants in a trial of a clinically effective zoster vaccine. J Infect Dis. 2009;200(7):1068–77.
5. Liesegang TJ. Corneal complications from herpes zoster ophthalmicus. Ophthalmology. 1985;92(3):316–24.
6. Li JY. Herpes zoster ophthalmicus: acute keratitis. Curr Opin Ophthalmol. 2018;29(4):328–33.
7. Kong CL, Thompson RR, Porco TC, Kim E, Acharya NR. Incidence rate of herpes zoster ophthalmicus: a retrospective cohort study from 1994 through 2018. Ophthalmology. 2020;127(3):324–30.
8. Davies EC, Pavan-Langston D, Chodosh J. Herpes zoster ophthalmicus: declining age at presentation. Br J Ophthalmol. 2016;100(3):312–4.
9. Nithyanandam S, Stephen J, Joseph M, Dabir S. Factors affecting visual outcome in herpes zoster ophthalmicus: a prospective study. Clin Exp Ophthalmol. 2010;38(9):845–50.
10. Jun LH, Gupta A, Milea D, Jaufeerally FR. More than meets the eye: varicella zoster virus-related orbital apex syndrome. Indian J Ophthalmol. 2018;66(11):1647–9.
11. Tsai MC, Cheng WL, Sheu JJ, Huang CC, Shia BC, Kao LT, Lin HC. Increased risk of dementia following herpes zoster ophthalmicus. PLoS One. 2017;12(11):e0188490.
12. Wu PH, Chuang YS, Lin YT. Does herpes zoster increase the risk of stroke and myocardial infarction? A comprehensive review. J Clin Med. 2019;8:4.
13. Zaal MJ, Völker-Dieben HJ, Wienesen M, D'Amaro J, Kijlstra A. Longitudinal analysis of varicella-zoster virus DNA on the ocular surface associated with herpes zoster ophthalmicus. Am J Ophthalmol. 2001;131(1):25–9.
14. Wenkel H, Rummelt V, Fleckenstein B, Naumann GO. Detection of varicella zoster virus DNA and viral antigen in human eyes after herpes zoster ophthalmicus. Ophthalmology. 1998;105(7):1323–30.
15. Kaufman SC. Anterior segment complications of herpes zoster ophthalmicus. Ophthalmology. 2008;115(2-Suppl):S24–32.
16. Moshirfar M, Murri MS, Shah TJ, Skanchy DF, Tuckfield JQ, Ronquillo YC, Birdsong OC, Hofstedt D, Hoopes PC. A review of corneal endotheliitis and endotheliopathy: differential diagnosis, evaluation, and treatment. Ophthalmol Ther. 2019;8(2):195–213.
17. Sakai JI, Usui Y, Suzuki J, Kezuka T, Goto H. Clinical features of anterior uveitis caused by three different herpes viruses. Int Ophthalmol. 2019;39(12):2785–95.

18. Porzukowiak TR, Ly K. In vivo confocal microscopy use in endotheliitis. Optom Vis Sci. 2015;92(12):e431–6.
19. Hoeksema L, Jansonius NM, Los LI. Risk factors for secondary glaucoma in herpetic anterior uveitis. Am J Ophthalmol. 2017;181:55–60.
20. Kedar S, Jayagopal LN, Berger JR. Neurological and ophthalmological manifestations of varicella zoster virus. J Neuroophthalmol. 2019;39(2):220–31.
21. Wilson DA, Yen-Lieberman B, Schindler S, Asamoto K, Schold JD, Procop GW. Should varicella-zoster virus culture be eliminated? A comparison of direct immunofluorescence antigen detection, culture, and PCR, with a historical review. J Clin Microbiol. 2012;50(12):4120–2.
22. Lee H, Cho HK, Kim KH. Seroepidemiology of varicella-zoster virus in Korea. J Korean Med Sci. 2013;28(2):195–9.
23. Pavan-Langston D. Herpes zoster antivirals and pain management. Ophthalmology. 2008;115(2-Suppl):S13–20.
24. Lo DM, Jeng BH, Gillespie C, Wu M, Cohen EJ. Current practice patterns and opinions on the management of recent-onset or chronic herpes zoster ophthalmicus of zoster eye disease study investigators. Cornea. 2019;38(1):13–7.
25. Pflugfelder SC, Massaro-Giordano M, Perez VL, Hamrah P, Deng SX, Espandar L, Foster CS, Affeldt J, Seedor JA, Afshari NA, Chao W, Allegretti M, Mantelli F, Dana R. Topical recombinant human nerve growth factor (cenegermin) for neurotrophic keratopathy: a multicenter randomized vehicle-controlled pivotal trial. Ophthalmology. 2020;127(1):14–26.
26. Oxman MN, Levin MJ, Johnson GR, Schmader KE, Straus SE, Gelb LD, Arbeit RD, Simberkoff MS, Gershon AA, Davis LE, Weinberg A, Boardman KD, Williams HM, Zhang JH, Peduzzi PN, Beisel CE, Morrison VA, Guatelli JC, Brooks PA, Kauffman CA, Pachucki CT, Neuzil KM, Betts RF, Wright PF, Griffin MR, Brunell P, Soto NE, Marques AR, Keay SK, Goodman RP, Cotton DJ, Gnann JW Jr, Loutit J, Holodniy M, Keitel WA, Crawford GE, Yeh SS, Lobo Z, Toney JF, Greenberg RN, Keller PM, Harbecke R, Hayward AR, Irwin MR, Kyriakides TC, Chan CY, Chan IS, Wang WW, Annunziato PW, Silber JL, Shingles Prevention Study Group. A vaccine to prevent herpes zoster and postherpetic neuralgia in older adults. N Engl J Med. 2005;352(22):2271–84.
27. Lal H, Cunningham AL, Godeaux O, Chlibek R, Diez-Domingo J, Hwang SJ, Levin MJ, McElhaney JE, Poder A, Puig-Barberà J, Vesikari T, Watanabe D, Weckx L, Zahaf T, Heineman TC, ZOE-50 Study Group. Efficacy of an adjuvanted herpes zoster subunit vaccine in older adults. N Engl J Med. 2015;372(22):2087–96.
28. Hwang CW Jr, Steigleman WA, Saucedo-Sanchez E, Tuli SS. Reactivation of herpes zoster keratitis in an adult after varicella zoster vaccination. Cornea. 2013;32(4):508–9.
29. Jastrzebski A, Brownstein S, Ziai S, Saleh S, Lam K, Jackson WB. Reactivation of herpes zoster keratitis with corneal perforation after zoster vaccination. Cornea. 2017;36(6):740–2.

Savitri Sharma

15.1 Introduction

Infectious conjunctivitis and keratitis may be caused by several groups of organisms including bacteria, viruses, fungi, and parasites Viruses cause up to 80% of conjunctivitis [1–4]. Many cases may be misdiagnosed as bacterial conjunctivitis and the accuracy of clinical diagnosis is 50% compared to laboratory confirmation [5]. Up to 90% of acute viral conjunctivitis are caused by adenoviruses with herpes simplex virus, varicella zoster virus, enteroviruses, coxsackieviruses, and other viruses [6]. Conjunctivitis has been described in viral infections such as measles, mumps, and Zika virus infection [7, 8]. Apart from viruses, several species of bacteria such as *Neisseria gonorrhoeae, Streptococcus pneumoniae, Haemophilus influenzae, Streptococcus pyogenes,* and *Staphylococci* are associated with conjunctival infection, especially in children. Concomitant with urethritis *N. gonorrhoeae* can cause bilateral purulent conjunctivitis with or without corneal involvement in adults. Isolated fungal infections of the conjunctiva are rare. Earlier classified with protozoa Microsporidia are now considered a parafungus and have been reported to be associated with keratoconjunctivitis that is clinically similar to adenovirus infection [9]. *Chlamydia trachomatis* is an obligate intracellular parasite that is responsible for several forms of conjunctivitis such as trachoma and inclusion conjunctivitis (adult and neonatal). Among the parasites, *Onchocerca volvulus* may cause conjunctival and corneal lesions by invasion and subsequent death of the microfilariae [10].

As listed in Table 15.1, various types of bacteria can potentially cause keratitis. The relative frequency of different bacteria as causative agents in keratitis may be geographical location based as well as risk factor and host dependent. The incidence of pneumococcal keratitis, which is commonly associated with chronic

S. Sharma (✉)
Jhaveri Microbiology Centre, L V Prasad Eye Institute, Hyderabad, Telangana, India
e-mail: savitri@lvpei.org

© Springer Nature Singapore Pte Ltd. 2021
S. Das, V. Jhanji (eds.), *Infections of the Cornea and Conjunctiva*,
https://doi.org/10.1007/978-981-15-8811-2_15

Table 15.1 Various genera of bacteria associated with bacterial keratitis

– Gram-negative aerobic/facultative anaerobic bacilli:	– *Pseudomonas* – *Escherichia* – *Citrobacter* – *Klebsiella* – *Serratia* – *Proteus* – *Haemophilus*
– Gram-negative anaerobic bacilli:	– *Bacteroides* – *Fusobacterium*
– Gram-negative aerobic cocci and coccobacilli:	– *Neisseria* – *Moraxella* – *Acinetobacter*
– Gram-positive aerobic/facultative anaerobic cocci:	– *Micrococcus* – *Staphylococcus* – *Streptococcus* – *Aerococcus*
– Gram-positive aerobic bacilli:	– *Bacillus*
– Gram-positive anaerobic bacilli:	– *Clostridium*
– Actinomycetes and related organisms (aerobic):	– *Arachnia* – *Bifidobacterium* – *Mycobacterium* – *Nocardia* – *Streptomyces* – *Corynebacterium*
– Actinomycetes and related organisms (anaerobic):	– *Actinomyces* – *Propionibacterium*
– Gram-positive anaerobic cocci:	– *Peptostreptococcus*

dacryocystitis [11], has decreased in developed countries as a result of modern anti-biotics and refinement in techniques for dacryocystorhinostomy [12]. *Staphylococcus* species continue to be the predominant cause of bacterial keratitis and in several reports *Staphylococcus epidermidis* or coagulase negative staphylococci (CONS) are the leading causes [13, 14]. *Pseudomonas* species is especially associated with daily or extended wear soft contact lenses related keratitis [15]. It is one of the commonest gram-negative bacteria causing microbial keratitis. Bacteria less frequently causing keratitis include *Corynebacterium* species [16], *Propionibacterium acnes* [17], *Bacillus* species [18, 19], *Neisseria gonorrhoeae, Listeria monocytogenes* [20], species of *Enterobacteriaceae* family [21], etc. *Nocardia* species are an important cause of keratitis [22]. Atypical mycobacteria such as *Mycobacterium fortuitum* [23], *Mycobacterium chelonae, Mycobacterium abscessus, Mycobacterium gordonae*, and *Mycobacterium avium-intracellulare* are infrequent causes of keratitis associated with corneal trauma or surgery. There are several reports of post excimer laser photorefractive keratectomy (PRK) and post excimer laser *in situ* keratomilieusis (LASIK) keratitis cases [24]. Caused by *Borrelia burgdorferi* a rare non-syphilitic spirochetal infection of the cornea has been reported [25]. Patients may develop bacterial infection of the cornea post penetrating keratoplasty. Unlike conjunctivitis, fungi are a common cause of keratitis. A large variety of species have been reported (Table 15.2).

The commonest virus causing keratitis worldwide is herpes simplex virus (HSV). The HSV infection is usually a recurrent disease and the immunologic response associated with the episode. Sunlight, trauma (including surgery), heat, abnormal body temperature, menstruation, other infectious diseases, and emotional stress, etc., have been implicated in the activation of HSV infection. Recurrent epithelial keratitis occurs by reactivation of live virus leading to clinical manifestations such as dendritic and geographic ulcers. The dendritic or geographic ulcer may completely resolve leading to stromal scarring. One quarter of the patients may develop stromal disease, which may be infectious or immunological [26].

Table 15.2 Types of fungal species associated with fungal keratitis

– Hyaline septate filamentous fungi:	– *Fusarium species* – *Aspergillus* species – *Acremonium* species – *Beauveria* species – *Cylindrocarpon* species – *Geotrichum candidum* – *Neurospora* species – *Penicillium* species – *Paecilomyces* species – *Pseudallescheria boydii* – *Sphaeropsis subglobosa* – *Scopulariopsis* species – *Ustilago* species – *Volutella* species
– Dematiaceous septate filamentous fungi:	– *Alternaria* species – *Bipolaris* species – *Curvularia* species – *Cladosporium* species – *Drechslera* species – *Exserohilum* species – *Exophiala jeanselmei* – *Lasiodiplodia theobromae* – *Macrophomina phaseolina* – *Phialophora* species
– Yeasts and yeast-like fungi:	– *Candida* species – *Cryptococcus* species – *Rhodotorula* species – *Trichosporon* species
– Dimorphic fungi:	– *Blastomyces dermatitidis* – *Paracoccidoides brasiliensis* – *Sporothrix schenkii*
– Hyaline aseptate/sparsely septate filamentous fungi:	– *Rhizopus* – *Mucor* – *Pythium*[a]

[a]Parafungus

Acanthamoeba and Microsporidia are two keratitis-causing parasites, the latter being currently classified as parafungus. *Acanthamoeba* keratitis occurs in immunocompetent, healthy young individuals. While contact lens wear is the commonest risk factor for *Acanthamoeba* keratitis in the United States the common risk factor in patients of *Acanthamoeba* keratitis seen in developing countries is history of corneal trauma or exposure to contaminated water [27, 28].

Laboratory tests for diagnosis of conjunctival and corneal infections include direct microscopy, culture, antigen detection by direct or indirect fluorescent antibody (DFA, IFA) methods, conventional or real-time polymerase chain reaction (PCR), etc. Point-of-care tests are available for the detection of adenovirus and herpes simplex virus infections.

15.2 Role of Microbiology in the Diagnosis of Conjunctival and Corneal Infections

Diagnosis for any infectious condition begins in the clinics with the observation of clinical features that might be suggestive of a particular etiology. Microbiological investigations are aimed at either confirming or negating the clinical suspicion. They are indicated in situations where clinical features on their own may not be confirmatory. Excellent reviews have pointed out that most cases of conjunctivitis are self-limiting [29, 30] and obtaining clinical samples for microbiological investigations are reserved for neonatal conjunjuntivitis, recurrent conjunctivitis, conjunctivitis recalcitrant to therapy, severe purulent discharge, etc. The decision to procure clinical specimens for culture, antigen detection, or molecular tests is based on the likelihood of benefit to the patient. Interpretation of the tests requires understanding of the normal flora of the conjunctiva and the lids. In clinic rapid viral antigen testing is available for adenovirus and has a sensitivity of 86% and specificity of 94% [31]. This test can prevent unnecessary use of antibiotics limiting development of antibiotic resistance apart from saving considerable amount of money. An immunochromatographic assay kit for office-based herpes simplex virus detection has been mainly used in the diagnosis of HSV keratitis [32].

Generally, microbiological investigation of keratitis is indicated in sight-threatening (>1–2 mm) ulcers, in ulcers wherein an atypical organism is suspected, and in any ulcer that is not responding to therapy. However, in tropical and subtropical parts of the world where the prevalence of fungal keratitis is high, it is recommended to investigate all corneal ulcers. The methodology of sample collection and processing is described below.

15.3 Clinical Sample Collection

It is important to collect samples for the diagnosis of conjunctivitis from the conjunctival sac and for keratitis from the cornea. Tears or serum samples are rarely helpful in the diagnosis of corneal or conjunctival infections. Some of the crucial guidelines include that the samples be collected carefully without contamination, without causing discomfort or pain to the patient and using appropriate technique in consultation with the microbiologist.

Some of the requirements for collection of samples include topical anesthetic eye drop (0.5% proparacaine hydrochloride), sterile cotton/dacron/calcium alginate swab, surgical blade number 15, Kimura spatula, glass slides (preferably cleaned with alcohol, hot air oven sterilized, wrapped in aluminum foil), and glass cover slips (preferably cleaned with alcohol). Culture media (liquid and solid), phosphate buffered saline pH 7.2, 95% ethyl alcohol and acetone for fixation, etc., are other requirements based on the intended investigations. Viral transport medium would be needed if viral culture is intended.

It is best to collect two conjunctival swabs if conjunctival discharge is present and send to the laboratory in sterile tubes. Moistened (with sterile saline or any liquid media) swabs may be used for optimum recovery of the organisms. While one swab could be used for making smears for direct microscopy, the other can be used for inoculation of culture media. Solid media could be inoculated initially followed by liquid media ending with breaking off the nonhandled distal end of the swab into the liquid medium. For viral culture, a dacron swab with conjunctival sample is agitated in cold viral transport medium. Wooden shaft of cotton or calcium alginate swab may inhibit viral growth. A conjunctival scraping under topical anesthesia using blade number 15 provides a good sample for direct microscopy from cases with minimal discharge with or without pseudomembrane.

The corneal sample is best collected using Kimura spatula or blade number 15 under topical anesthesia under slit lamp magnification in the clinic. Multiple scrapings are transferred on to glass slides and inoculated on culture media. If taken out of the refrigerator, the culture media should preferably be warmed to room temperature before use. The corneal scrapings are transferred on the solid media in multiple "C" shaped strokes. Slides and inoculated media are transferred to the laboratory in closed containers for immediate processing. An alternative method of collection of corneal sample using a single-sample device (Eswab, Copan Diagnostics, Inc) has been described that was comparable with the conventional method in the diagnosis of bacterial keratitis [33].

15.4 Sample Processing and Direct Smear Examination

In general, no transport medium (except for virus or *Chlamydia* culture) is recommended for conjunctival and corneal samples. Although McLeod et al. have described Amies transport medium without charcoal [34] to be effective transport medium, comparable to direct processing, in the investigation of fungal and bacterial keratitis, validation of this method by other investigators is lacking. Other useful samples in the investigation of microbial keratitis associated with contact lens wear would include contact lenses, contact lens cases, and contact lens solutions. These samples are directly processed for culture of bacteria, fungi, or parasites in appropriate media and smears are generally not made. Special procedures are required for

Table 15.3 Direct smear examination methods for the diagnosis of conjunctival and corneal infections

Type of sample	Type of organism/antigen to be detected	Staining methods for smears
Eye lash	• Parasites (Demodex, Lice)	• Saline/Glycerol Wet Mount
Conjunctival swabs/scrapings	• Bacteria, Fungi, Microsporidia	• Gram, Giemsa, KOH + Calcofluor White, Ziehl-Neelsen Stain
	• Viral antigens	• Direct/indirect immunofluorescence or immunoperoxidase assay
Corneal scrapings	• Bacteria, fungi, parasite (*Acanthamoeba*, Microsporidia)	• Gram, Giemsa, KOH + Calcofluor White, Lactophenol Cotton Blue, Gomori Methenamine Silver, Ziehl-Neelsen Stain
	• Viral antigens	• Direct/indirect immunofluorescence or immunoperoxidase assay

the collection of samples for the detection of parasites and viruses. Samples such as corneal buttons/biopsies need to be transported to the laboratory in sterile dry containers where they may be cut/minced into tiny pieces and inoculated on different culture media. Transport in normal saline is fraught with possibility of contamination. Direct smear examination methods that may be used for detection of various organisms from conjunctiva and cornea are shown in Table 15.3. Sample is transferred from the blade/spatula/swab to a glass slide over an area of approximately 1 cm circle marked on the reverse with a marker. While the specimen is thinly spread for dry smears (Gram, Giemsa, Gomori methenamine silver, etc.), it needs to be placed in the circle and covered with a coverslip without spreading, for wet smears (potassium hydroxide-KOH, calcofluor white-CFW, lactophenol cotton blue-LPCB, etc.). Preparation of at least two smears is recommended, which helps in confirmation of the findings. We prefer a combination of KOH + CFW, Gram, and Giemsa stained smears, which has provided us a high sensitivity and specificity for the detection of bacteria, fungi, microsporidia, and *Acanthamoeba* along with details of inflammatory cells in corneal scrapings. Fungi being uncommon in conjunctivitis, routine use of KOH + CFW is not justified for conjunctival samples. They are usually examined by Gram and Giemsa stains. A common binocular laboratory light microscope is adequate for the examination of the smears except when fluorescent stain such as calcofluor white is used which requires a fluorescence microscope. Ziehl-Neelsen stain using 20% H_2SO_4 or 1% H_2SO_4 (modified Ziehl-Neelsen stain or Kinyoun's stain) can be employed on the corneal scrapings when the Gram stain is suggestive of either mycobacteria (unstained, poorly stained bacilli in Gram stain) or *Nocardia* (thin, beaded, branching filaments). Gram stained smear can be decolorized and subjected to these special stains obviating the need to collect an additional scraping.

For polymerase chain reaction (PCR) the samples are placed in sterile phosphate buffered saline pH 7.2 and submitted to the laboratory where they may be retained at −20 °C until tested.

A rapid diagnosis of viral infection can be established by observing stained smears of corneal scrapings, conjunctival scrapings/swabs. Nonspecific staining techniques used for this purpose include Giemsa, Papanicolaou, and Hematoxylin-eosin stain [35]. Multinucleated giant cells, koilocytic changes, and intranuclear/intracytoplasmic inclusions, and types of inflammatory cells are some of the crucial information that can be obtained.

Conjunctival samples stained with Gram stain and KOH + CFW showing gram-positive cocci and microsporidial spores are shown in Fig. 15.1a–d. Corneal scrapings stained with Gram stain and Ziehl-Neelsen (ZN) stain showing gram-positive cocci, gram-positive bacilli, fungal filaments, budding yeast cells, *Pythium* filaments, *Acanthamoeba* cysts, microsporidia spores, etc., are shown in Fig. 15.2a–n. Figure 15.2m shows aseptate filaments of *Pythium* in the corneal scraping stained with Gomori methenamine silver (GMS) stain. Apart from fungal filaments, KOH + CFW is a highly sensitive stain for the observation of *Acanthamoeba* cysts, *Pythium*, yeast, and microsporidial spores (Fig. 15.3a–d and Fig. 15.1c). A gram stained smear can be decolorized with acetone and restained with either ZN or GMS

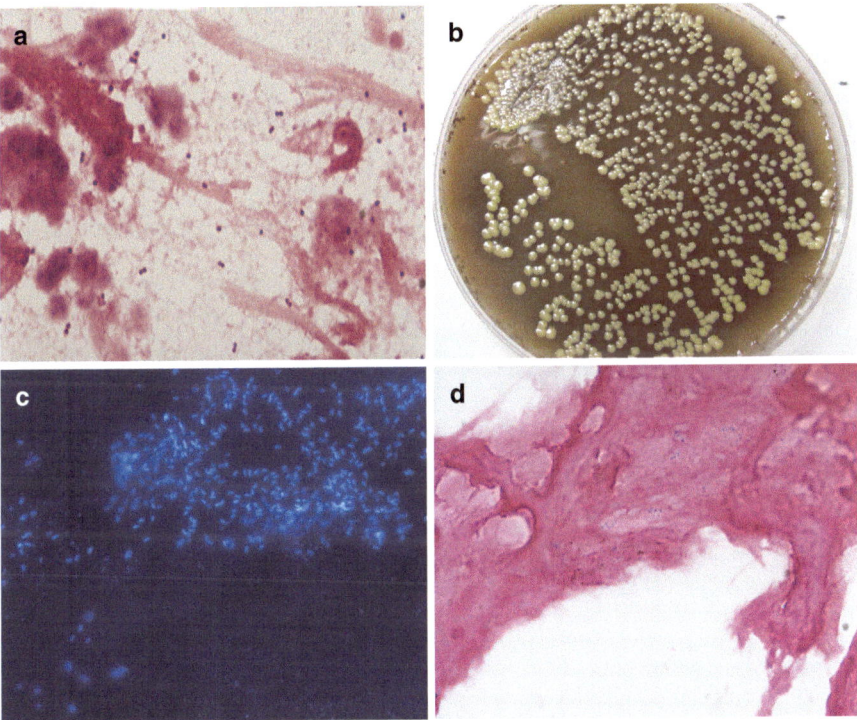

Fig. 15.1 (a) Conjunctival swab from a patient with purulent conjunctivitis showing spherical gram-positive cocci in singles, pairs, and in groups; (b) Confluent growth of golden yellow glistening colonies of *Staphylococcus aureus* on chocolate agar (37 °C, 24 h); (c) Conjunctival scraping showing microsporidial spores under fluorescence microscope (KOH + CFW, ×400); (d) Conjunctival scraping showing microsporidial spores with stippled gram-positive staining (Gram stain, ×1000)

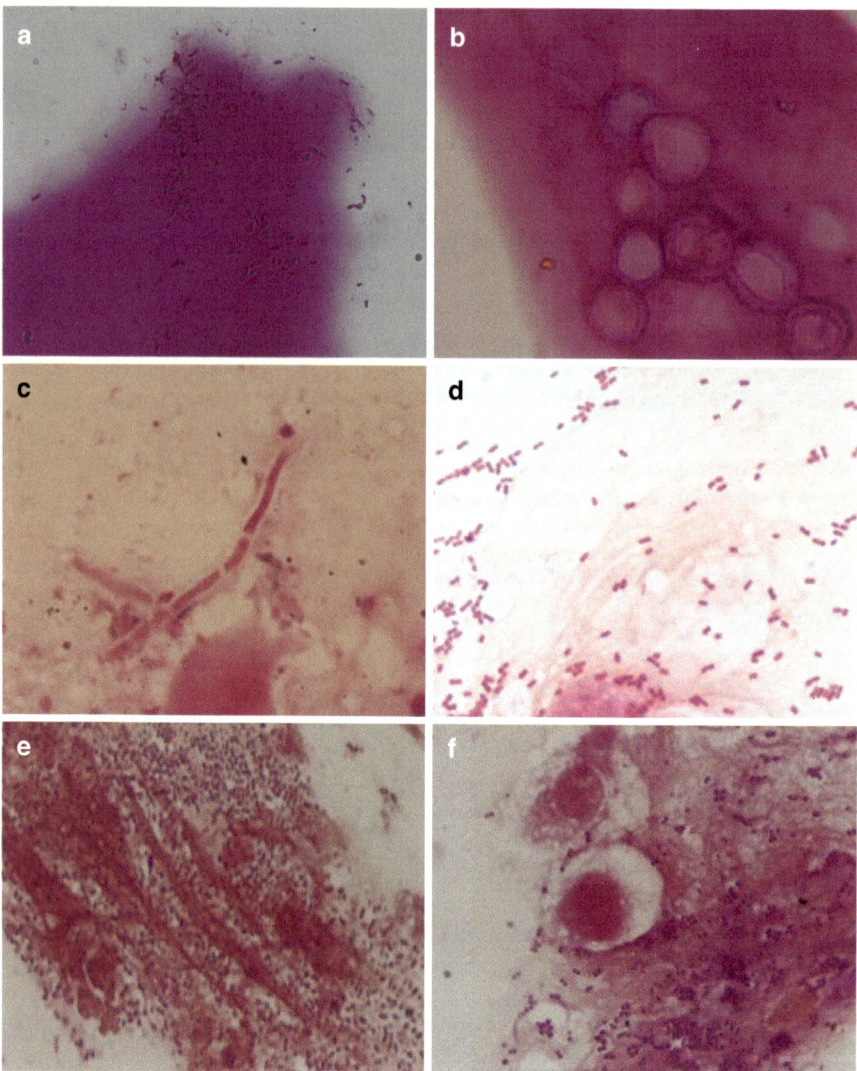

Fig. 15.2 Corneal scrapings showing: (**a**) Gram-positive beaded bacilli arranged in Chinese letter pattern suggestive of *Corynebacterium species* (Gram stain, ×1000); (**b**) Double walled *Acanthamoeba* cysts (Gram stain, ×1000); (**c**) septate, hyaline fungal filaments (Gram stain, ×1000); (**d**) Box-like gram-negative bacilli in pairs suggestive of *Moraxella species* (Gram stain, ×1000); (**e**) capsulated gram-positive cocci in pairs, suggestive of *Streptococcus pneumoniae* (Gram stain, ×1000); (**f**) Spherical gram-positive cocci in groups and short chains suggestive of *Staphylococcus* species (Gram stain, ×1000); (**g**) Microsporidial spores stained gram-positive (Gram stain, ×1000); (**h**) Budding yeast cells stained gram-positive (Gram stain, ×1000); (**i**) Gram-positive, thin, branching, beaded filaments suggestive of actinomycetes (Gram stain, ×1000); (**j**) Thin branching acid-fast filaments confirmatory of *Nocardia* species (Kinyoun stain, ×1000); (**k**) Poorly stained/unstained, beaded, gram-positive bacilli of *Mycobacterium species* (Gram stain, ×1000); (**l**) Slender acid-fast bacilli confirmatory of *Mycobacterium species*; (**m**) Aseptate, broad, branching filaments with ribbon-like folds suggestive of *Pythium species* (Gomori methenamine silver stain, ×400); (**n**) Broad, aseptate, branching filaments suggestive of *Pythium species* (Gram stain, ×1000)

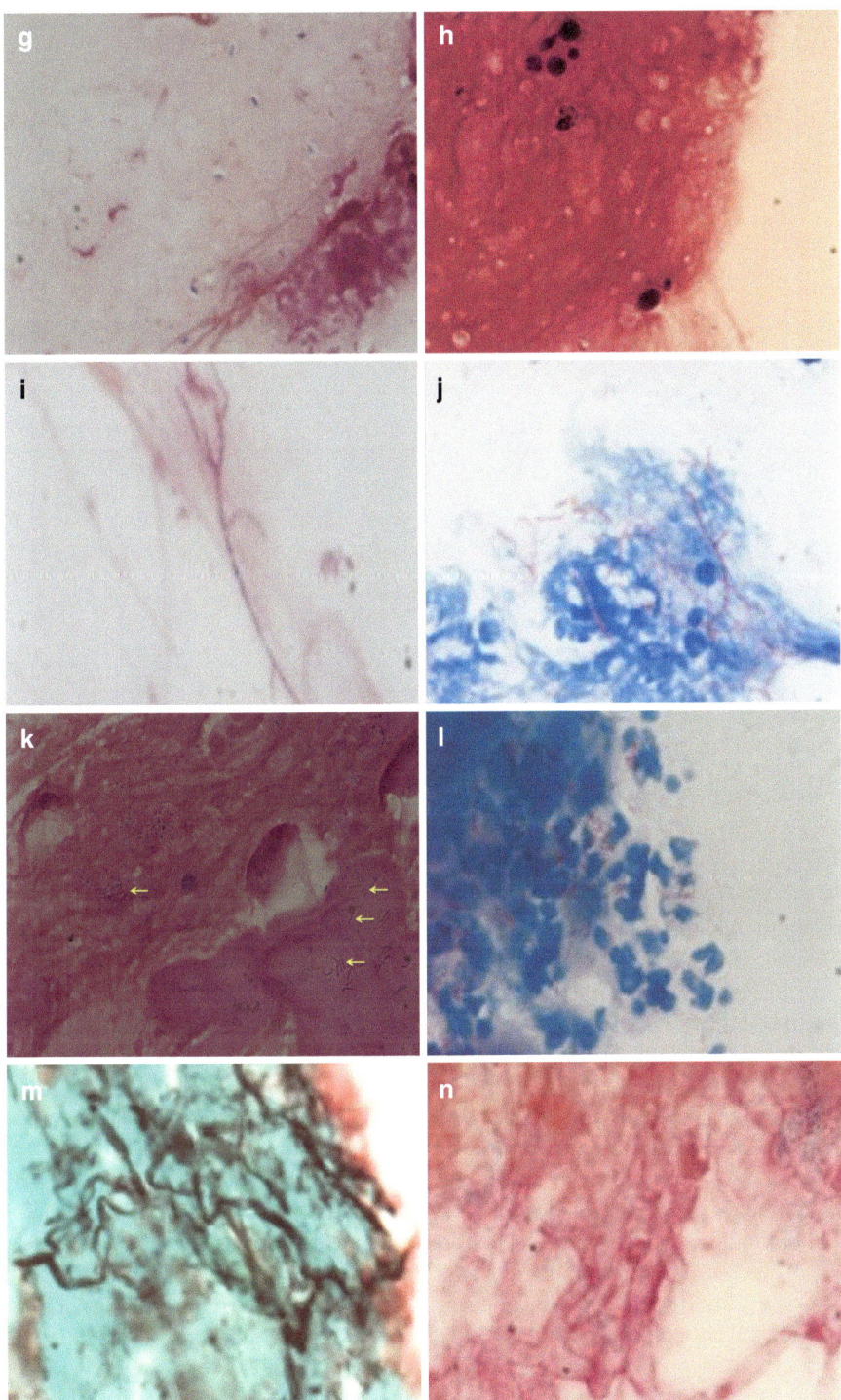

Fig. 15.2 (continued)

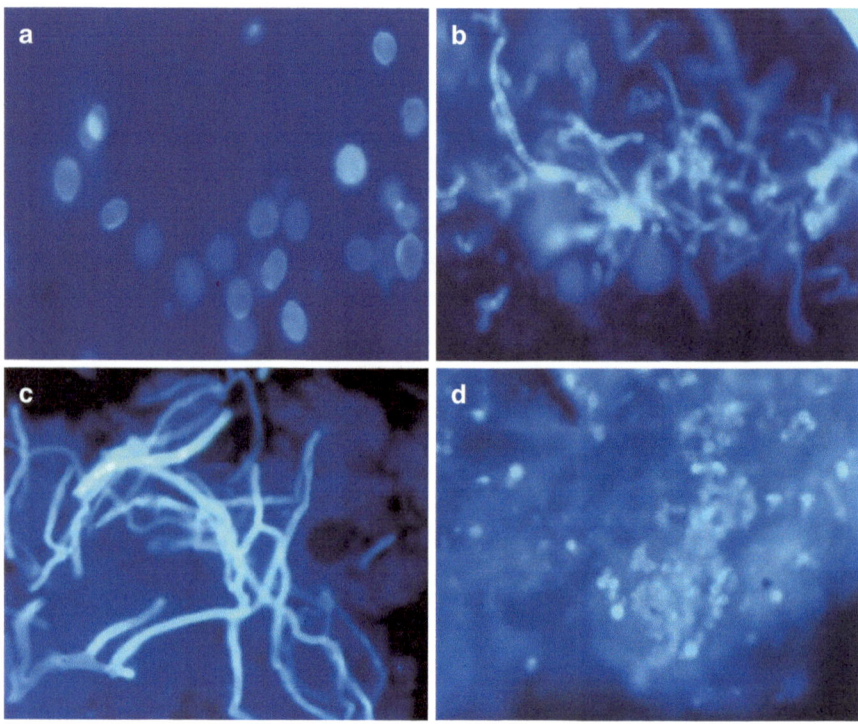

Fig. 15.3 Corneal scrapings stained with potassium hydroxide and calcofluor white (KOH + CFW) and observed under fluorescence microscope (total magnification ×400) showing: (**a**) *Acanthamoeba* cysts with characteristic hexagonal shape and double cyst wall; (**b**) septate, fungal filaments; (**c**) aseptate fungal filaments suggestive of *Pythium species*; and (**d**) round budding yeast cells

stain. Intranuclear inclusions are more efficiently seen in Papanicolaou stain than Giemsa stained smears; however, Giemsa stain is good for differentiating cell types. These staining techniques are rapid and inexpensive; however, they are often non-specific and have low sensitivity in the diagnosis of viral infections.

Specific cytology techniques used for viral diagnosis are techniques that indirectly suggest the presence of viral antigen in the clinical sample. Detection of cell associated viral antigen in a corneal scraping or conjunctival scraping is very useful in the diagnosis of viral infection. Corneal scraping should be made into a smear on glass slide and fixed in cold acetone (4 °C) prior to immunofluorescence assay. The commonly used assays constitute direct and indirect immunofluorescence and indirect immunoperoxidase assays for the diagnosis of HSV, VZV keratitis, and adenoviral keratoconjunctivitis. Figure 15.4 shows apple green fluorescence in the corneal cells positive for HSV 1 antigen by indirect immunofluorescence assay. These tests are rapid, specific, and sensitive, especially when suitable monoclonal or purified polyclonal antibodies are used. Relatively higher sensitivity and lower specificity is achieved with purified polyclonal antibody tests while monoclonal antibodies show high specificity but lower sensitivity. Indirect immunoperoxidase (IP) assay has

Fig. 15.4 Corneal scraping under fluorescence microscopy showing apple green fluorescence suggestive of presence of herpes simplex virus-1 antigen in the epithelial cells (indirect immunofluorescence assay). *Reagents*: Polyclonal rabbit antibody anti-herpes simplex virus type 1, and polyclonal swine anti-rabbit immunoglobulin conjugated with fluorescein isothiocyanate (FITC)

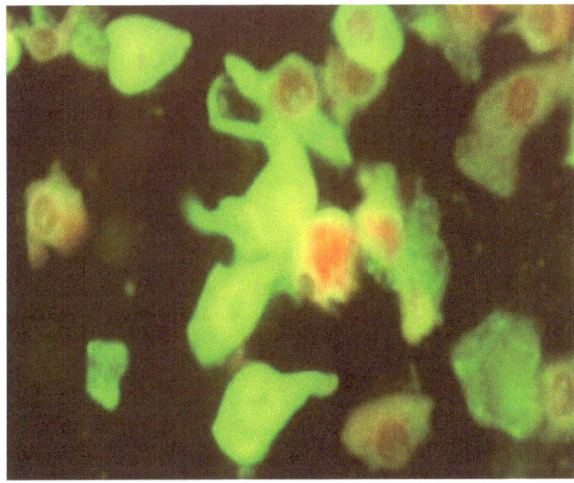

Table 15.4 Culture media for the diagnosis of conjunctivitis/nonviral keratitis

Media	(1) Blood agar—aerobic
	(2) Chocolate agar
	(3) Brain heart infusion broth
	(4) Thioglycollate broth
	(5) Robertson's cooked meat broth
	(6) Non-nutrient agar
	(7) Sabouraud dextrose agar
Optional media	(1) Blood agar—anaerobic
	(2) Potato dextrose agar
	(3) Lowenstein-Jensen medium

distinct advantage over indirect immunofluorescence (IF) assay. The former provides a permanent preparation for records and utilizes an ordinary light microscope for observation while the latter has the inherent problem of quenching (fading) of fluorescence and requires an expensive fluorescence microscope. While the IF technique provides better results with frozen tissue sections IP technique can be done on paraffin embedded tissue sections.

15.5 Culture of Bacteria, Fungi, and Parasites (*Acanthamoeba*)

We recommend a common procedure for the culture of bacteria, fungi, and *Acanthamoeba* from corneal scrapings, for the clinical features of nonviral keratitis caused by these organisms could overlap. Different media that could be used for culture of common organisms from the corneal and conjunctival samples along with the incubation temperature and period required for incubation are given in Table 15.4. Culture of viruses requires cell lines and a separate protocol as shown in Table 15.5.

Table 15.5 Methods of transportation of specimens to the virology laboratory for investigation of viral conjunctivitis/keratitis

(A) Corneal scrapings
(1) Smear on glass slide, air dry, and send for staining/IF/IP
(2) Transfer in a vial (0.5–1 ml) of viral transport medium (VTM) and send for culture. It can be stored at 4 °C without freezing
(3) Transfer on a cellulose acetate membrane, air dry, fix in acetone/methanol, and send for staining/IF/IP
(4) Transfer in 1 ml of PBS/MEM/HBSS and send for PCR
(B) Corneal impression smear on glass slide or cellulose acetate membrane, air dry, fix in acetone/methanol/15 min, and send for staining/IF/IP
(C) Corneal/conjunctival swab
(1) Use dacron/cotton swab to collect material and transfer in VTM and send for culture. It can be stored at 4 °C without freezing
(D) Corneal button
(1) Place in VTM and send for culture
(2) Place in 10% buffered formalin and send for histopathology
(3) Place in PBS/MEM/HBSS and send for PCR

The number and type of media may be chosen as per the availability of the samples and clinical suspicion. However, we recommend use of media that would allow growth of bacteria, fungi, and *Acanthamoeba* in all clinically determined nonviral keratitis. For the investigation of conjunctivitis one could restrict to media for bacteria and fungi. All media are incubated aerobically at 37 °C except Sabouraud dextrose agar and potato dextrose agar that require 25–27 °C (BOD incubator). Chocolate agar is incubated in 3–5% CO_2 in a candle jar or CO_2 incubator. Owing to presence of oxygen reducing agents anaerobic organisms can be grown in thioglycollate broth and Robertson's cooked meat medium incubated aerobically in conventional bacteriological incubator. To grow anaerobes on blood agar it needs to be incubated in anaerobic chamber or anaerobic jar with gas pack.

All media are incubated for minimum of 1 week (can be extended to 2 weeks) and examined daily for growth. Bacteria such as *Nocardia* species, atypical mycobacteria, and *Acanthamoeba* grow slowly and require prolonged incubation. Although most fungi associated with eye infections are saprophytes and grow within a week, they may require incubation for 2–3 weeks for proper sporulation and identification. It is advisable to extend the incubation period for fungus or *Acanthamoeba* in presence of suggestive clinical features or detection of the organisms in direct microscopy.

Size, color, texture, consistency, and number of colonies on the inoculation marks on solid media are recorded. An approximate semiquantitative growth estimation may be recorded as one plus (<10 colonies), two plus (10–20 colonies), and three plus or confluent (>20 colonies) growth. While bacterial and fungal colonies are examined with unaided eyes, handheld magnifying lens may be used to observe small colonies. Observation of *Acanthamoeba* growth, on the other hand, requires use of light microscope. We prefer to place the non-nutrient agar plates (with lid on) under 4× or 10× objective lens of the microscope to avoid contamination due to repeated opening of plate. The refractile, irregular structures of trophozoites with acanthopodia appear in the vicinity of the corneal scraping inoculation mark on the surface of the medium. One may be able to see the characteristic track marks made by the migration of the trophozoites on the *E.coli* lawn. Normally a trophozoite can be seen at the end of each track. With passing time the trophozoites are seen to convert into cysts. Unlike bacteria and fungi no colonies are formed by *Acanthamoeba* that are visible to unaided eye.

Production of turbidity indicates growth in liquid medium that need to be subcultured (transfer with loop on to a solid medium) and Gram stained for identification. Since it is common for culture media that are made in the laboratory to get contaminated, utmost quality control in the form of prior incubation and batch testing with known standard strains are required. In addition, it is helpful to follow certain guidelines to determine the significance of growth on culture media from conjunctival and corneal samples.

The growth of bacteria or fungus in culture is considered significant if the growth is more than 10 colonies (++) or confluent on the site of inoculation on solid media (Fig. 15.5b), or the organism was seen in direct microscopy (Fig. 15.5a), or if the same organism is grown in more than one medium.

Fig. 15.5 (**a**) Gram stain of corneal scraping showing slender gram-negative bacilli suggestive of *Pseudomonas* species and (**b**) Confluent growth of *Pseudomonas aeruginosa* on chocolate agar (37 °C, 48 h)

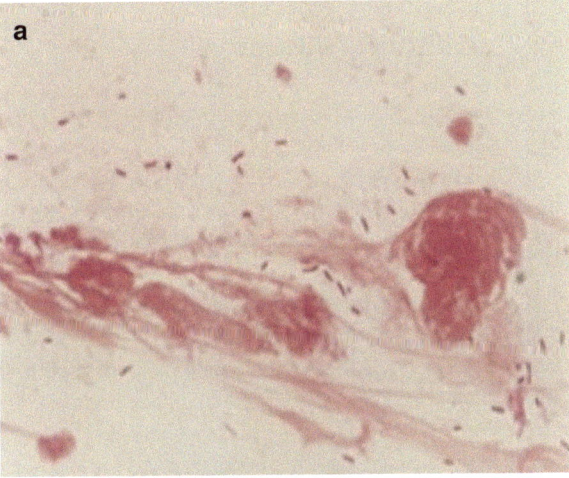

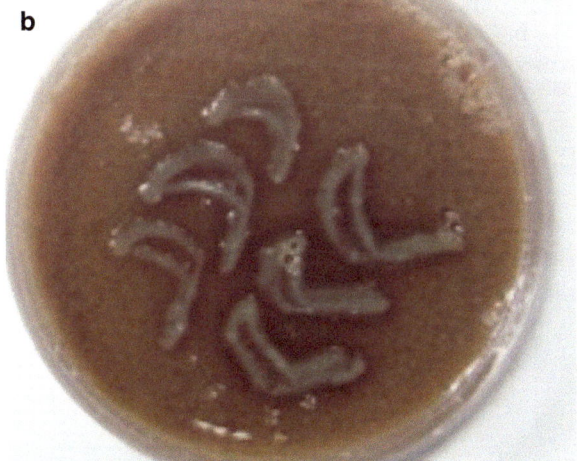

15.6 Identification of Bacteria and Fungi

Standard microbiological procedures are adequate to establish the genus and species of the bacterial or fungal isolates from corneal and conjunctival samples. Most microbiology laboratories follow conventional biochemical tests. However, these are now being replaced with modern automated systems such as Vitek 2 compact system, matrix-assisted laser desorption ionization-time of flight mass spectrometry (MALDI-ToF-MS) for the identification of bacteria and yeast. Generally, a combination of conventional and automated methods may be needed. Filamentous fungi continue to be identified on the basis of colony characteristics and microscopic features. Several websites such as "doctor fungus," "mycology online," and Atlas of Clinical Fungi are helpful in morphological identification, apart from standard textbooks. Role of DNA sequencing of conserved genes in the identification of organisms is fast catching up in many laboratories and has become routine in some. Special tests may be required for identification of some species (zoospore formation by *Pythium insidiosum*) [36].

15.7 Culture of Viruses

Currently, isolation of viruses is not considered a preferred method for the diagnosis of viral infections, for the expense, expertise, and time that it entails. The sample for viral culture needs to be collected in an appropriate transport medium and sent to the laboratory while kept in ice pack. Methods of transport would vary according to the type of sample collected. Hank's balanced salt solution or 2 Sucrose Phosphate broth may be used [35].

Classically described techniques of virus isolation of embryonated eggs and animal inoculation are no more favored by most virology laboratories for routine diagnosis of viral infections. Immortal cell lines such as HeLa, Vero, HEp 2, MRC-5, and human corneal epithelial cell line have been used for isolation of herpes simplex virus from corneal scrapings [37].

Viral growth in cell lines is determined either by characteristic cellular changes, i.e., cytopathic effect (CPE) or by IF or IP techniques, which detect viral antigens in the infected cell lines. Initiation of CPE may take several days but antigens can be detected even before CPE occurs, thereby rendering the latter a more rapid method. For rapid detection of virus antigens in cultured cells the often used technique is that of shell vial technique. It is a modification of conventional tissue culture technique wherein entry of virus into the monolayer of susceptible cells (on a cover slip in a vial) is facilitated by centrifugation (spin amplification) of the vial containing cells and the clinical sample. The virus growth occurs in a shorter period (18–72 h) by this method and additionally, both IF and IP techniques can be performed easily on the cover slips retrieved from the vials for antigen detection.

Serologic tests for herpes simplex virus neutralizing antibody or complement-fixing immunoglobulins may show a rising antibody titer during primary viral infection but have no value in recurrent infection. Since majority of the adult population is latently infected with herpes simplex virus, serological test is useful only when negative to rule out an infection.

15.8   Antibiotic Susceptibility Testing

In most laboratories the antimicrobial susceptibility testing of bacterial isolates is done by Kirby Bauer disc diffusion method, a qualitative assay, using CLSI (Clinical and Laboratory Standards Institute) guidelines [38]. CLSI (earlier known as NCCLS-National Committee for Clinical Laboratory Standards) is an US-based international, interdisciplinary, nonprofit, nongovernmental organization approved by FDA-USA and recommended by the world health organization (WHO). Bacterial isolates to be tested for susceptibility are made into a standard suspension and a lawn culture is made usually on Mueller Hinton agar over which commercially available antibiotic discs are placed followed by incubation. The drug diffuses radially in the medium producing a circular zone of inhibition if the organism is susceptible and smaller/no zone if resistant (Fig. 15.6b). Quality control includes standardization of the bacterial suspension, adequate thickness of the medium, appropriate incubation conditions, and accurate measurement of the zone of inhibition. The size of the zone of inhibition obtained is interpreted by referring to standard zone diameter interpretative chart that labels an organism as either susceptible, intermediate, or resistant to the antibiotics based on clinical breakpoints. The European equivalent organisation is EUCAST (European Committee for Antimicrobial Susceptibility Testing) which sets breakpoints for European Medicines Agency. Apart from clinical breakpoints for the interpretation of

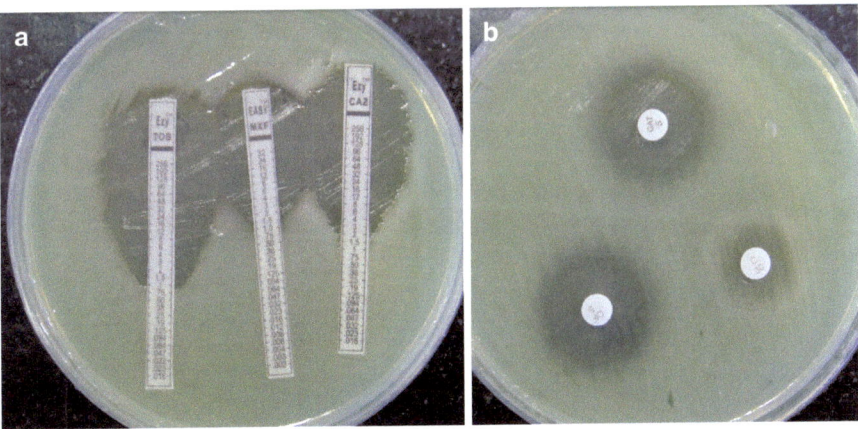

Fig. 15.6 Antibiotic susceptibility testing of *Pseudomonas aeruginosa* on Mueller Hinton agar by (**a**) E test showing elliptical zone of inhibition against the strip of antibiotic containing different concentrations of antibiotic along the strip and by (**b**) disc diffusion method showing zone of inhibition around the antibiotic discs

susceptibility tests it also provides epidemiological cutoffs for newer antibiotics. Although some differences exist between them both CLSI and EUCAST guidelines are acceptable across the world. Periodic attempts are made by the committees to harmonize the two systems. While the documents of CLSI guidelines come with a cost the EUCAST guidelines are free of cost on the website. Since the antibiotic disc content used in disc diffusion assays is based on serum level of the drug achievable by standard systemic therapy and does not represent the ocular levels of antibiotics, measurement of minimum inhibitory concentration (MIC) of the drug is considered a better parameter. Also, an infection caused by an organism resistant to an antibiotic by the test may respond to the drug for the reason that higher concentration of antibiotic can be delivered directly at the site of infection in the eye unlike systemic treatment.

MIC of a drug can be determined by several methods, Vitek 2 compact system being commonly used. Currently, many laboratories also use E test to determine MIC of drugs against bacteria and yeast [39, 40]. Earlier known as Epsilometer test, E test is a manual *in vitro* quantitative test to measure MIC of drugs with the ease of performing disc diffusion test. It employs a ready to use (commercially available from bioMerieux, France) plastic strip containing predefined gradient of an antibiotic. The strip is applied to the surface of an agar plate inoculated with the standard suspension of a test strain and the plate is incubated. The duration and temperature of incubation are predetermined based on the intrinsic growth characteristics of the organism. The MIC value is read from the scale in terms of µg/mL where the ellipse edge intersects the strip (Fig. 15.6a).

Certain drugs such as ceftazidime, vancomycin, piperacillin-tazobactam, colistin, and imipenem require MIC testing for confirmation of resistance indicated on the basis of Kirby Bauer disc diffusion assay. CLSI based broth microdilution method is used for testing susceptibility of filamentous fungi to antifungal drugs [41]. Although CLSI guidelines are available for testing MIC of yeast [42], aerobic actinomycetes (Mycobacteria, *Nocardia*) [43], and filamentous fungi [41], breakpoints for interpretation of the results are not available for all ocular fungi and actinomycetes. The testing methodology and guidelines are evolving concurrently with the increasing understanding of antifungal therapy for eye infections. Antifungal susceptibility testing is performed by very few laboratories and remains in the realm of research rather than routine owing to difficulty in testing and interpretation. Moreover, the panel of antifungal drugs available for therapy of ocular infections is too small to justify routine testing.

15.9   Molecular Methods

Microbiological tests for the diagnosis of infectious diseases have taken a leap in sensitivity and specificity by virtue of molecular techniques. These techniques basically detect the DNA of the organisms in clinical samples. They can also be used for detection of RNA. Presently they are the most sought after techniques for the detection of organisms that are difficult or expensive to culture or are unculturable. They seem to be ideal for the diagnosis of viral infections for precisely these reasons. Apart from viral infections they have a big role to play in the diagnosis of corneal or conjunctival infections caused by Microsporidia, *Acanthamoeba*, *Propionibacterium acnes*, atypical mycobacteria, *Chlamydia trachomatis*, etc. Apart from detection of microbial DNA or RNA for diagnosis, these methods are extremely useful in the identification of organisms by DNA sequencing, a methodology that has opened up doors for recognition of heretofore unknown organisms. The commonly used methods include polymerase chain reaction (PCR) and real-time PCR that are briefly described below. Role of next generation sequencing (targeted or unbiased) of microbial DNA and RNA has added a greater dimension to the understanding of infectious diseases.

15.9.1 Polymerase Chain Reaction

Polymerase chain reaction (PCR) is capable of amplifying DNA of organisms that may or may not be viable. Therefore, samples from patients treated with antibiotics can also be used for the detection of DNA of the organisms. Primers are designed to either help detect a particular organism or a group of organisms. Primers specific for a targeted organism have an overall limited value, however, are useful when clinical features point at specific organism such as *Mycobacterium tuberculosis*, herpes simplex virus, cytomegalovirus, and herpes zoster virus.

Panbacterial, universal, or eubacterial PCR targets conserved region of 16S rRNA gene and can be used for the diagnosis of bacterial keratitis. The detection limit by nested PCR can be as low as one organism. A multiplex PCR with gram-negative and gram-positive specific primers has also been described [44]. Several studies have reported application of panfungal PCR in the diagnosis of infectious keratitis. Primers based on 18S rRNA, ITS, or 28S rRNA genes have been used [45–47]. These PCR tests are reported to be highly specific and sensitive to the detection level of 1 fg of fungal DNA.

Generally, a second step is required to identify the species of bacteria or fungus following panbacterial and panfungal PCRs. Methods such as sequencing of the amplified DNA or hybridization with specific probes can be used. Sequence of the amplified DNA is compared with similar sequences in databases using BLASTn program of the National Centre for Biotechnology Information (NCBI, GenBank database). A score of 97% and similarity of 98% allows the genus recognition and a score of 99% or more may assign a species name. Phylogenetic analysis further confirms the species in relation to known sequences available in the database. It allows comparison with type strains available.

Hybridization technique constitutes transfer of amplified DNA on a membrane (dot blot assay), to which are added labeled (radioactive isotopes, fluorophores, haptens like biotin or digoxigenin or an enzyme) specific probes. The probes are usually a short strand of oligonucleotide specific for hybridization with complementary sequence of either one or a group of organisms. In DNA chip technology, complementary sequences to signature genes of specific organisms or groups of organisms are dotted on the chip, to which is added multiplex PCR amplified biotin labeled denatured DNA (of the sample) that would hybridize to complementary DNA on the chip. In the next step enzyme labeled streptavidin would reveal the specific gene by color development on addition of the substrate [48].

Bacterial and fungal genome can be differentiated by their genetic fingerprint produced by use of restriction enzymes on the amplicons using PCR based Restriction Fragment Length Polymorphism (PCR-RFLP). The number of fragments is proportionate to the number of restriction sites in the genome and is specific for particular species [49]. With the availability of commercial agencies that help in sequencing at a reasonable cost, DNA sequencing is preferred over RFLP and hybridization techniques by most microbiologists. DNA sequencing and phylogenetic analysis allows recognition of unknown organisms [36].

In recent times, next generation sequencing (NGS) is evolving as a technology for precise identification of organisms. Unbiased metagenomic deep RNA sequencing has been applied to identify pathogens causing conjunctivitis [50].

Application of real-time qualitative or quantitative PCR in the diagnosis of infectious keratitis is increasing by the day. Quantitative PCR (qPCR) determines the amount of absolute or relative DNA in the sample. Real-time PCR requires a special thermocycler that measures fluorescence, which is produced in proportion to the amplification of the DNA, cycle by cycle. Commercial kits (herpes simplex virus, herpes zoster virus, cytomegalovirus, *Mycobacterium tuberculosis,* etc.) are available for diagnostic application of this technique. Being quantitative this test has a potential prognostic value to determine therapeutic response. Automated real-time PCR has been employed for rapid diagnosis of adenoviral keratoconjunctivitis [51]. Assessment of prevalence and clinical outcome of HSV type-1 [52], and quantitation in tear fluid and aqueous humor has been done using real-time PCR [53]. Several studies have shown the wide application of this test in the understanding of HSV keratitis such as detection of large number of HSV DNA copies in herpetic epithelial keratitis compared to stromal keratitis [54], and detection of HSV DNA in tears and saliva of 98% of tested asymptomatic individuals [55]. This technique was useful to demonstrate that Cytomegalovirus (CMV) is an important cause of corneal edema (endotheleitis) [56] and is the method of choice for the diagnosis of CMV endotheleitis [56].

Molecular techniques in the hands of microbiologists are evolving rapidly and are majorly impacting the understanding of infectious diseases of the eye. NGS of ocular samples has not only shown that healthy conjunctiva harbors many more genera of fungi than can be deciphered using culture techniques, but it has also unraveled dysbiosis in the fungal microbiome of conjunctiva and cornea in patients with fungal keratitis [57, 58]. Studies from L V Prasad Eye Institute, India have reported alterations in bacterial and fungal gut microbiome in patients with bacterial and fungal keratitis using NGS technology with far-reaching implications of possible role of probiotics in the control of these infections [59, 60]. More work in this direction is obviously warranted to understand the significance of the findings.

15.10 Conclusion

Accurate diagnosis of infectious diseases of the conjunctiva and cornea requires a well-equipped microbiology laboratory and well-trained staff. While conventional methods of microscopy and culture of clinical samples remain the gold standard enormous progress has been made with application of molecular methods in the diagnosis, which should be utilized when feasible along with appropriate interpretations that are clinically relevant.

References

1. Stenson S, Newman R, Fedukowicz H. Laboratory studies in acute conjunctivitis. Arch Ophthalmol. 1982;100(8):1275–7.
2. Rönnerstam R, Persson K, Hansson H, Renmarker K. Prevalence of chlamydial eye infection in patients attending an eye clinic, a VD clinic, and in healthy persons. Br J Ophthalmol. 1985;69(5):385–8.
3. Uchio E, Takeuchi S, Itoh N, Matsuura N, Ohno S, Aoki K. Clinical and epidemiological features of acute follicular conjunctivitis with special reference to that caused by herpes simplex virus type 1. Br J Ophthalmol. 2000;84(9):968–72.
4. Fitch CP, Rapoza PA, Owens S, Murillo-Lopez F, Johnson RA, Quinn TC, Pepose JS, Taylor HR. Epidemiology and diagnosis of acute conjunctivitis at an inner-city hospital. Ophthalmology. 1989;96(8):1215–20.
5. O'Brien TP, Jeng BH, McDonald M, Raizman MB. Acute conjunctivitis: truth and misconceptions. Curr Med Res Opin. 2009;25(8):1953–61.
6. Akçaya E, Çarhanb A, Hondurc G, Tufand ZK, Durue N, Kılıçf S, Ensaria EN, Uğurlua N, Çağıla N. Molecular identification of viral agents associated with acute conjunctivitis: a prospective controlled study. Braz J Infect Dis. 2017;21(4):391–5.
7. Koch A, Krönert C, Lotti T, Vojvodic A, Wollina U. Adult measles—case reports of a highly contagious disease. Open Access Maced J Med Sci. 2019;7(18):3009–12.
8. Crespillo-Andújar C, Díaz-Menéndez M, Trigo E, Arsuaga M, de la Calle F, Lago M, de Guevara MCL, Barreiro P, Montero D, Garcia-Bujalance S, Alvarado EA, de la Calle M, Sánchez-Seco MP, de Ory F, Vazquez A, Arribas JR, La Paz-Carlos III, Hospital Multidisciplinary Working Group on Zika Virus Disease. Characteristics of Zika virus infection among international travelers: a prospective study from a Spanish referral unit. Travel Med Infect Dis. 2020;33:101543.
9. Das S, Sharma S, Sahu SK, Nayak SS, Kar S. New microbial spectrum of epidemic keratoconjunctivitis: clinical and laboratory aspects of an outbreak. Br J Ophthalmol. 2008;92(6):861–2.
10. Sakla AA, Donnelly JJ, Lok JB, Khatami M, Rockey JH. Punctate keratitis induced by subconjunctivally injected microfilariae of Onchocerca lienalis. Arch Ophthalmol. 1986;104(6):894–8.
11. Aasuri MK, Reddy MK, Sharma S, Rao GN. Co-occurrence of pneumococcal keratitis and dacryocystitis. Cornea. 1999;18(3):273–6.
12. O'Brien TP. Bacterial keratitis, Chapter 94. In: Krachmer JH, Mannis MJ, Holland EJ, editors. Cornea: cornea and external diseases, clinical diagnosis and management. St. Louis: Mosby; 1997. p. 1139–89.
13. McClellan KA, Bernard PJ, Billson FA. Microbial investigations in keratitis at the Sydney Eye Hospital. Aust N Z J Ophthalmol. 1989;17(4):413–6.
14. Sharma S, Kunimoto DY, Garg P, Rao GN. Trends in antibiotic resistance of corneal pathogens: Part I. An analysis of commonly used ocular antibiotics. Indian J Ophthalmol. 1999;47(2):95–100.
15. Adams CP Jr, Cohen EJ, Laibson PR, Galentine P, Arentsen JJ. Corneal ulcers in patients with cosmetic extended-wear contact lenses. Am J Ophthalmol. 1983;96(6):705–9.

16. Rubinfeld RS, Cohen EJ, Arentsen JJ, Laibson PR. Diphtheroids as ocular pathogens. Am J Ophthalmol. 1989;108(3):251–4.
17. Jones DB, Robinson NM. Anaerobic ocular infections. Trans Sect Ophthalmol Am Acad Ophthalmol Otolaryngol. 1977;83(2):309–31.
18. Vanbijsterveld OP, Richards RD. Bacillus infections of the cornea. Arch Ophthalmol. 1965;74:91–5.
19. Choudhuri KK, Sharma S, Garg P, Rao GN. Clinical and microbiological profile of Bacillus keratitis. Cornea. 2000;19(3):301–6.
20. Zaidman GW, Coudron P, Piros J. Listeria monocytogenes keratitis. Am J Ophthalmol. 1990;109(3):334–9.
21. Lass JH, Haaf J, Foster CS, Belcher C. Visual outcome in eight cases of Serratia marcescens keratitis. Am J Ophthalmol. 1981;92(3):384–90.
22. Perry HD, Nauheim JS, Donnenfeld ED. Nocardia asteroides keratitis presenting as a persistent epithelial defect. Cornea. 1989;8(1):41–4.
23. Turner L, Stinson I. Mycobacterium fortuitum; as a cause of corneal ulcer. Am J Ophthalmol. 1965;60:329–31.
24. Szerenyi K, McDonnell JM, Smith RE, Irvine JA, McDonnell PJ. Keratitis as a complication of bilateral, simultaneous radial keratotomy. Am J Ophthalmol. 1994;117(4):462–7.
25. Baum J, Barza M, Weinstein P, Groden J, Aswad M. Bilateral keratitis as a manifestation of Lyme disease. Am J Ophthalmol. 1988;105(1):75–7.
26. Wilhelmus KR, Coster DJ, Donovan HC, Falcon MG, Jones BR. Prognostic indicators of herpetic keratitis. Analysis of a five-year observation period after corneal ulceration. Arch Ophthalmol. 1981;99(9):1578–82.
27. Davamani F, Gananaselvan J, Anandakannank SN, Sundararaj T. Studies of the prevalence of acanthamoeba keratitis in and around Chennai. Indian J Med Microbiol. 1998;16(4):152–3.
28. Sharma S, Garg P, Rao GN. Patient characteristics, diagnosis, and treatment of non-contact lens related Acanthamoeba keratitis. Br J Ophthalmol. 2000;84(10):1103–8.
29. Høvding G. Acute bacterial conjunctivitis. Acta Ophthalmol. 2008;86(1):5–17.
30. Azari AA, Barney NP. Conjunctivitis: a systematic review of diagnosis and treatment. JAMA. 2013;310(16):1721–9.
31. Sambursky R, Tauber S, Schirra F, Kozich K, Davidson R, Cohen EJ. The RPS adeno detector for diagnosing adenoviral conjunctivitis. Ophthalmology. 2006;113(10):1758–64.
32. Inoue Y, Shimomura Y, Fukuda M, Miyazaki D, Ohashi Y, Sasaki H, Tagawa Y, Shiota H, Inada N, Okamoto S, Araki-Sasaki K, Kimura T, Hatano H, Nakagawa H, Nakamura S, Hirahara A, Tanaka K, Sakuma H. Multicentre clinical study of the herpes simplex virus immunochromatographic assay kit for the diagnosis of herpetic epithelial keratitis. Br J Ophthalmol. 2013;97(9):1108–12.
33. Pakzad-Vaezi K, Levasseur SD, Schendel S, Mark S, Mathias R, Roscoe D, Holland SP. The corneal ulcer one-touch study: a simplified microbiological specimen collection method. Am J Ophthalmol. 2015;159(1):37–43.
34. McLeod SD, Kumar A, Cevallos V, Srinivasan M, Whitcher JP. Reliability of transport medium in the laboratory evaluation of corneal ulcers. Am J Ophthalmol. 2005;140(6):1027–31.
35. Sharma S, Sreedharan A. Diagnostic procedures in infectious keratitis, Chapter 08. In: Nema HV, Nema N, editors. Diagnostic procedures in ophthalmology. New Delhi: Jaypee Brothers Medical Publishers (P) Ltd; 2009. p. 316–32.
36. Sharma S, Balne PK, Motukupally SR, Das S, Garg P, Sahu SK, Arunasri K, Manjulatha K, Mishra DK, Shivaji S. Pythium insidiosum keratitis: clinical profile and role of DNA sequencing and zoospore formation in diagnosis. Cornea. 2015;34(4):438–42.
37. Araki-Sasaki K, Ohashi Y, Sasabe T, Hayashi K, Watanabe H, Tano Y, Handa H. An SV40-immortalized human corneal epithelial cell line and its characterization. Invest Ophthalmol Vis Sci. 1995;36(3):614–21.
38. Weinstein MP, Patel JB, Bobenchik AM, Campeau S, Cullen SK, Galas MF, Gold H, Humphries RM, Lewis JS II, Limbago B, Mathers AJ, Mazzulli T, Richter SS, Satlin M,

Schuetz AN, Swenson JM, Tamma PD. Performance standards for antimicrobial susceptibility testing. M100. 28th ed. Wayne, PA: Clinical and Laboratory Standards Institute; 2019.

39. Reddy AK, Reddy RR, Paruvelli MR, Ambatipudi S, Rani A, Lodhi SAK, Reddy JML, Reddy KR, Pandey N, Videkar R, Sinha MK, Majji AB, Deb-Jorder N, Sahu AK, Myneni J, Abraham A. Susceptibility of bacterial isolates to vancomycin and ceftazidime from patients with endophthalmitis: is there a need to change the empirical therapy in suspected bacterial endophthalmitis? Int Ophthalmol. 2015;35(1):37–42.

40. Motukupally SR, Nanapur VR, Chathoth KN, Murthy SI, Pappuru R, Mallick A, Sharma S. Ocular infections caused by Candida species: type of species, in vitro susceptibility and treatment outcome. Indian J Med Microbiol. 2015;33(4):538–46.

41. Rex JH, Alexander BD, Andes D, Arthington-Skaggs B, Brown SD, Chaturvedi V, Espinel-Ingroff A, Ghannoum MA, Motyl MR, Ostrosky-Zeichner L, Pfaller MA, Sheehan DJ, Walsh TJ. Reference method for broth dilution antifungal susceptibility testing of filamentous fungi. M38-A2, 28(16). Wayne, PA: Clinical and Laboratory Standards Institute; 2008.

42. Rex JH, Alexander BD, Andes D, Arthington-Skaggs B, Brown SD, Chaturvedi V, Ghannoum MA, Espinel-Ingroff A, Knapp CC, Ostrosky-Zeichner L, Pfaller MA, Sheehan DJ, Walsh TJ. Reference method for broth dilution antifungal susceptibility testing of yeasts. M27-A3, 28(14). Wayne, PA: Clinical and Laboratory Standards Institute; 2008.

43. Woods GL, Brown-Elliott BA, Conville PS, Desmond EP, Hall GS, Lin G, Pfyffer GE, Ridderhof JC, Siddiqi SH, Wallace RJ Jr, Warren NG, Witebsky FG. Susceptibility testing of mycobacteria, nocardiac, and other aerobic actinomycetes. 2nd ed. Wayne, PA: Clinical and Laboratory Standards Institute; 2011.

44. Carroll NM, Jaeger EE, Choudhury S, Dunlop AA, Matheson MM, Adamson P, Okhravi N, Lightman S. Detection of and discrimination between gram-positive and gram-negative bacteria in intraocular samples by using nested PCR. J Clin Microbiol. 2000;38(5):1753–7.

45. Bagyalakshmi R, Therese KL, Madhavan HN. Application of semi-nested polymerase chain reaction targeting internal transcribed spacer region for rapid detection of panfungal genome directly from ocular specimens. Indian J Ophthalmol. 2007;55(4):261–6.

46. Ghosh A, Basu S, Datta H, Chattopadhyay D. Evaluation of polymerase chain reaction-based ribosomal DNA sequencing technique for the diagnosis of mycotic keratitis. Am J Ophthalmol. 2007;144(3):396–403.

47. Vengayil S, Panda A, Satpathy G, Nayak N, Ghose S, Patanaik D, Khokhar S. Polymerase chain reaction-guided diagnosis of mycotic keratitis: a prospective evaluation of its efficacy and limitations. Invest Ophthalmol Vis Sci. 2009;50(1):152–6.

48. Basu S, Sharma S, Kar S, Das T. DNA chip-assisted diagnosis of a previously unknown etiology of intermediate uveitis-Toxoplasma gondii. Indian J Ophthalmol. 2010;58(6):535–7.

49. Lestin F, Kraak R, Podbielski A. Two cases of keratitis and corneal ulcers caused by Burkholderia gladioli. J Clin Microbiol. 2008;46(7):2445–9.

50. Lalitha P, Seitzman GD, Kotecha R, Hinterwirth A, Chen C, Zhong L, Cummings S, Lebas E, Sahoo MK, Pinsky BA, Lietman TM, Doan T. Unbiased pathogen detection and host gene profiling for conjunctivitis. Ophthalmology. 2019;126(8):1090–4.

51. Koidl C, Bozic M, Mossböck G, Mühlbauer G, Berg J, Stöcher M, Dehnhardt J, Marth E, Kessler HH. Rapid diagnosis of adenoviral keratoconjunctivitis by a fully automated molecular assay. Ophthalmology. 2005;112(9):1521–8.

52. Remeijer L, Duan R, van Dun JM, Wefers Bettink MA, Osterhaus AD, Verjans GM. Prevalence and clinical consequences of herpes simplex virus type 1 DNA in human cornea tissues. J Infect Dis. 2009;200(1):11–9.

53. Fukuda M, Deai T, Higaki S, Hayashi K, Shimomura Y. Presence of a large amount of herpes simplex virus genome in tear fluid of herpetic stromal keratitis and persistent epithelial defect patients. Semin Ophthalmol. 2008;23(4):217–20.

54. Kakimaru-Hasegawa A, Kuo CH, Komatsu N, Komatsu K, Miyazaki D, Inoue Y. Clinical application of real-time polymerase chain reaction for diagnosis of herpetic diseases of the anterior segment of the eye. Jpn J Ophthalmol. 2008;52(1):24–31.

55. Kaufman HE, Azcuy AM, Varnell ED, Sloop GD, Thompson HW, Hill JM. HSV-1 DNA in tears and saliva of normal adults. Invest Ophthalmol Vis Sci. 2005;46(1):241–7.
56. Kandori M, Inoue T, Takamatsu F, Kojima Y, Hori Y, Maeda N, Tano Y. Prevalence and features of keratitis with quantitative polymerase chain reaction positive for cytomegalovirus. Ophthalmology. 2010;117(2):216–22.
57. Prashanthi GS, Jayasudha R, Chakravarthy SK, Padakandla SR, SaiAbhilash CR, Sharma S, Bagga B, Murthy SI, Garg P, Shivaji S. Alterations in the ocular surface fungal microbiome in fungal keratitis patients. Microorganisms. 2019;7(9):E309.
58. Shivaji S, Jayasudha R, Prashanthi GS, Chakravarthy SK, Sharma S. The human ocular surface fungal microbiome. Invest Ophthalmol Vis Sci. 2019;60(1):451–9.
59. Jayasudha R, Chakravarthy SK, Prashanthi GS, Sharma S, Garg P, Murthy SI, Shivaji S. Alterations in gut bacterial and fungal microbiomes are associated with bacterial Keratitis, an inflammatory disease of the human eye. J Biosci. 2018;43(5):835–56.
60. Chakravarthy SK, Jayasudha R, Ranjith K, Dutta A, Pinna NK, Mande SS, Sharma S, Garg P, Murthy SI, Shivaji S. Alterations in the gut bacterial microbiome in fungal Keratitis patients. PLoS One. 2018;13(6):e0199640.

Role of Histopathology in the Diagnosis of Corneal and Conjunctival Infections

Geeta K. Vemuganti, Somasheila I. Murthy, and Dilip K. Mishra

16.1 Introduction

Microbial keratitis is an important cause of ocular morbidity worldwide. While the outcome obviously depends on early diagnosis, prompt and effective treatment, it is also influenced largely by various host and agent factors [1]. Some of the common causes of corneal infections include bacterial, fungal, viral, and protozoan, which can be diagnosed by clinical examination with final confirmation from microbiological demonstration in smears and/or cultures from tissue samples. In advanced cases, surgical procedures such as corneal biopsy, penetrating keratoplasty, or even evisceration of the eye are required either for therapeutic or diagnostic indications. These tissues thus provide an opportunity for the pathologists not only to confirm the etiological diagnosis but also to contribute to the understanding of the disease process. Therefore, histological evaluation and molecular methods aid in diagnosis and improve our understanding of the disease pathogenesis in the cornea and conjunctiva. This chapter provides a brief outline of clinical features and treatment of specific infections with emphasis on histopathology and molecular methods of diagnosis.

G. K. Vemuganti (✉)
School of Medical Sciences, University of Hyderabad, Hyderabad, Telangana, India

S. I. Murthy
Cornea & Anterior Segment Service, The Cornea Institute, L V Prasad Eye Institute, Hyderabad, Telangana, India
e-mail: smurthy@lvpei.org

D. K. Mishra
Ophthalmic Pathology Service, L V Prasad Eye Institute, Hyderabad, Telangana, India
e-mail: dilipkumarmishra@lvpei.org

© Springer Nature Singapore Pte Ltd. 2021
S. Das, V. Jhanji (eds.), *Infections of the Cornea and Conjunctiva*,
https://doi.org/10.1007/978-981-15-8811-2_16

16.2   Handling of Corneal Specimens

The specimens of corneal tissues may be obtained for diagnostic purposes, therapeutic purposes, or both. These include:

- Corneal biopsy
- Keratoplasty specimens: penetrating keratoplasty, lamellar keratoplasty, or graft specimens
- Evisceration: corneal scleral rim and scooped out intraocular contents

The most common fixative used in histopathology is 10% buffered formalin (the commercially available 40% Formaldehyde solution is considered as 100%) which stabilizes the protein, oil, and the carbohydrate [1–4]. "Corneal buttons could also be fixed in a fixative called Perenyi's fluid: (100 ml prepared by mixing of 40 ml of 10% nitric acid, 30 ml each of absolute alcohol and 0.5% chromic acid)".

Corneal button: Gross examination of the corneal button includes size, thickness, surface and margins for irregularities, translucency, perforation, vascularization, thinning, ulceration, or deposits. Endothelial surface is examined for the presence of adherent uveal tissue and formation of exudates or membranes. After placing the corneal tissue on a flat surface with the endothelial surface up, it is bisected into half using a sharp blade. Care must be taken to cut the cornea along the region of scarring, infiltrates, or any pathology identified on gross examination. The other half is retained for future studies while half is submitted for routine processing. In cases of therapeutic keratoplasty, half of the corneal button is submitted for microbiologic studies and the rest of the tissue is processing for histopathologic studies. Embedding of the corneal tissue is similar to skin biopsy or mucosal biopsy, i.e., by edge embedding.

Routine hematoxylin and eosin (H&E) staining along with periodic acid Schiff (PAS) stain is done on all sections. These stains highlight basement membrane, Descemet's membrane (DM), and other structures such as fungal filaments. In addition, special stains such as Grocott-Gomori Methenamine Silver stain (GMS) and Acid Fast (AF) stain, etc., are utilized as per the suspected clinical diagnosis or histologic findings.

While reviewing the corneal tissues that have been embedded like an edge, the appearance of cornea is similar to the features seen on slit lamp examination and changes in the epithelium, Bowman's layer (BL), stroma, DM, and endothelium should all be recorded.

16.3   General Histologic Changes in Corneal Infections

Although the severity and rate of progression differs in different infections, corneal infections typically undergo a cycle of epithelial ulceration, infiltration of the stroma by lymphocytes, plasma cells, and polymorphonuclear (PMN) cells followed by BL destruction, necrosis, and even full-thickness cornea perforation. While acute infections such as fungal and bacterial demonstrate collection of infiltrates in anterior two third of stroma, in chronic infections, changes related to repair such as partial regeneration of the epithelial, stromal edema, new vessel formation, and the accumulation of giant cells along with transformation of stromal keratocytes to myofibroblasts are noted. These changes ultimately lead to remodeling of the stroma and scarring.

16.4 Histopathology of Corneal Infections

16.4.1 Bacterial Keratitis

Epithelial ulceration with destruction of Bowman's and anterior part of the stroma and florid infiltration with PMNs are noted prominently. These PMNs are known to release collagenolytic enzymes as host response against the bacteria, which in turn liberate bacterial endotoxins. In the case of relentless progression, perforation with iris incarceration is noted. Such a response is termed pseudo-cornea. Some of the specimens display the presence of refractile wavy unstained material with scalloping margins on the surface, which corresponds to Cyanoacrylate glue. This is noted best in the scanner view after lowering the condenser. Bacteria on histologic sections are appreciated when present in colonies and with the use of Grams stain (Fig. 16.1a, b). Some of the atypical and rare presentation of bacterial keratitis includes infectious crystalline keratopathy (ICK), mostly seen in grafts or in patients using topical corticosteroid eye drops. In these cases, multiple large colonies of bacteria are noted with little or no stromal inflammation. The local immune compromised state in cornea facilitates the bacteria to flourish in colonies and also develop a protective biofilm. In advanced cases however there could be severe inflammation of the stroma. The term ICK is derived from the clinical appearance

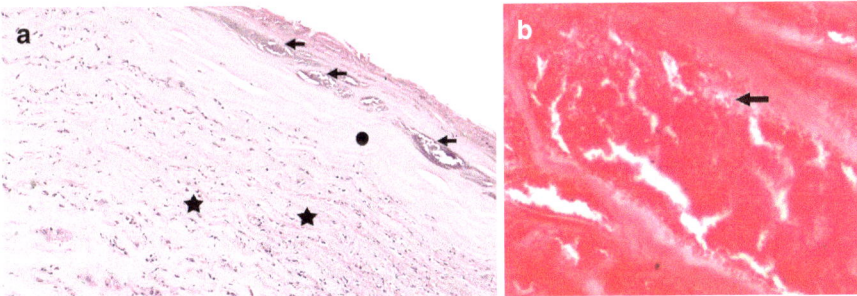

Fig. 16.1 (**a**) A case of bacterial keratitis presenting as infectious crystalline keratopathy which worsened and underwent keratoplasty. The epithelium is ulcerated and the stroma shows multiple bacterial colonies (arrows) with no inflammatory cells whereas mixed inflammatory cells seen away from the bacterial colonies (star) with clear zone of stroma in between (solid circle); (Haematoxylin & Eosin stain, ×200); (**b**) On Gram staining, the colonies are seen as Gram variable bacterial colonies (arrow) in anterior stroma. (Gram's stain, ×1000)

of these colonies which appears as spindle-like or needle-like extensions, hence the term "crystalline." Some of the organisms implicated in ICK are *Streptococcus* sp. and candida.

16.4.2 Fungal Keratitis

Apart from ulceration, edema, and severe inflammation, the location of the fungi and the duration of the disease can change the location of the infiltrates. Early disease has patchy, focal infiltrates restricted to the anterior two thirds of the stroma. Apparently disconnected lesions from the primary focus are often noted, corresponding to the characteristic clinical finding of satellite lesions seen in fungal infections.

With prolonged disease, the infiltrates coalesce and extend both horizontally and vertically into the deeper stroma, similar to the clinical spectrum of advancing disease. There is loss of the tissue architecture and extensive destruction, necrosis, and perforation (Fig. 16.2a). In a few cases, fungal filaments may be seen in close approximation over the DM and also can be noted crossing the intact DM into the anterior chamber. In severe forms where there is extensive tissue destruction, only the DM may be seen corresponding to clinical finding of descemetocele, or there can be fragmented DM with surrounding disorganized cellular architecture (Fig. 16.2b). Atypical presentations include deep lesions with exudates in the anterior chamber and unaffected looking anterior stroma, which could closely mimic a stromal viral keratitis with superadded mycotic keratitis. The clinical significance of this finding is that in such cases, corneal biopsy, unless is deep and targeted to the lesion, may be negative for fungus on histologic examination. In 14% of cases, the findings of granulomatous inflammation as giant cell reaction has been noted [3]. On H&E staining (Fig. 16.3a), fungal filaments are noted as unstained tubular septate structures or in case where they are cut through transverse axis they are present as rounded empty structures with a lumen. Special stains such as PAS and GMS make these prominent (Fig. 16.3b). The hyphae filaments measure up to 10 µm in

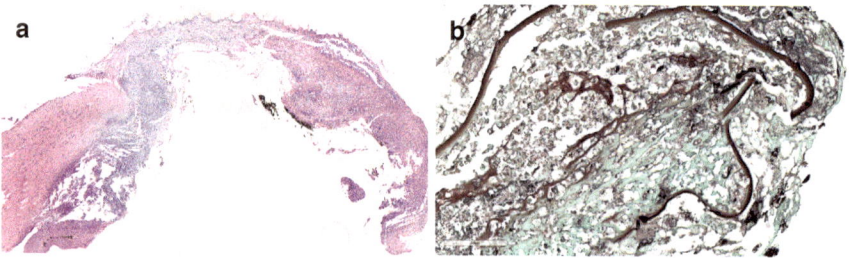

Fig. 16.2 (a) The corneal tissue of fungal keratitis shows total loss of tissue architecture, neutrophilic exudates, necrosis, and perforation (Haematoxylin & Eosin stain, ×100); (b) Fragmented DM within disorganized necrotic tissue and fungal filaments on the DM (GMS, ×400)

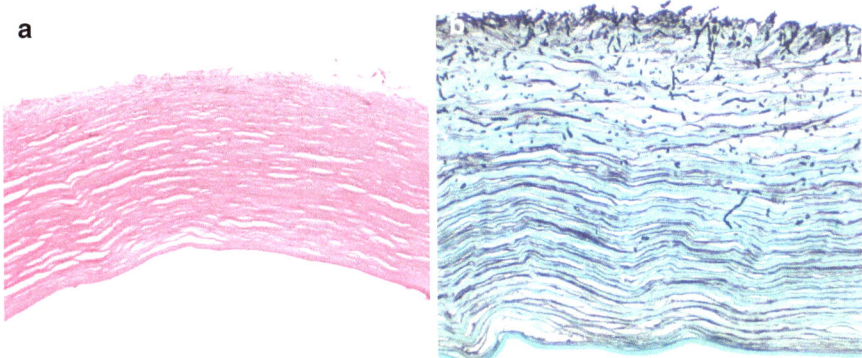

Fig. 16.3 (**a**) Corneal button showing unstained tubular fungal filaments in the anterior to mid stroma fungal filaments are noted as unstained tubular septate structures (Haematoxylin & Eosin stain, ×200); (**b**) The fungal filaments are prominently noted as black stained filamentous structures, or oval in transverse section, noted to penetrate into mid stroma (GMS stain, ×200)

diameter and are of different lengths. Most often these filaments appear short as they are broken or end-on, traversing through the entire cornea and the DM.

The sensitivity of histopathological detection of fungus is about 66%. The reasons for these include lack of intact filaments in the late stages of disease especially as these case receive prolonged medical therapy [3], or due to sampling errors such as the tissue may not be representative of the affected portion of the cornea which was sent for processing. While screening the specimen for fungal filaments, the likelihood of finding these is higher in the areas of the specimen where the inflammation is the least. This negative correlation between inflammation and location of the fungal filaments implies that in vivo the fungus has a higher probability of being located beyond the areas of the visible infiltrates. Dematiaceous fungus is a pigmented fungus which appears as a dry and elevated plaque-like pigmented infiltrate on the cornea [4]. Histopathologically, this appears as a dense carpet-like accumulation of filaments, easily identifiable even on routine stains. There is variable pigmentation and usually minimal tissue disorganization or inflammation.

16.4.3 Viral Keratitis

Herpes simplex virus (HSV) 1, 2 are known to cause keratitis. The clinical manifestations are dendritic ulcer, necrotizing stromal keratitis, immune stromal keratitis, viral endotheliitis, and also keratouveitis [5]. Scarring and vascularization are commonly noted clinically, requiring keratoplasty for visual rehabilitation and these grafts are prone to failure due to rejection. The specimens received in pathology include keratoplasty specimens primarily, and some cases of perforated or severe necrotizing stromal keratitis.

16.4.3.1 Necrotizing Stromal Keratitis (NSK)

Clinically, this is a destructive inflammation, due to host response to invasion by live virus.

Histopathology of NSK

The epithelium may show ulceration. There are neutrophilic infiltrates in stroma based on the severity, can be either diffuse or focal in nature or can also be noted as coalescent abscesses. Some of the features pointing towards a viral etiology (but not pathognomonic) include mononuclear infiltrates, multinucleated giant cells (MNG) inclusion bodies in the epithelial cells and rarely in deep stroma. Due to endothelial cell being affected, often there are folds in the DM and edema. In some cases, we can also note stromal loss and necrosis with descemetocele formation or perforation with giant cell reaction around Descemet's membrane (Fig. 16.4). In other cases, especially chronic or recurrent cases, a prominent feature noted is vascularization progressing towards the site of active inflammation. The antigen has been isolated from epithelial cells, keratocytes (less often), in the MNGs and the endothelial cells. Electron microscopy can detect intact viruses.

16.4.3.2 Immune Stromal Keratitis (ISK)

Recurrence of infection is the hallmark of immune keratitis, occurring in 20% of population with ocular Herpes. Primarily it is believed to be immune mediated. However, direct invasion and active replication of virus has also been implicated [6].

Histopathology of ISK

In contrast to NCK, the epithelium is intact. Stroma shows edema and mixed inflammatory infiltrates, which could be focal, multifocal, or diffuse. Rapid neovascularization with arborizing branches either patent or as ghost vessels with perivascular cuffing is commonly noted. Presence of epithelial hyperplasia, down growths, pannus formation, BL fragmentation, stromal scar tissue, myofibroblastic transformation of keratocytes, lipid keratopathy, duplication of DM, and retrocorneal membrane formation are all other indicators of chronicity.

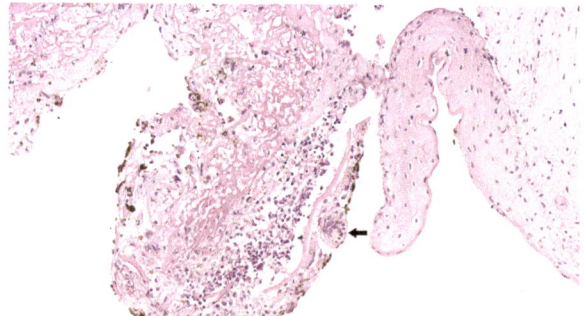

Fig. 16.4 A case of severe viral stromal keratitis with stromal necrosis, pseuodocornea formation, Multinucleated giant cell reaction around Descemet's membrane (Haematoxylin & Eosin stain, ×200)

16.4.4 Acanthamoeba Keratitis

Acanthamoeba keratitis was first recognized in association with contact lens wear in 1973. However, since then this entity has been reported in association with trauma, and exposure to soil and contaminated water. The hallmark finding in this infection is the presence of cysts as well as trophozoites, amid epithelial and Bowman's layer destruction, stromal infiltration, and keratocytic apoptosis [7]. While trophozoites are noted as oval to elongated basophilic structures larger than keratocytic nuclei and located within collagen lamella, the cysts are more oval, and show classic double-walled staining well with H&E or PAS and GMS (Fig. 16.5a, b). The nucleus in the cyst is located paracentral. It is important to recall here that unlike the appearance of trophozoites on corneal scrapings which appear much larger than the cysts; the trophozoites in formalin fixed paraffin embedded tissues appear smaller than cysts. This is attributed to the dehydration step involved in tissue processing, to which the cysts are more resistant and hence appear larger. Apart from moderate to severe inflammatory infiltration, granulomatous inflammation, new blood vessels, and apoptotic loss of keratocytes have also been reported, especially in advanced cases associated with scleritis [8].

16.4.5 Nocardia Keratitis

These are filamentous and beaded bacilli, of the order Actinomycetales. Not a frequent cause of infectious keratitis [9], more often: *Nocardia asteroides* (commonest), *N. gypsoides, N. brasiliensis, N. caviae, and N. farcini* have been implicated. Nocardia is notoriously recalcitrant and an indolent infection. Based on its clinical appearance of wreath-like raised infiltrates and chronicity, it is misdiagnosed as mycotic keratitis or other infectious keratitis. Similar to fungal infection, common predisposing factors include use of corticosteroids, prior ocular surgery such as LASIK or cataract surgery (due to surgical contamination by contaminated instruments such as blades), contact lens wear, and most commonly injury with soil [10, 11].

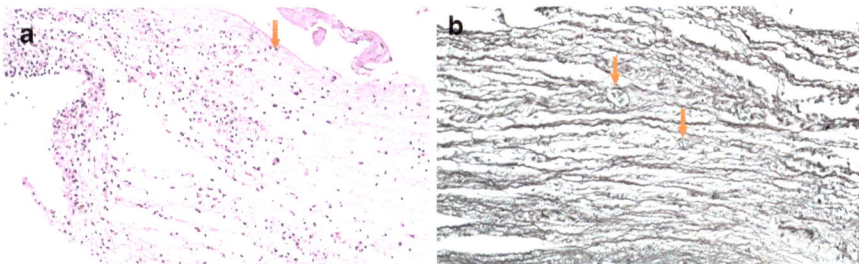

Fig. 16.5 (**a**) Acanthamoeba keratitis with mixed inflammatory infiltrates in stroma and few oval cysts of Acanthamoeba (Haematoxylin & Eosin stain, ×200); (**b**) Double-walled oval retractile cysts of Acanthamoeba (orange arrow) (GMS, ×200)

The corneal specimen could be either a biopsy specimen, such as in a case of cataract surgical wound, or amputated flap in post-LASIK infection. Nocardia has also been noted after lamellar or penetrating keratoplasty. Histopathologically, apart from epithelial ulceration and severe stromal destruction and inflammation, one can note clusters of thin branching filament-like organism in Gram stained specimens. In the case of post-LASIK and post-PRK infections; these can be noted in the necrotic areas. As these are acid fast, 1% modified Ziehl-Neelsen stained preparation is seen at 1000× magnification (oil immersion). The bacilli are noted as bright red staining bodies. Dense population of colonies of organisms implies the use of corticosteroids which promote the growth of this infection by inhibiting the inflammatory response. Unlike fungus, these organisms do not breach the Descemet's membrane.

16.4.6 Atypical Mycobacterial Keratitis

Atypical mycobacteria or nontuberculous mycobacteria (NTM) were described by Turner and Stinson as keratitis due to *Mycobacterium fortuitum* in 1965. Predisposing factors are trauma, retained corneal foreign body, and after surgery. It has also been reported as infectious crystalline keratopathy in grafts. This organism was also implicated in post-LASIK outbreaks of infection [12, 13]. Due to these outbreaks, 64% of all bacterial infections following LASIK is due to NTM. The most common species are *M. chelonea* and *M. fortuitum* (both are rapid growers) [13].

Ulceration of the epithelium, necrosis and tissue loss of stroma, and presence of severe acute and chronic inflammation are seen, including granulomatous inflammation. Concomitant use of corticosteroids in some cases leads to suppression of granulomatous inflammation, with the consequence that severe and prolonged keratitis is seen clinically [12]. On histological examination, cases pretreated with steroids would show stromal thinning and scanty infiltration. NTM are noted as dense colonies within the corneal stromal pockets or within amputated LASIK flaps (Fig. 16.6a, b) [13].

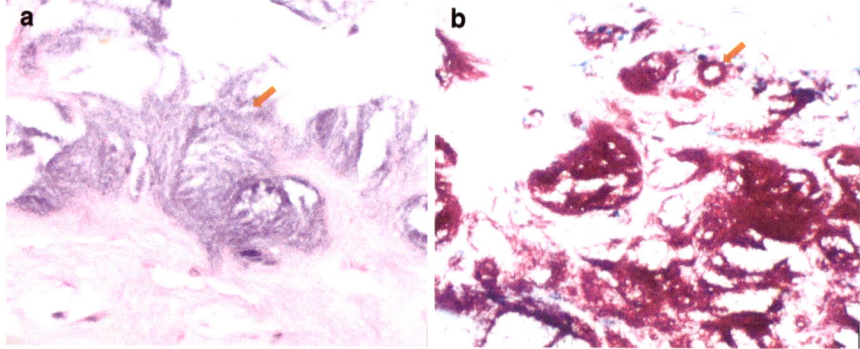

Fig. 16.6 (**a**) Corneal biopsy specimen of amputated LASIK flap shows bluish colonies of slender bacteria (Haematoxylin & Eosin stain, ×400); (**b**) These colonies of non-tubercular bacilli stain bright red with special stains (1% acid fast stain, ×1000)

16.4.7 Microsporidial Keratitis

Microsporidial stromal keratitis is an emerging cause of keratitis [14]. There are two clinical presentations of ocular microsporidial infections: corneal stromal keratitis and keratoconjunctivitis variant.

The cornea may show varying degrees of inflammation depending on prior use of steroids. Unless looked for carefully, these spores, which are approximately 2–4 μm, can be overlooked as they take up stain variably. Classically they are rice-grain like oval or rounded with a band like horizontal girdle. Rarely the spores can be found to traverse the Descemet's membrane and reach the anterior chamber and found in the exudates. Several stains can be used to easily delineate the spores such as Calcoflour white (CFW) with 10% Potassium Hydroxide, GMS, 1% Acid fast stain (Fig. 16.7a, b), and Masson's trichrome. Of these, 1% acid fast stain is easy and economical with good inter-observable agreement [15].

16.4.8 Pythium Keratitis

Pythium sp. is an algae which only recently has been reported as a cause of infectious keratitis, closely mimicking fungal keratitis both clinically and microbiologically *P. insidiosum*, belongs to the kingdom Stramenopila, is a fungus-like, aquatic oomycete mainly found in temperate, tropical, and subtropical climate [16]. Clinically these lesions invade the cornea and spread in a tentacle-like or reticular spread, with dot-like opacities in the active edges, which is one of the hallmark features to differentiate it from fungus. As it lacks chitin and ergosterol, there is no response to antifungals and the infection can rapidly progress to invade the entire cornea and spread to limbus, necessitating therapeutic keratoplasty [17]. These organisms are best identified as aseptate ribbon-like broad filaments with right angle bends on KOH-CFW preparation. Histopathology shows ulceration of the

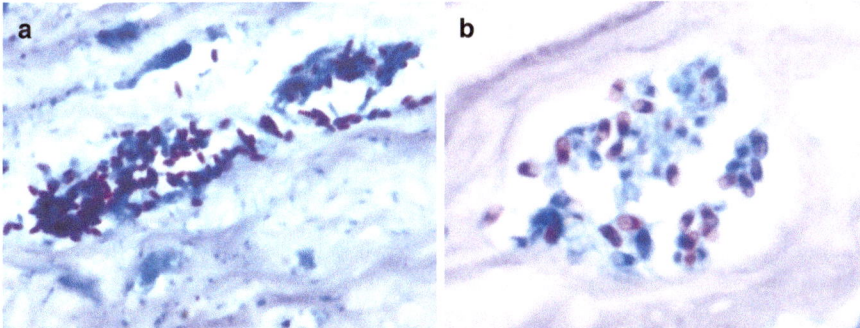

Fig. 16.7 (a) The typical appearance of brightly staining microsporidial spores in stroma cleft-like spaces (1% acid fast stain, ×1000); (b) The spores show variable staining with AFB with the classical waistband-like appearance (1% acid fast stain, ×1000)

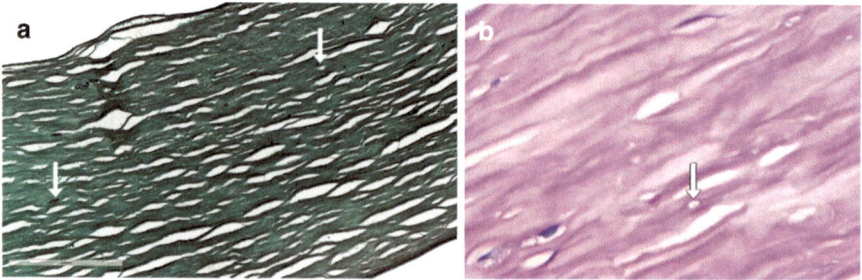

Fig. 16.8 (**a**) Aseptate hyphae and cut ends (arrows) of hyphae of Pythium in stroma (GMS, ×200); (**b**) Poorly and faint stained oocyte of Pythium (arrow) in stroma (Periodic Acid Schiff stain, ×400)

epithelium with stromal destruction and inflammation ranging from moderate to severe. Similar to the findings noted in fungal keratitis, in this infection too the load of Pythium filaments is maximum in areas where inflammation is scanty. The organisms are noted as wide filaments with admixed narrower structures. The DM is uncommonly involved. The oocyte is stained poorly to well-stained (variable) with PAS (Fig. 16.8a, b) and stains well with Potassium hydroxide-sulfuric acid stain [18]. Whereas fungal filaments stain well with PAS and GMS but not with Potassium hydroxide-sulfuric acid stain.

16.4.9 Miscellaneous Infections and Infection-Like Conditions

16.4.9.1 *Treponema pallidum*

Interstitial keratitis [19, 20] due to syphilis is much less frequent. In congenital syphilis, corneal edema and inflammation can be noted in pediatric patients, between the ages of 5–15. Most of these cases resolve with topical corticosteroids. Histological study is documented of only a few cases. There is presence of corneal edema, WBC infiltration—either diffuse or localized—in the mid and posterior stroma. Prominent vascularization is present. As the disease becomes chronic, fibrous pannus with ghost vessels, scarring, and DM thickening depict healed lesions. *Treponema pallidum* organisms have not been isolated from these.

16.4.9.2 *Mycobacterium tuberculosis*

Phlyctenular keratitis [19, 20] is a presumed classical ocular manifestation of systemic tuberculosis. These are seen clinically as a peripheral or limbal corneal inflammatory lesion with a leash of blood vessels. Histologically, the lesion involves the stroma usually only anteriorly, with a focus of subacute and chronic inflammatory cells. There may be mild stromal necrosis and later on scar tissue in chronic stage. Tubercle bacilli have not been identified in these lesions and it appears to be a hypersensitivity reaction.

16.4.9.3   *Mycobacterium leprae*

Corneal disease is frequently seen in long-standing leprosy, either directly as an infection due to lepra bacilli or secondary to chronic ocular changes like exposure keratopathy [19, 20]. Histologically, lepromatous leprosy produces a nonulcerating diffuse granulomatous stromal infiltration characterized by infiltration with foamy histiocytes and giant cells. These cells contain lepra bacilli, picked up on acid fast staining.

16.4.9.4   *Onchocerciasis*

Infection by *Onchocerciasis volvulus* [19, 20] is one of the leading causes of blindness worldwide. Microfilaria has been observed in all ocular tissues and migrates easily to the cornea. Histologically, intact microfilaria with scant inflammation is noted. In cases of degenerated organisms, intense eosinophilic response is noted with secondary changes in all layers of cornea, like epithelial edema, bullae, replacement of Bowman's layer by inflammatory pannus and stromal vascularization and fibrosis.

16.4.9.5   Shield Ulcer

In chronic seasonally exacerbated allergic inflammatory condition of Vernal keratoconjunctivitis, the ocular surface especially the tarsal and/or bulbar conjunctiva is severely inflamed and results in punctate epitheliopathy [21–23]. Subsequent coalescence of punctate erosions results in epithelial defect with a characteristic shape which is known as shield ulcer. It is not a true ulcer as the bed of the epithelial defect is clean initially and devoid of inflammatory cells, later a fibrin plaque gets deposited which prevents reepithelialization of shield ulcer [23]. Secondary infection of these epithelial defects may give rise to true ulcers.

16.4.9.6   Tunnel Infection

Infection of the sclerocorneal wound after cataract surgery is referred to as tunnel infections. When there is persistence of tunnel infection, deroofing of the tunnel and submitting the tissues for histopathologic examination is usually rewarding (Fig. 16.9) and identifies the organisms [24].

Fig. 16.9 Tunnel infection with yeast in a case of cataract surgery (Periodic Acid Schiff stain, ×1000)

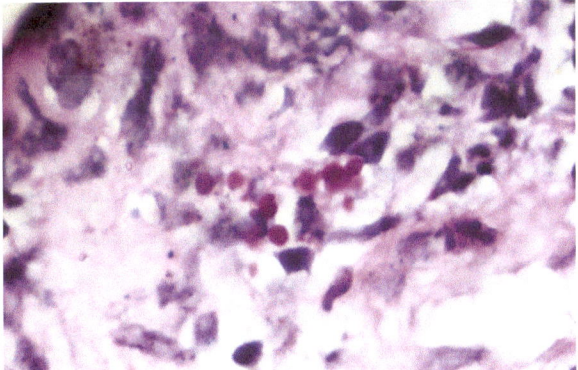

16.4.9.7 Infectious Crystalline Keratopathy

This condition presents with a crystal needle-like appearance in the corneal stroma which may occur with any organism but has been described more commonly in bacterial infection. They appear as fine, branch-like gray-white opacifications and usually not associated with inflammation. Histologically these lesions are colonies of bacteria with minimal or no inflammatory response which is believed to be the sequestration of the bacteria against host detection due to the secretion of the biofilm over the bacterial colonies. Diagnostic testing such as gram stains, acid fast stains, routine bacterial and fungal cultures, as well as mycobacterial cultures, confirms the nature of the organism [25].

16.4.9.8 Mixed Infections

Rarely in immune-compromised conditions, the corneal infections may be due to more than one organism, e.g., fungus and bacteria, acanthamoeba and bacteria, and hence care should be taken to identify both morphologies with the help of special stains and correlated with microbiologic findings.

16.5 Molecular Diagnosis

Nucleic acid-based testing has revolutionized our approach to diagnosis and therapy in a wide variety of conditions including infections. These assays are based on isolation of DNA or RNA, followed by hybridization or amplification methods or a combination of the two. DNA probe-based assays are particularly well suited for in situ hybridization in tissues and for culture confirmation. However, they are less sensitive than DNA amplification techniques such as polymerase chain reaction (PCR). An overview of principals and applications of molecular diagnostic techniques such as PCR, fluorescent in situ hybridization (FISH), microarray, and DNA chip technology can be found elsewhere [26].

While the corneal scrapings and biopsy can be submitted to molecular pathology directly, the DNA extracted from the formalin fixed paraffin embedded tissue sections forms another valuable source of material to be tested and correlated with clinical and histologic findings. Availability of commercially available kits have made it possible to evaluate the archived material, with reasonable results.

These methods have been applied to diagnose viral infections, microsporidial infection, atypical mycobacterium, *Mycobacterium* causing lepromatous lesions [27, 28]. In addition to aiding in diagnosis, molecular techniques also improve our understanding of the disease process. For example, corneal tissue from HSV seropositive patients (with no clinical manifestation of the disease) was shown to have the presence of HSV DNA as well as viable HSV in culture [29]. This finding strengthened the understanding about the potential of latent HSV to induce donor-to-host infection in corneal recipients.

16.6   Tips for Diagnosis of Corneal Infections

(a) Good orientation of the corneal button, use of PAS stain, and examination of all the layers of cornea is the minimal requirement for interpreting corneal infections.

(b) To a large extent, if accurate and necessary clinical information is present, two major groups of histopathological characteristics are required. Firstly, assessment of characteristics of the inflammation such as the distribution, severity, and areas of inflammation is needed. Secondly, the presence of associated features such as granulomatous inflammation, necrosis, and vascularization. All of this put together can provide 60–70% of information towards the etiologic agents.

(c) For accurate identification and positive confirmation of the microbiological agent results of special stains, such as GMS, AF stain, and Grams, are needed.

(d) Polymerase chain reaction would then help either when all above methods fail or as another method of identification of the organism, such as microsporidia [30], fungal [31], nocardia [32], acanthamoeba [33], mycobacterium [34], and eubacterial PCRs [35]. This is especially useful also in the detection of viral keratitis [36].

16.7   Conjunctival Infections

Conjunctival infections or conjunctivitis rarely presents as a specimen for histopathology examination. Some of the rare unresolved cases that present include chronic infections or inflammation involving the palpebral conjunctiva, limbus, lid margin, or caruncle presenting as an ulcer, ulcero-nodular lesions may require a biopsy for confirmation of diagnosis. Some of such cases in our experience have been mycobacterial infections affecting the palpebral conjunctiva and limbus which were diagnosed by the presence of necrotizing, granulomatous lesions, and were positive for acid fast bacilli [37]. Other rare cases of subconjunctival nodular granulomatous lesions which on excision and biopsy prove to be fungal infections have been reported [38, 39].

16.8   Conclusion

As corneal infections are infrequently seen by the general pathologist, histopathological diagnosis is challenging both to the clinician and the pathologist. Being familiar with the features to be expected in each infection and the use of appropriate histochemistry and molecular methods could go a long way to reach a tissue diagnosis and enable the clinician to institute prompt therapy.

Acknowledgments The work of Somasheila I. Murthy and Dilip K. Mishra was supported by the Hyderabad Eye Research Foundation. The authors acknowledge Mr. G. Chenchu Naidu and Mr. B. Sreedhar Rao (Pathology Department) and Mr. G. P. Naresh (Photography Department).

References

1. Huang AJW, Wichiensin P, Yang MC. Bacterial keratitis. Chapter 81. In: Krachmer JH, Mannis MH, Holland EJ, editors. Cornea: fundamentals, diagnosis and management. St Louis: Mosby Elsevier; 2011. p. 1005–33.
2. Srinivasan M. Fungal keratitis. Curr Opin Ophthalmol. 2004;15(4):321–7.
3. Vemuganti GK, Garg P, Gopinathan U, Naduvilath TJ, John RK, Buddi R, Rao GN. Evaluation of agent and host factors in progression of mycotic keratitis: a histologic and microbiologic study of 167 corneal buttons. Ophthalmology. 2002;109(8):1538–46.
4. Garg P, Vemuganti GK, Chatarjee S, Gopinathan U, Rao GN. Pigmented plaque presentation of dematiaceous fungal keratitis: a clinicopathologic correlation. Cornea. 2004;23(6):571–6.
5. Holland EJ, Schwartz GS. Classification of herpes simplex virus keratitis. Cornea. 1999;18(2):144–54.
6. Holbach LM, Font RL, Naumann GO. Herpes simplex stromal and endothelial keratitis. Granulomatous cell reactions at the level of Descemet's membrane, the stroma, and Bowman's layer. Ophthalmology. 1990;97(6):722–8.
7. Vemuganti GK, Sharma S, Athmanathan S, Garg P. Keratocyte loss in Acanthamoeba keratitis: phagocytosis, necrosis or apoptosis? Indian J Ophthalmol. 2000;48(4):291–4.
8. Vemuganti GK, Pasricha G, Sharma S, Garg P. Granulomatous inflammation in Acanthamoeba keratitis: an immunohistochemical study of five cases and review of literature. Indian J Med Microbiol. 2005;23(4):231–8.
9. Sridhar MS, Gopinathan U, Garg P, Sharma S, Rao GN. Ocular nocardia infections with special emphasis on the cornea. Surv Ophthalmol. 2001;45(5):361–78.
10. Garg P, Sharma S, Vemuganti GK, Ramamurthy B. A cluster of Nocardia keratitis after LASIK. J Refract Surg. 2007;23(3):309–12.
11. Javadi MA, Kanavi MR, Zarei-Ghanavati S, Mirbabaei F, Jamali H, Shoja M, Mahdavi M, Naghshgar N, Yazdani S, Faramarzi A. Outbreak of Nocardia keratitis after photorefractive keratectomy: clinical, microbiological, histopathological, and confocal scan study. J Cataract Refract Surg. 2009;35(2):393–8.
12. de la Cruz J, Pineda R 2nd. LASIK-associated atypical mycobacteria keratitis: a case report and review of the literature. Int Ophthalmol Clin. 2007;47(2):73–84.
13. Garg P, Bansal AK, Sharma S, Vemuganti GK. Bilateral infectious keratitis after laser in situ keratomileusis: a case report and review of the literature. Ophthalmology. 2001;108(1):121–5.
14. Vemuganti GK, Garg P, Sharma S, Joseph J, Gopinathan U, Singh S. Is microsporidial keratitis an emerging cause of stromal keratitis? A case series study. BMC Ophthalmol. 2005;5:19.
15. Joseph J, Vemuganti GK, Garg P, Sharma S. Histopathological evaluation of ocular microsporidiosis by different stains. BMC Clin Pathol. 2006;6:6.
16. Gaastra W, Lipman LJ, De Cock AW, Exel TK, Pegge RBG, Scheurwater J, Vilela R, Mendoza L. Pythium insidiosum: an overview. Vet Microbiol. 2010;146(1–2):1–16.
17. Bagga B, Sharma S, Madhuri Guda SJ, Nagpal R, Joseph J, Manjulatha K, Mohamed A, Garg P. Leap forward in the treatment of Pythium insidiosum keratitis. Br J Ophthalmol. 2018;102(12):1629–33.
18. Mittal R, Jena SK, Desai A, Agarwal S. Pythium insidiosum keratitis: histopathology and rapid novel diagnostic staining technique. Cornea. 2017;36(9):1124–32.
19. Spencer WH. Cornea. In: Spencer WH, editor. Ophthalmic pathology: an atlas and textbook. Philadelphia: WB Saunders; 1996. p. 202–6.
20. Barney NP. Cornea color atlas. Arch Ophthalmol. 1997;115(1):137.

21. Barney NP. Vernal and atopic keratoconjunctivitis. In: Krachmer JH, Mannis MH, Holland EJ, editors. Cornea: fundamentals, diagnosis and management. St Louis: Mosby Elsevier; 2011. p. 573.

22. Iqbal A, Jan S, Babar TF, Khan MD. Corneal complications of vernal catarrh. J College Phys Surg Pakistan JCPSP. 2003;13(7):394–7.

23. Rahi AH, Buckley R, Grierson I. Chapter 23: Pathology of corneal plaque in vernal keratoconjunctivitis. In: O'Connor GR, Chandler JW, editors. Advances in immunology and immunopathology of eye. New York: Massom; 1985. p. 91–4.

24. Roy A, Sahu SK, Padhi TR, Das S, Sharma S. Clinicomicrobiological characteristics and treatment outcome of sclerocorneal tunnel infection. Cornea. 2012;31(7):780–5.

25. Porter AJ, Lee GA, Jun AS. Infectious crystalline keratopathy. Surv Ophthalmol. 2018;63(4):480–99.

26. Netto GJ, Saad RD, Dysert PA 2nd. Diagnostic molecular pathology: current techniques and clinical applications, part I. Proc (Bayl Univ Med Cent). 2003;16(4):379–83.

27. Fyfe JA, McCowan C, O'Brien CR, Globan M, Birch C, Revill P, Barrs VRD, Wayne J, Hughes MS, Holloway S, Malik R. Molecular characterization of a novel fastidious mycobacterium causing lepromatous lesions of the skin, subcutis, cornea, and conjunctiva of cats living in Victoria, Australia. J Clin Microbiol. 2008;46(2):618–26.

28. Shamsi FA, Chaudhry IA, Moraes MO, Martinez AN, Riley FC. Detection of Mycobacterium leprae in ocular tissues by histopathology and real-time polymerase chain reaction. Ophthalmic Res. 2007;39(2):63–8.

29. Robert PY, Adenis JP, Denis F, Alain S, Ranger Rogez S. Herpes simplex virus DNA in corneal transplants: prospective study of 38 recipients. J Med Virol. 2003;71(1):69–74.

30. Reddy AK, Balne PK, Gaje K, Garg P. PCR for the diagnosis and species identification of microsporidia in patients with keratitis. Clin Microbiol Infect. 2011;17(3):476–8.

31. Vengayil S, Panda A, Satpathy G, Nayak N, Ghose S, Patanaik D, Khokhar S. Polymerase chain reaction-guided diagnosis of mycotic keratitis: a prospective evaluation of its efficacy and limitations. Invest Ophthalmol Vis Sci. 2009;50(1):152–6.

32. Rodríguez-Nava V, Couble A, Devulder G, Flandrois JP, Boiron P, Laurent F. Use of PCR-restriction enzyme pattern analysis and sequencing database for hsp65 gene-based identification of Nocardia species. J Clin Microbiol. 2006;44(2):536–46.

33. Schroeder JM, Booton GC, Hay J, Niszl IA, Seal DV, Markus MB, Fuerst PA, Byers TJ. Use of subgenic 18S ribosomal DNA PCR and sequencing for genus and genotype identification of acanthamoebae from humans with keratitis and from sewage sludge. J Clin Microbiol. 2001;39(5):1903–11.

34. Hermans PW, van Soolingen D, Dale JW, Schuitema AR, McAdam RA, Catty D, van Embden JD. Insertion element IS986 from Mycobacterium tuberculosis: a useful tool for diagnosis and epidemiology of tuberculosis. J Clin Microbiol. 1990;28(9):2051–8.

35. Hykin PG, Tobal K, McIntyre G, Matheson MM, Towler HM, Lightman SL. The diagnosis of delayed post-operative endophthalmitis by polymerase chain reaction of bacterial DNA in vitreous samples. J Med Microbiol. 1994;40(6):408–15.

36. Aurelius E, Johansson B, Sköldenberg B, Staland A, Forsgren M. Rapid diagnosis of herpes simplex encephalitis by nested polymerase chain reaction assay of cerebrospinal fluid. Lancet. 1991;337(8735):189–92.

37. Chaurasia S, Ramappa M, Murthy SI, Vemuganti GK, Fernandes M, Sharma S, Sangwan VS. Chronic conjunctivitis due to Mycobacterium tuberculosis. Int Ophthalmol. 2014;34(3):655–60.

38. Hampton DE, Adesina A, Chodosh J. Conjunctival sporotrichosis in the absence of antecedent trauma. Cornea. 2002;21(8):831–3.

39. Yamagata JPM, Rudolph FB, Nobre MCL, Nascimento LV, Sampaio FMS, Arinelli A, Freitas DF. Ocular sporotrichosis: a frequently misdiagnosed cause of granulomatous conjunctivitis in epidemic areas. Am J Ophthalmol Case Rep. 2017;23(8):35–8.

Role of In Vivo Confocal Microscopy in the Diagnosis of Microbial Keratitis

17

Dipika V. Patel

17.1 Introduction

Tissue sampling and microbiological culture are imperative in the diagnosis of infectious keratitis. However, isolating the causative organism may be difficult, particularly in cases of atypical keratitis where reported culture-positive rates are low and some cultures may take days to weeks to become positive. Delay in diagnosis and appropriate treatment may have a detrimental effect on visual prognosis. In vivo confocal microscopy (IVCM) is a noninvasive tool that potentially enables rapid diagnosis of infective keratitis, particularly in atypical cases.

17.2 In Vivo Confocal Microscopy

IVCM enables noninvasive *en face* imaging of the living human cornea at the cellular level. The underlying principle behind IVCM is that light is passed through an aperture and focused onto a small area of the cornea. The reflected light is focused via a second aperture arranged such that out of focus light is eliminated. Because the illumination and detection paths share the same focal plane, the term "confocal" is used [1].

A variety of types of IVCM have been developed, with variations in the type of illuminating light and aperture. The tandem scanning confocal microscope (Tandem Scanning Corporation, Reston, USA) used white light as the illumination source in combination with a spinning pinhole disc while the slit scanning confocal

D. V. Patel (✉)

Department of Ophthalmology, Faculty of Medical and Health Sciences, University of Auckland, Auckland, New Zealand
e-mail: dipika.patel@auckland.ac.nz

© Springer Nature Singapore Pte Ltd. 2021
S. Das, V. Jhanji (eds.), *Infections of the Cornea and Conjunctiva*,
https://doi.org/10.1007/978-981-15-8811-2_17

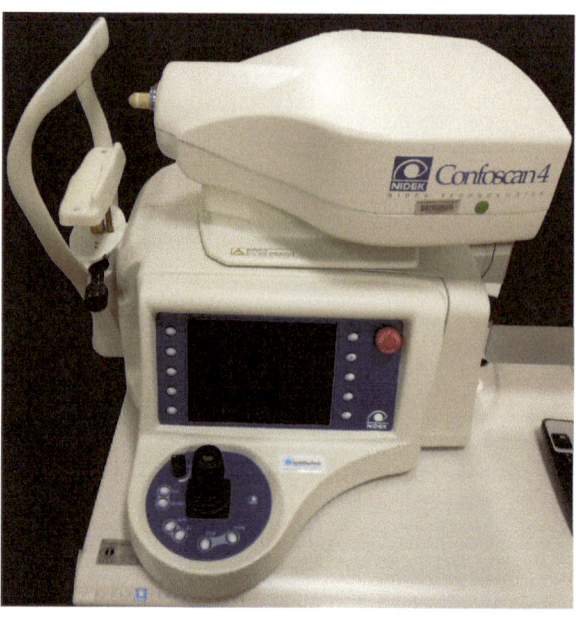

Fig. 17.1 Confoscan 4
in vivo confocal
microscope (Nidek
Technologies,
Padova, Italy)

microscope (Confoscan, Nidek technologies, Padova, Italy) used a white light illumination source in combination with a scanning slit (Fig. 17.1). Although these type of IVCM are available in some centers, they are no longer commercially available.

The Heidelberg Retina Tomograph Rostock Corneal Module (RCM) (Heidelberg Engineering GmBH, Germany) is currently the only commercially available IVCM (Fig. 17.2). The RCM is a laser scanning IVCM that utilizes a 670 nm red wavelength Helium–Neon diode laser source.

17.3   Image Acquisition Modes

17.3.1 Slit Scanning IVCM

The Confoscan 4 has two image acquisition modes, in which scanning is performed through the z-axis of the cornea either automatically (full-thickness scan of the cornea with selectable scan step size) or semi-automatically (selectable scan depth and step size). The minimum step size is 1.5 μm and the maximum scan depth is 800 μm. This microscope does not provide the option of disabling z-scanning while still acquiring images. A fixation target within the lens can be selected either centrally or at one of eight peripheral positions. The illumination intensity may be adjusted within a range of 1–100 at any time during the examination.

Fig. 17.2 The Heidelberg Retina Tomograph 3 with Rostock Corneal Module in vivo confocal microscope (Heidelberg Engineering GmBH, Germany)

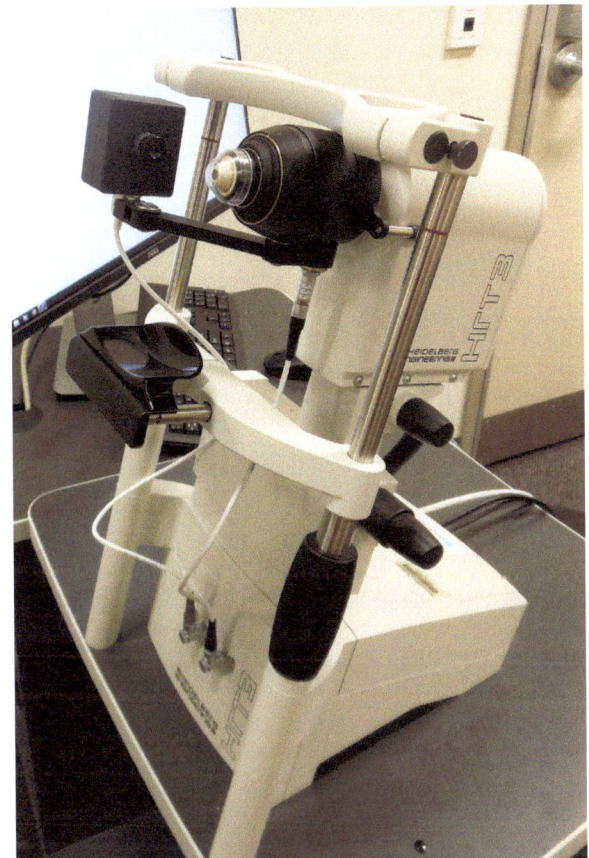

17.3.2 Laser Scanning IVCM

The RCM offers greater operator flexibility for in vivo corneal examination compared to other types of IVCM. Three examination modes are available.

17.3.2.1 Section Mode

The section mode enables acquisition and storage of a single image at a time. The cornea may thus be scanned manually in the X-Y-Z axes and images acquired at the desired points by pressing a foot pedal. Manual scanning in the z-axis may be performed through a range of 0–1500 μm. The author has found this to be the most versatile mode for clinical corneal examination. In particular, this technique enables imaging to be targeted to regions of interest such as the edge of a corneal infiltrate.

17.3.2.2 Volume Mode

The volume mode allows acquisition of 40 images in consecutive focal planes 2 μm apart. Therefore, 80 μm of cornea can be scanned automatically in the z-axis.

17.3.2.3   Sequence Mode

In the sequence mode, a series of 100 images are acquired at a selectable rate between 1 and 30 frames per second. The result is a movie, 3–100 s in duration. During acquisition, the objective lens may either remain stationary or be manually scanned in the X-Y-Z axes.

Images may be stored in JPEG or TIF file format. The dimensions of acquired images represent 400 µm × 400 µm of the cornea and the optical lateral and axial resolution is as low as 2 µm and 4 µm, respectively [1].

17.4   Clinical Examination Technique

17.4.1 Slit Scanning IVCM

The objective lens tip and the chin and head rests are disinfected using sterile wipes containing 70% isopropyl alcohol. The patient's eyes are then anesthetized using topical anesthetic drop.

Viscotears (Carbomer 980, 0.2%, Novartis, North Ryde, NSW, Australia) is used as a coupling agent between the objective lens and the cornea. A pea sized drop of this viscous gel is placed on the tip of the objective lens, ensuring it is homogenous and free of bubbles.

Once the patient has been made comfortable, with the chin on the chin rest and the forehead pressed firmly against the forehead bar, they are instructed to look straight ahead.

A joystick is used to move the microscope head electronically. The objective lens is first grossly aligned with the eye undergoing examination. Fine adjustments are then made to align the lens tip with the central cornea. The lens tip is subsequently advanced forwards until the gel touches the corneal surface, then further still, until the corneal endothelium comes into view. At this stage, further fine adjustments in the X-Y plane may be required to achieve good centration. Once centered, the lens is advanced just beyond the endothelium, into the anterior chamber, and image acquisition commenced.

17.4.2 Laser Scanning IVCM

The initial step in examination using RCM is preparation of the objective lens tip. A homogenous, bubble-free, pea-sized, drop of Viscotears is placed on the lens tip. A sterile disposable cap is then mounted over the lens tip, such that the gel forms a meniscus between the objective lens and the cap. The focal plane adjustment wheel is then adjusted until a bright reflection is observed, indicating that the lens is focussed within the front of the cap. The depth setting is then reset to zero.

The patient's eyes are anesthetized using topical anesthetic drop, and Viscotears is used in the eyes for lubrication. The patient is seated comfortably, with the chin on the chin rest and the forehead pressed firmly against the forehead bar. Alignment is further aided by use of a CCD camera attachment enabling live imaging of the cornea from the temporal side during examination. Adjustment of the position of the lens tip in the X-Y-Z axes can only be performed manually. The cornea is applanated by the lens cap, and applanation should be maintained throughout the examination, carefully avoiding corneal compression. Examination using the selected mode may then be commenced.

17.5   The Healthy Cornea

Due to its high resolution and magnification, IVCM allows imaging of corneal cells and their nuclei. Superficial epithelial cells are visible as polygonal cells of various size and reflectivity, with visible cell nuclei which are surrounded by a dark band. Basal epithelial cells measure 10–15 μm in diameter and form a regular mosaic with dark cell bodies and bright cell borders (Fig. 17.3a). Bowman's layer appears as an amorphous homogenous layer. Subbasal nerves are visible at the level of Bowman's layer as well-defined reflective linear branching structures (Fig. 17.3b).

Stromal keratocytes (Fig. 17.3c e) are imaged as well-defined bright, oval-round, objects against a dark background. In the midstroma, keratocytes have a more regular oval shape, while posterior stromal keratocytes appear more elongated and spindle shaped than anteriorly. Stromal nerves appear as thick, reflective linear structures of various orientations, which branch in a dichotomous pattern.

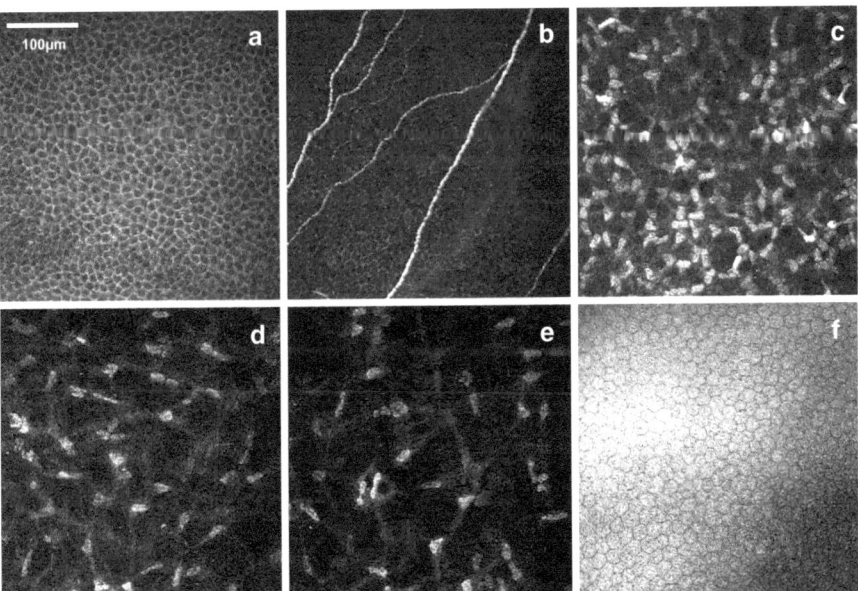

Fig. 17.3 Laser scanning in vivo confocal microscopy images of a normal human cornea showing: (**a**) the basal epithelium, (**b**) subbasal nerve plexus, (**c**) anterior stroma, (**d**) mid-stroma, (**e**) posterior stroma, and (**f**) endothelium

Endothelial cells are seen as a regular array of mainly hexagonal cells that exhibit bright cell bodies and dark cell borders (Fig. 17.3f).

17.6 Nonspecific Signs of Infection

17.6.1 Leukocytes

Corneal infiltration by leukocytes may occur in response to corneal injury, inflammation, or infection. When imaged by IVCM, leukocytes appear as bright spots (Fig. 17.4a) that may be visible within the epithelium, at the level of Bowman's layer, within the stroma, or on the endothelium.

17.6.2 Langerhans Cells

On IVCM, Langerhans cells located at the level of Bowman's layer and basal epithelium appear as hyperreflective particles with a diameter of up to 15 μm [2]. In the healthy cornea, these cells appear as either cell bodies with small/no processes (immature phenotype). Maturation of Langerhans cells may be induced by corneal injury, inflammation, or infection and the mature phenotype is characterized by cell bodies bearing long dendritic processes (Fig. 17.4b).

The presence of leukocytes and mature Langerhans cells are nonspecific signs and are not diagnostic of any particular disease. However, it has been reported that infective keratitis of different etiologies is associated with the infiltration of different morphological subtypes of inflammatory cells on IVCM. Smedowski et al. [3]

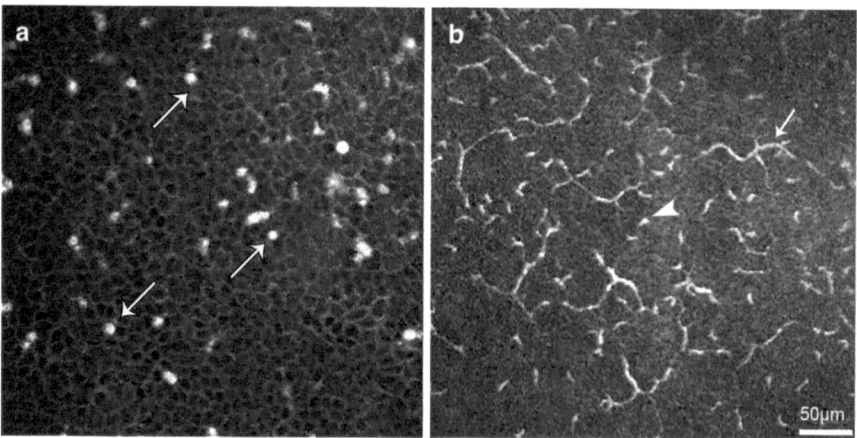

Fig. 17.4 Laser scanning in vivo confocal microscopy images: (**a**) at the level of the basal epithelium in a patient with corneal graft rejection showing leukocytes (arrows) and (**b**) at the level of Bowman's layer showing immature (arrowhead) and mature (arrow) Langerhans cells

identified two basic types of inflammatory cell morphologies: round and non-round cells. The round cells (type 1 cells) are small (<10 µm), oval-shaped cells with no visible fibrils. The non-round cells were subdivided into four subtypes: small (<50 µm), elongated cells with short fibrils (type 2 cells); large (>50 µm) dendriform cells with an elongated, thin cell body and long, thin fibrils (type 3 cells); giant (>100 µm) dendriform cells with an elongated, thin cell body and short, thin fibrils (type 4 cells); and giant (50–100 µm) multi-shaped cells with a thick cell body and short, thick fibrils that might also contain long cilia (type 5 cells) [3].

17.7   *Acanthamoeba* Keratitis

Acanthamoeba cysts may appear as double-walled cysts, signet rings, and bright spots of less than 30 µm in diameter when imaged by IVCM (Fig. 17.5) [4]. The similarity in appearance between *Acanthamoeba* cysts and inflammatory cells, which also appear as bright spots, may lead to erroneous diagnosis.

The predominant inflammatory cell type on IVCM in *Acanthamoeba* keratitis is the non-round type 5 cell (giant multi-shaped cells with a thick cell body and short, thick fibrils) and these cells were not observed in any other type of keratitis. Additionally, it was reported that the density of infiltrating cells in *Acanthamoeba* keratitis was three times lower than in fungal keratitis [3].

Chidambaram et al. [5] showed that bright spots and double-walled cysts were most commonly observed (89% and 83% of patients, respectively), whereas the signet ring appearance was only observed in 17% of cases. They also noted that the cysts appeared to group together in lines or clusters and that prior corticosteroid use

Fig. 17.5 Laser scanning in vivo confocal microscopy image of a cornea with *Acanthamoeba* keratitis showing a double-walled cyst (arrow) and bright spots (arrowhead)

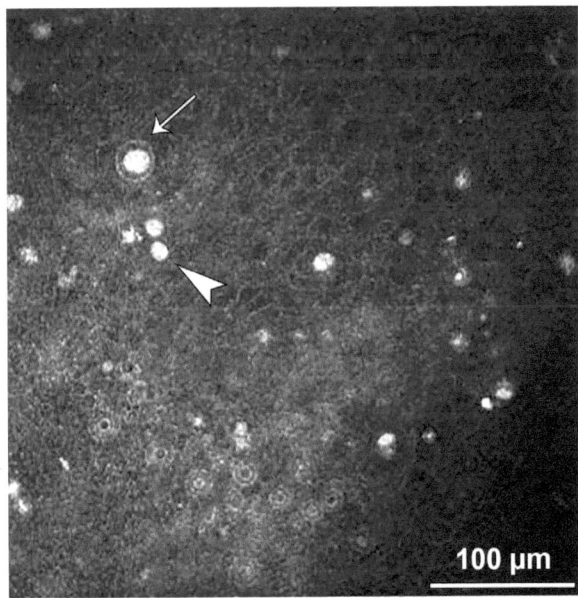

was more strongly associated with the formation of clusters, rather than lines, of cysts [5].

IVCM images of trophozoites have been described as ovoid or irregularly shaped structures, more than 30 μm in size, with spiny surface structures suggestive of acanthopodia [4, 6]. However, trophozoites are often difficult to distinguish from keratocytes; therefore, IVCM descriptions of their appearance remain controversial.

The aforementioned variability in IVCM signs highlights the importance of using standardized diagnostic criteria when using IVCM in the diagnosis of *Acanthamoeba* keratitis. Additionally, the experience of examiners has been shown to be an important aspect of diagnostic accuracy [7].

There is some variation in the reported sensitivity and specificity of IVCM in the diagnosis of *Acanthamoeba* (Table 17.1). This variation may be related to differences in type of IVCM, diagnostic criteria, reference standard, and observer experience.

Table 17.1 Summary of studies investigating the diagnostic accuracy of *in vivo* confocal microscopy in the diagnosis of acanthamoeba keratitis

	Diagnostic criteria	Sensitivity (%)	Specificity (%)	Masked observers	Observer experience
Tu et al. [8]	Cysts or trophozoites, on IVCM	92.9	77.3	No	Experienced
Kanavi et al. [6]	Cysts or trophozoites, on IVCM	100	84	Not reported	Not reported
Goh et al. [9]	Double-walled cysts, signet rings, and round/oval hyperreflective spots	100	100	Not reported	Experienced
Füst et al. [10]	Bright spots on IVCM	100	50	Not reported	Not reported
	Cysts, trophozoites, or signet rings on IVCM	67	94		
De Craene et al. [4]	Trophozoite-like hyperreflective objects	10.9	100	Yes	Trained physicians
	Round or ovoid hyperreflective objects with no double wall	73.9	48.2		
	Round or ovoid hyperreflective objects with hyporeflective halo	8.7	100		

Table 17.1 (continued)

	Diagnostic criteria	Sensitivity (%)	Specificity (%)	Masked observers	Observer experience
Chidambaram et al. [11]	Cysts on IVCM	88.2	98.2	Yes	2–5 years experience
Kheirkhah et al. [12]	Cysts on IVCM	59	92.7	Yes	Inexperienced
Kheirkhah et al. [12]	Cysts on IVCM	69.7	97.1	Yes	Experienced

De Craene et al. [4] examined 12 different signs on IVCM images of 50 Acanthamoeba PCR-positive patients. These were compared with a control group of infectious and immune keratitis that can mimic *Acanthamoeba* keratitis. Four types of images were associated significantly with PCR-positive *Acanthamoeba* keratitis: bright spots (round or ovoid hyperreflective objects with no double wall; diameter, <30 µm); target images (hyperreflective objects with hyporeflective halo; diameter, <30 µm); clusters of hyperreflective objects (diameter, <30 µm); and trophozoite-like objects (diameter, >30 µm). Specificity of both target and tropho-zoite images was 100%. This figure was 98.2% for clusters and 48.2% for bright spots. If the diagnosis of *Acanthamoeba* keratitis was made on presence of target images, clusters, or trophozoite images (at least 1 of the 3 features), the positive predictive value of confocal microscopy was 87.5% and the negative predictive value was 58.5% [4].

In an early study using slit scanning IVCM, Tu et al. [8] reported a sensitivity of 92.9% and a specificity of 77.3% in strictly culture-positive patients. However, the observers were not masked in this study. Similarly, Kanavi et al. [6] reported sensitivity of 100% and specificity of 84% in corneal/contact lens case culture-positive cases, although observer experience and masking were not reported.

Using laser scanning IVCM, Goh et al. [9] reported 100% sensitivity and specificity in patients with definite acanthamoeba keratitis (positive IVCM, PCR, and/or culture and resolution with treatment) and 88.9% sensitivity and 100% specificity in patients with clinical *Acanthamoeba* keratitis (clinical signs and response to treatment). Füst et al. [10] highlighted the importance of diagnostic criteria and noted that in cases where bright spots (without or with any of the other three structures) were present in the IVCM, sensitivity was 100% and specificity was 50%. When excluding the cases where the only signs of *Acanthamoeba* were the bright spots, and only the cases where cysts, trophozoites, or signet rings were also present were considered, the sensitivity was 67% and the specificity was 94% [10]. The importance of identifying double-walled cysts, signet rings, or trophozoites was further highlighted by De Craene et al. [4] who reported that these features are 100% specific for acanthamoeba. Despite their relatively low sensitivity (less than 11%), these features were pathognomonic of the disease [4].

Chidambaram et al. [11] pooled five graders of varying levels of experience (2–5 years) and reported a sensitivity of 88.2% and a specificity of 98.2% for the diagnosis of *Acanthamoeba* keratitis using laser scanning IVCM. Hau et al. [7] noted that the longer the duration of *Acanthamoeba* keratitis, the higher the likelihood that a correct diagnosis was made by the observers in grading the IVCM images. They also showed a twofold difference in sensitivity between the most experienced and the least experienced observer, indicating higher diagnostic accuracy with experience [7]. The relationship between observer experience and diagnostic accuracy was further supported by Kheirkhah et al. [12]

A retrospective study by Huang et al. [13] used IVCM to image eyes with *Acanthamoeba* keratitis at five corneal locations (one central and four peripheral) and quantified the density and maximum depth of *Acanthamoeba* cysts. Eyes with *Acanthamoeba* keratitis requiring therapeutic keratoplasty were more likely to have a deeper and more diffuse penetration of cysts in the cornea, and a higher density of cysts at presentation compared with those resolving with medical treatment. They also reported that 200–250 μm depth separated the eyes with good and poor prognosis [13].

The effect of medical therapy on cyst density has also been studied. In a small retrospective study, Wang [14] et al. reported a mean cyst density in the central cornea at presentation of 99.0 ± 64.9 cells/mm^2 (range, 38–255/mm^2). Cyst density significantly decreased at a rate of 5.3% for each month of anti-amoebic treatment [14].

17.8 Fungal Keratitis

Filamentous and yeast fungal elements in the cornea are readily imaged by IVCM. On IVCM, *Fusarium* hyphae are visible as hyperreflective lines 200–300 μm in length and 3–5 μm in width, with branches at 90° angles (Fig. 17.6) [15]. *Aspergillus* hyphae have similar dimensions and morphology to *Fusarium* hyphae on IVCM (Fig. 17.7). An early small study reported the branching angle for *Aspergillus* hyphae to be 45°, and may therefore be a potentially distinguishing feature [15]. However, a subsequent study in a large cohort of 98 patients showed no significant difference in the branching angle between *Fusarium* hyphae (59.7°) and *Aspergillus* hyphae (63.3°) [16]. Similarly, a recent study of 65 patients with culture-positive fungal keratitis reported mean branching angles of 49.91 ± 14.41 μm for *Fusarium spp.* and 49.11 ± 16.23 μm for *Aspergillus spp.* The mean hyphal diameter was 3.09 ± 0.45 μm for Aspergillus spp. and 2.87 ± 0.39 μm for *Fusarium spp.* [17]. It may therefore be concluded that although IVCM remains a valuable tool to detect fungal filaments in corneal ulcers, it cannot be used to distinguish *Fusarium spp* from *Aspergillus spp.* [16].

The IVCM features of *Candida albicans* are elongated particles measuring 10–40 μm in length and 5–10 μm in width, thought to resemble candida pseudofilaments [15]. Interestingly, 49% of eyes with fungal keratitis exhibit a honeycomb distribution of inflammatory cells in the anterior stroma on IVCM compared to 20% of eyes with non-fungal microbial keratitis [5]. Smedowski et al. [3] noted that the predominant inflammatory cell type on IVCM in fungal keratitis was the non-round type 3 cell (large dendriform cells with an elongated, thin cell body and long, thin fibrils) distributed within the epithelial and subepithelial layers. The pathognomonic

Fig. 17.6 Laser scanning in vivo confocal microscopy image showing fusarium hyphae (arrow)

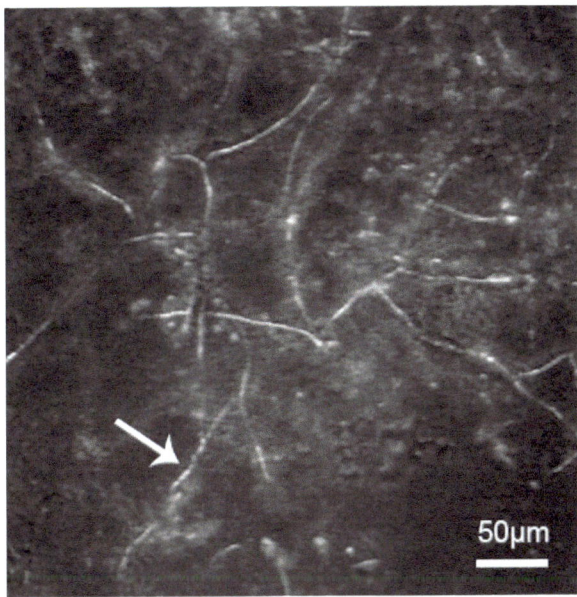

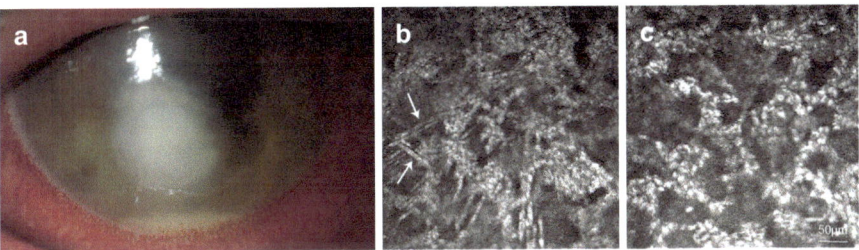

Fig. 17.7 (**a**) Slit-lamp photograph of a patient with *Aspergillus* keratitis. (**b**) Laser scanning in vivo confocal microscopy image showing *Aspergillus* hyphae (arrows), and (**c**) A honeycomb distribution of inflammatory cells in the stroma

signs of fungal keratitis were non-round type 4 cells (giant dendriform cells with an elongated, thin cell body and short, thin fibrils) that were not observed in any other type of keratitis [3].

As well as reporting IVCM morphological features, studies have also investigated the sensitivity and specificity of IVCM in the diagnosis of fungal keratitis (Table 17.2). Using slit scanning IVCM, Kanavi [6] et al. reported a sensitivity of 94% and specificity of 78% for the diagnosis of fungal keratitis by experienced observers. In a large prospective study, Chidambaram [11] et al. reported a sensitivity of 85.7% and specificity of 81.4% for the diagnosis of fungal keratitis using laser scanning IVCM. Interestingly, having access to a clinical image of the ulcer resulted in a greater sensitivity for fungal detection (89.8% sensitivity) [11]. A subsequent retrospective reliability study by Kheirkhah [18] et al. assessed the effect of observer experience on diagnostic accuracy and showed that the level of experience had a

Table 17.2 Summary of studies investigating the diagnostic accuracy of *in vivo* confocal microscopy in the diagnosis of fungal keratitis

	Diagnostic criteria	Sensitivity (%)	Specificity (%)	Masked observers	Observer experience
Kanavi et al. [6]	High contrast hyphae-like structures	94	78	Not reported	Not reported
Chidambaram et al. [11]	Fungal filaments	85.7	81.4	Yes	2–5 years experience
Kheirkhah et al. [18]	Filamentous elements	42.9	87.5	Yes	Inexperienced
Kheirkhah et al. [18]	Filamentous elements	71.4	89.6	Yes	Experienced
Wu et al. [19]	Automatic hyphae detection	89.29	95.65	Yes	Computer

significant impact on sensitivity (71.4% and 42.9% for experienced and inexperienced observers respectively) but not on specificity (89.6% and 87.5% for experienced and inexperienced observers respectively) [18].

In an attempt to enhance diagnostic accuracy, by removing the effects of subjectivity and experience associated with human observers, researchers have investigated using an automatic hyphae detection system based on image recognition. When a dataset of IVCM images obtained from 56 cases of fungal keratitis were analysed, the specificity of the image recognition-based automatic hyphae detection was 95.65% and the sensitivity was 89.29% [19].

Using an alternative approach, Liu [20] et al. developed a novel convolutional neural network framework for the automatic diagnosis of fungal keratitis from laser scanning IVCM images using data augmentation and image fusion and reported a diagnostic accuracy of 99.95%.

Hyphal density has been reported to be a useful indicator when monitoring the effect of treatment [17]. Chidambaram [21] et al. recently further identified the following IVCM features as indicators for poor outcomes in patients with fungal keratitis.

(a) A stellate appearance of interconnected cellular processes with absence of visible nuclei (thought to represent activated keratocytes), if present in the corneal stroma in baseline images, or development of this appearance in the final visit IVCM images.
(b) The presence of an inflammatory cell infiltrate forming a honeycomb distribution in IVCM images at the final visit.
(c) Detection of fungal hyphae in final visit IVCM images.
(d) The appearance of dendritiform cells in the stroma at the final visit (postulated to represent dendritic cells or macrophages or fibroblasts), when not present at the baseline visit.

IVCM may therefore be a useful adjunct to clinical examination for monitoring response to treatment in patients with fungal keratitis.

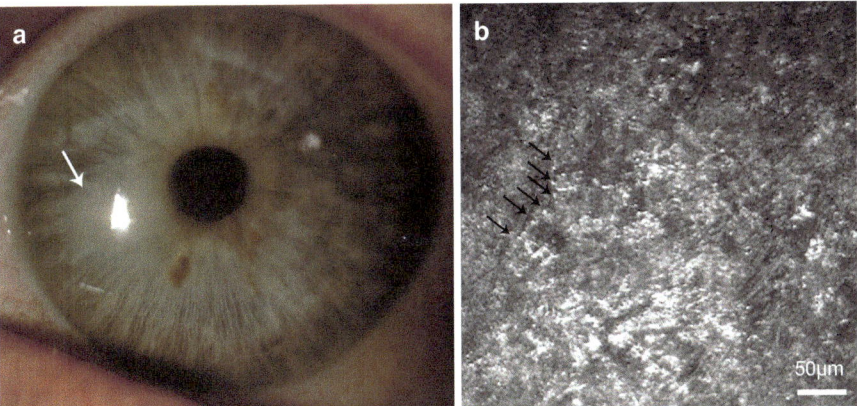

Fig. 17.8 (**a**) Slit-lamp photograph of a patient with microsporidia keratitis. (**b**) Laser scanning in vivo confocal microscopy image showing hyperreflective dots in the stroma

17.9 *Microsporidia* Keratitis

Microsporidia keratitis is rare and may be clinically confused with herpes simplex keratitis or *Acanthamoeba* keratitis. IVCM in cases of microsporidial keratitis have shown epithelial rosette formation with intracellular bright ovoid bodies [22, 23].

In patients with stromal involvement, IVCM shows linearly aligned hyperreflective dots (diameter 2–5 μm) interspersed between keratocytes in the anterior and mid-stroma (Fig. 17.8) [23, 24]. Sagoo [24] et al. reported a case of microsporidia keratitis in which the loss of presumed spores imaged by IVCM mirrored the clinical response to therapy, suggesting a role for IVCM in monitoring treatment effect.

17.10 *Nocardia* Keratitis

Clinically, *Nocardia* keratitis may be misdiagnosed as mycotic or mycobacterial keratitis. *Nocardia* are filamentous and branched gram-positive rod bacteria. Due to its large filamentous structure, *Nocardia* is one of the few bacterial causes of keratitis that can be visualized on IVCM.

Using slit scanning IVCM, Vaddavalli [25] et al. reported the presence of thin beaded filamentous structures that demonstrate right-angled branching in eyes with Nocardia keratitis. *Nocardia* filaments were best seen at the edge of the infiltrate.

In a subsequent study using laser scanning IVCM, Chidambaram [5] et al. only observed these features in one of three patients with confirmed *Nocardia* keratitis. The authors, therefore, suggested that it may not always be possible to rely on direct visualization of thin beaded filaments in IVCM images of Microbial Keratitis to make the diagnosis of *Nocardia* keratitis, particularly in the presence of significant stromal edema or inflammation [5]. Diagnostic accuracy is also reduced due to the similarity in appearance of fungal hyphae and *Nocardia* filaments on IVCM [7].

17.11 CMV Endotheliitis

IVCM appearances of cytomegalovirus (CMV) endotheliitis were first described by Shiraishi [26] et al. in a case report of a patient with CMV endotheliitis diagnosed by polymerase chain reaction (PCR). Laser scanning IVCM showed focal groups of enlarged endothelial cells with visible bright nuclei surrounded by dark halos. This appearance was thought to resemble an "owl's eye." Further studies [27, 28] have confirmed these observations and Kobayashi [28] et al. also showed that these lesions disappear after successful treatment.

The presence of the coin-shaped lesions on slit-lamp biomicroscopy and owl's eye morphology on IVCM is thought to be pathognomonic of CMV endotheliitis [27]. IVCM is therefore a useful noninvasive adjunctive tool for the diagnosis of CMV corneal endotheliitis.

17.12 Conclusions

Multiple studies have demonstrated the value of IVCM in the rapid detection of atypical infections such as acanthamoeba or fungal keratitis. However, the optical resolution limits of IVCM (2 μm) preclude its use in detecting bacterial or viral pathogens.

Limitations of IVCM in diagnosing microbial keratitis include similarities between inflammatory and pathogenic organisms, difficulty in interpreting equivocal images, and reliance on observer experience when interpreting images. Therefore, IVCM should not be used as a stand-alone tool in diagnosing keratitis, but as an adjunctive tool.

In addition to its role in diagnosis, IVCM has been shown to be useful in assessing prognosis and monitoring the effects of treatment.

References

1. Patel DV, McGhee CN. Contemporary in vivo confocal microscopy of the living human cornea using white light and laser scanning techniques: a major review. Clin Exp Ophthalmol. 2007;35(1):71–88.
2. Zhivov A, Stave J, Vollmar B, Guthoff R. In vivo confocal microscopic evaluation of Langerhans cell density and distribution in the normal human corneal epithelium. Graefes Arch Clin Exp Ophthalmol. 2005;243(10):1056–61.
3. Smedowski A, Tarnawska D, Orski M, Wroblewska-Czajka E, Kaarniranta K, Aragona P, Wylegala E. Cytoarchitecture of epithelial inflammatory infiltration indicates the aetiology of infectious keratitis. Acta Ophthalmol. 2017;95(4):405–13.
4. De Craene S, Knoeri J, Georgeon C, Kestelyn P, Borderie VM. Assessment of confocal microscopy for the diagnosis of polymerase chain reaction-positive Acanthamoeba keratitis: a case-control study. Ophthalmology. 2018;125(2):161–8.
5. Chidambaram JD, Prajna NV, Palepu S, Lanjewar S, Shah M, Elakkiya S, Macleod D, Lalitha P, Burton MJ. In vivo confocal microscopy cellular features of host and organism in bacterial, fungal, and Acanthamoeba keratitis. Am J Ophthalmol. 2018;190:24–33.

6. Kanavi MR, Javadi M, Yazdani S, Mirdehghanm S. Sensitivity and specificity of confocal scan in the diagnosis of infectious keratitis. Cornea. 2007;26(7):782–6.

7. Hau SC, Dart JK, Vesaluoma M, Parmar DN, Claerhout I, Bibi K, Larkin DF. Diagnostic accuracy of microbial keratitis with in vivo scanning laser confocal microscopy. Br J Ophthalmol. 2010;94(8):982–7.

8. Tu EY, Joslin CE, Sugar J, Booton GC, Shoff ME, Fuerst PA. The relative value of confocal microscopy and superficial corneal scrapings in the diagnosis of Acanthamoeba keratitis. Cornea. 2008;27(7):764–72.

9. Goh JWY, Harrison R, Hau S, Alexander CL, Tole DM, Avadhanam VS. Comparison of in vivo confocal microscopy, PCR and culture of corneal scrapes in the diagnosis of Acanthamoeba keratitis. Cornea. 2018;37(4):480–5.

10. Füst Á, Tóth J, Simon G, Imre L, Nagy ZZ. Specificity of in vivo confocal cornea microscopy in Acanthamoeba keratitis. Eur J Ophthalmol. 2017;27(1):10–5.

11. Chidambaram JD, Prajna NV, Larke NL, Palepu S, Lanjewar S, Shah M, Elakkiya S, Lalitha P, Carnt N, Vesaluoma MH, Mason M, Hau S, Burton MJ. Prospective study of the diagnostic accuracy of the in vivo laser scanning confocal microscope for severe microbial keratitis. Ophthalmology. 2016;123(11):2285–93.

12. Kheirkhah A, Satitpitakul V, Syed ZA, Müller R, Goyal S, Tu EY, Dana R. Factors influencing the diagnostic accuracy of laser-scanning in vivo confocal microscopy for Acanthamoeba keratitis. Cornea. 2018;37(7):818–23.

13. Huang P, Tepelus T, Vickers LA, Baghdasaryan E, Huang J, Irvine JA, Hsu HY, Sadda S, Lee OL. Quantitative analysis of depth, distribution, and density of cysts in Acanthamoeba keratitis using confocal microscopy. Cornea. 2017;36(8):927–32.

14. Wang YE, Tepelus TC, Gui W, Irvine JA, Lee OL, Hsu HY. Reduction of Acanthamoeba cyst density associated with treatment detected by in vivo confocal microscopy in Acanthamoeba keratitis. Cornea. 2019;38(4):463–8.

15. Brasnu E, Bourcier T, Dupas B, Degorge S, Rodallec T, Laroche L, Borderie V, Baudouin C. In vivo confocal microscopy in fungal keratitis. Br J Ophthalmol. 2007;91(5):588–91.

16. Chidambaram JD, Prajna NV, Larke N, Macleod D, Srikanthi P, Lanjewar S, Shah M, Lalitha P, Elakkiya S, Burton MJ. In vivo confocal microscopy appearance of Fusarium and Aspergillus species in fungal keratitis. Br J Ophthalmol. 2017;101(8):1119–23.

17. Tabatabaei SA, Soleimani M, Tabatabaei SM, Beheshtnejad AH, Valipour N, Mahmoudi S. The use of in vivo confocal microscopy to track treatment success in fungal keratitis and to differentiate between Fusarium and Aspergillus keratitis. Int Ophthalmol. 2020;40(2):483–91.

18. Kheirkhah A, Syed ZA, Satitpitakul V, Goyal S, Müller R, Tu EY, Dana R. Sensitivity and specificity of laser-scanning in vivo confocal microscopy for filamentous fungal keratitis: role of observer experience. Am J Ophthalmol. 2017;179:81–9.

19. Wu X, Tao Y, Qiu Q, Wu X. Application of image recognition-based automatic hyphae detection in fungal keratitis. Australas Phys Eng Sci Med. 2018;41(1):95–103.

20. Liu Z, Cao Y, Li Y, Xiao X, Qiu Q, Yang M, Zhao Y, Cui L. Automatic diagnosis of fungal keratitis using data augmentation and image fusion with deep convolutional neural network. Comput Methods Prog Biomed. 2020;187:105019.

21. Chidambaram JD, Prajna NV, Palepu S, Palepu S, Lanjewar S, Shah M, Elakkiya S, Lalitha P, Macleod D, Burton MJ. Cellular morphological changes detected by laser scanning in vivo confocal microscopy associated with clinical outcome in fungal keratitis. Sci Rep. 2019;9(1):8334.

22. Malhotra C, Jain AK, Kaur S, Dhingra D, Hemanth V, Sharma SP. In vivo confocal microscopic characteristics of microsporidial keratoconjunctivitis in immunocompetent adults. Br J Ophthalmol. 2017;101(9):1217–22.

23. Hsiao YC, Tsai IL, Kuo CT, Yang TL. Diagnosis of microsporidial keratitis with in vivo confocal microscopy. J Xray Sci Technol. 2013;21(1):103–10.

24. Sagoo MS, Mehta JS, Hau S, Irion LD, Curry A, Bonshek RE, Tuft SJ. Microsporidium stromal keratitis: in vivo confocal findings. Cornea. 2007;26(7):870–3.

25. Vaddavalli PK, Garg P, Sharma S, Thomas R, Rao GN. Confocal microscopy for Nocardia keratitis. Ophthalmology. 2006;113(9):1645–50.
26. Shiraishi A, Hara Y, Takahashi M, Oka N, Yamaguchi M, Suzuki T, Uno T, Ohashi Y. Demonstration of "owl's eye" morphology by confocal microscopy in a patient with presumed cytomegalovirus corneal endotheliitis. Am J Ophthalmol. 2007;143(4):715–7.
27. Peng RM, Guo YX, Xiao GG, Li CD, Hong J. Characteristics of corneal endotheliitis among different viruses by in vivo confocal microscopy. Ocul Immunol Inflamm. 2019;7:1–9.
28. Kobayashi A, Yokogawa H, Higashide T, Nitta K, Sugiyama K. Clinical significance of owl eye morphologic features by in vivo laser confocal microscopy in patients with cytomegalovirus corneal endotheliitis. Am J Ophthalmol. 2012;153(3):445–53.